A Cancer Survivor's Almanac

A Cancer Survivor's Almanac

Charting Your Journey

Third Edition

National Coalition for Cancer Survivorship
Edited by Barbara Hoffman, J.D.

WITH AN INTRODUCTION BY SAM DONALDSON

WILEY

John Wiley & Sons, Inc.

For general information about our other products and services, please contact our Customer Care Department within the United States at (800) 762-2974, outside the United States at (317) 572-3993 or fax (317) 572-4002.

Wiley also publishes its books in a variety of electronic formats. Some content that appears in print may not be available in electronic books.

ISBN 0-471-34669-1

Printed in the United States of America

10 9 8 7 6 5 4 3 2

Contents

Dedication to Natalie Davis Spingarn

by
Senator Joe Lieberman

This book is dedicated to Natalie Davis Spingarn, who dedicated her life to bringing comfort, courage, and joy into the lives of her fellow cancer patients.

I met Natalie in 1963, when she was the press secretary for the late Senator Abraham Ribicoff and I was a summer intern. Natalie made a great impression on me then and, quite a few years later, served as a senior intern in my own Senate office—where she contributed her intelligence, experience, and judgment to our efforts in the area of health policy.

Natalie was committed to bettering the real lives of real people. She never forgot on whose behalf she had the privilege to serve.

That is how she came to be one of the most potent advocates for cancer patients in the nation. For the last quarter century of her life, Natalie herself was fighting cancer. She was no doubt in pain much of the time. At times, she was certainly afraid.

Some who struggle against cancer understandably turn away from the disease, to prevent it from defining and controlling their lives. Natalie had a different reaction. She faced cancer down, took it on, learned everything she could about it, and worked hard—tirelessly, ceaselessly—to help others do the same.

In so doing, she helped lead a healthcare revolution that transformed, and is still transforming, our vision of cancer patients and their vision of themselves: where we once saw passive recipients of care, we now see men and women with the mettle, the might, and the right to participate in their treatment and demand the help they deserve.

I learned a great deal from Natalie's counsel, her articles, and her books. But what I will carry with me most is the way she lived her life: with purpose, humor, energy, and grace. Despite her longtime struggle with cancer, Natalie's life was not, in the end, defeated by the disease. She fought it and helped others fight it; her resistance produced a lasting victory.

Acknowledgments

This book was a collaborative effort in the true sense of the word. The dedicated staff of the National Coalition for Cancer Survivorship, especially Donna Doneski, Rebecca Gregory, Jennifer Greiner, Eric Gordon, Stacia Grosso, Susan Scherr, Bill Schmidt, Elizabeth Smart, and Courtney Workman, made this book a reality. We greatly appreciate Judith Blanchard, M.S.; Steven Friedman; Rebecca Gregory; Wendy Harpham, M.D.; Catherine Harvey, Ph.D.; Pamela J. Haylock, Ph.D.; and Grace Monaco, J.D., for their invaluable comments on several chapters. In addition to writing chapters, Elizabeth J. Clark, Ph.D.; Susan Leigh, R.N.; Catherine Logan-Carillo; Gena Love; and Ellen Stovall provided inspiration, research, and suggestions. Melissa Morgan meticulously checked the resources listed in Chapter 17.

For indulging our long hours at the computer and offering practical suggestions, our special thanks to our families, including Thelma Hoffman, Frank Hoffman, Paul Shapiro, Emily Shapiro, Sarah Shapiro, and Nancy Shapiro.

This third edition of *A Cancer Survivor's Almanac* rests on the foundation built by Fitzhugh Mullan, M.D., a cofounder of the National Coalition for Cancer Survivorship and coauthor of the first edition of the book. Philip Spitzer has generously served with unwavering faith in this project as our literary agent since 1989.

We are also grateful to:

- Rachel Dultz, M.D.; John Glick, M.D.; and Philip Wey, M.D., for their skill and compassion;
- Jan Smith Donaldson, for her fresh ideas and dedication;
- Elizabeth Goss, J.D., for her clear explanations of health law and policy;
- Debra Thaler-DeMers's family (her parents for the gift of life; Gabrielle and Joshua for their love, support, and the gift of their music; her mother for driving her to treatments; and her sister Terri, who suggested she become an oncology nurse);
- the cancer survivors who taught Georgia Decker about CAM therapies;
- Roseann Calacone for her endurance and support to Georgia Decker;
- the work of David Eisenberg, M.D., and associates;
- David Spiegel, M.D., for his work on the psychosocial treatment of cancer patients;
- Frances Marcus Lewis, Ph.D., R.N., for her pioneering research with cancer patients;

- Debi McCaffrey Boyle, R.N., M.S.N., A.O.C.N., for her visionary survivorship work and mentoring;
- Lois Loescher, Ph.D., R.N., for her generosity, support, and friendship; and
- Eleanor Jodun, who taught us about hope.

Finally, our special thanks to the supportive and professional staff of John Wiley & Sons, including Tom Miller, Elizabeth Zack, Lisa Considine, Kim Nir, and Kim Hendrickson.

Introduction

by
Sam Donaldson

This is a book for the living. And why not? More than nine million Americans living today are cancer survivors, a significant number of whom will go on about their business, working, raising a family, playing a little golf and such, enjoying retirement, and eventually be hit by a truck or suffer some other "routine" end.

Still, as those of us who have had to come to grips with a cancer diagnosis know, our first thoughts are often dark; we are frightened and at a loss how to proceed. In the summer of 1995, when I heard the biopsy results that I had a melanoma tumor in a lymph node area of my groin, I went home and told my wife I might have three months to live at the most. How I figured that out I don't know—I'm not a doctor—but that's what I thought. And as to treatment, I wasn't sure where to turn.

Every person suddenly drafted into the "cancer club" needs help with the physical, emotional, and practical matters associated with this dreadful disease. And that is why the National Coalition for Cancer Survivorship (NCCS) is such an important organization for so many of us. And why this book is so helpful.

We suddenly want scores of questions answered. For instance: In addition to our doctor, who can we turn to for knowledgeable advice? How do we find a second opinion? How do we evaluate a choice of therapies? What do we want from our family and friends in the way of emotional help and how do we let them know what we want? What will happen to our health insurance? Will we lose our job? And though cancer is no longer an automatic death sentence, what are the prudent legal and financial steps we should take in light of our diagnosis? These are just some of the crucial topics discussed in this book.

NCCS defines a cancer survivor as "anyone with a diagnosis of cancer, whether newly diagnosed or in remission or with recurrence or terminal cancer." It is the only survivor-led advocacy organization working exclusively on behalf of all cancer survivors, regardless of stage of survivorship, and the millions more touched by cancer. Founded in 1986, NCCS continues to lead the cancer survivorship movement by advocating nationally for quality cancer care for all Americans. It helps survivors through its public policy work and by creating educational resources like this book. This book was written by the most experienced and respected cancer survivors and professionals, most of whom have decades of experience educating and advocating for survivors.

After I was diagnosed I was very lucky to receive advice and help along the lines found in this book. Thanks to caring people like those at NCCS, I was pointed toward Dr. Steven Rosenberg at the National Cancer Institute. He looked at my biopsy report, studied my CAT scan, and examined me. "I think you have a good chance to lead a healthy life of normal length," he told me. "I don't believe you," I blurted out in reply.

Now, here I am eight years later thanking my lucky stars that Dr. Rosenberg was the expert and I wasn't. You, too, can live with cancer. Read on.

Part One

Taking Care
of Your
Medical Needs

Chapter One

Understanding Cancer, Its Treatment, and the Side Effects of Treatment

by Patricia Ganz, M.D.

*A*S YOU BEGIN YOUR JOURNEY—Each of you is part of a growing community of cancer patients who are pioneers experiencing the benefits and difficulties of survivorship. As you journey through the phases of cancer survivorship, you often will be the one to provide information and education to your family, friends, and even physicians about the medical and physical effects of your treatment. Knowing as much as possible about your disease, its treatments, and its potential effects on your body can empower you to take charge of your health and help you make the most of your survivorship experience.

While this chapter could not be comprehensive, it is a starting point for developing your personal educational agenda. Resources referred to throughout this chapter and this book will help you learn what you need to know about cancer and find the information you need.

You may find yourself in unfamiliar territory as you begin your journey as a cancer survivor. Part of the challenge is a new vocabulary and a technical environment that a patient cannot avoid. As you learn about this new environment, you will be empowered with greater control over managing your condition and meeting your needs for health care.

WHAT IS CANCER?

Cancer is the general term used to describe a large group of diseases whose hallmark is the uncontrolled growth of cells in the tissue in which the cancer arises. Before a single cell commits itself to a malignant and irreversible course, a long precancerous period exists in which cells may appear normal but have already acquired some of the genetic changes that will become cancer. From this single cancer cell, over the course of many years, a malignant tumor becomes clinically detectable. The whole process, from the beginning of the earliest changes in the DNA to the detection of a clinically apparent cancer, may take as long as 20 years.

The goals of current cancer screening and prevention efforts are (1) to detect cancers in a premalignant phase—for example, colon polyps—and either to remove them or to prevent the conversion of genetically abnormal cells into malignant cells through the use of medications; and (2) to detect cancers when they are localized and have not spread outside the tissue of origin. Other approaches, such as immunizations against infections that may precede cancer—such as hepatitis B—may in fact reduce the incidence of some cancers—liver cancer, for example.

Cancer cells at first grow locally, but they eventually invade and destroy the surrounding tissues. Cancer cells also have a propensity to spread to other parts of the body through the lymph system or bloodstream. In general, the smaller and more localized the tumor, the better the prognosis. However, some cancers, such as leukemia and lymphoma, are widespread at diagnosis in most cases.

In general, most newly diagnosed cancer patients go through a series of staging tests, including blood work, x-rays, and scans, to determine the extent of the disease. Your doctor is the best person to consult regarding the details of your illness and treatment; however, it may be useful for you to understand the stage or extensiveness of your disease, as that information will be important to understanding your prognosis—the likely outcome of treatment for your disease.

WHAT IS CANCER TREATMENT?

After you have been diagnosed with cancer, a treatment plan for your unique medical situation will be developed based on all of the information that has been gathered through blood tests, radiological studies, surgery, and microscopic and biochemical evaluations of your cancer. The treatment plan that your doctors develop will have a specific goal. In general, the possibilities include cure, long-term control of the cancer, or symptomatic relief only.

CURE—Cure is the goal for a wide range of cancers today. Over half of newly diagnosed cancer patients will be cured of their disease. *Cure,* from the medical point of view, means that all of the cancer can be removed successfully by surgery, or completely eliminated from the body through the use of medications or radiation treatments. Cure also implies that the likelihood of the cancer returning at a later date—either in the same local area or somewhere else—is extremely low. *Curative intent* treatment means that the initial treatment plan is chosen with the expectation that the patient will be cured.

Although some people have focused on five years of disease-free survival as the equivalent of cure, others may have a very high likelihood of long-term cure after as few as two years of treatment. On the other hand, some may be at risk for recurrent cancer for much longer than five years. Today, curative intent treatment is a realistic goal for many newly diagnosed cancer patients.

LONG-TERM CONTROL—Long-term control of cancer is the treatment goal for some cancer patients. The aim of long-term control is to modify the course of the disease, usually by temporarily eliminating the cancer, slowing its growth, and controlling its symptoms. In many cases, the cancer becomes resistant to the treatment and returns. Chronic leukemias, myeloma, and some non-Hodgkin's lymphomas are examples of cancers for which treatment provides long-term control.

SYMPTOM RELIEF–Symptom relief only (sometimes called *palliation*) is the treatment goal for most patients with advanced cancers. These cancers, in general, demonstrate only a minor response to chemotherapy or radiation, and are too extensive to be removed with surgery. Chemotherapy and radiation are used frequently with advanced cancers, but primarily for symptom relief rather than elimination of the cancer. In addition to anticancer treatment, measures for pain relief and medication for depression, anxiety, and any other symptoms caused by the cancer are usually included in the treatment plan.

TREATMENT PHASES

INITIAL DIAGNOSTIC AND TREATMENT PHASE–This phase starts with your first encounter with the doctor to report new symptoms or to undergo tests, including a biopsy of the cancer. A biopsy is the removal of a small piece of tissue that can be examined under a microscope. Next comes a meeting with a number of experts to make the initial treatment plan. For most cancers, a delay of a few weeks to complete various diagnostic tests and to meet with doctors should be expected. This period often is the best time to define the treatment plan that will give you the best chance of cure or long-term survival. On rare occasions, treatment is started immediately.

When cancer is diagnosed, it usually has existed in a subclinical form for many years. For this reason, you should not be afraid to delay treatment to obtain a second opinion. If the cancer has spread, it did so before the cancer was first detected. Taking a few weeks to seek appropriate opinions and to define the best treatment plan will not hurt, and indeed may help, your chance of doing well.

MAINTENANCE PHASE–The maintenance phase of treatment is a time when treatment is continued but usually on a less intensive schedule. The goal of this treatment is to keep your condition stable and under control, while continuing to kill any remaining cancer cells. For example, maintenance therapy is commonly given to children with acute lymphocytic leukemia (ALL). For some kinds of cancer treatment, this approach may include giving high doses of chemotherapy as a final booster before discontinuing treatments.

FOLLOW-UP CARE–The follow-up care phase is the time after completion of surgery, radiation therapy, chemotherapy, or a combination of treatments, when it is thought that the cancer has been eradicated completely. During this phase you will be recovering from the short-term effects of treatment and beginning to resume a more normal life, with fewer doctors' appointments. Initially you may see your doctor every one or two months, and then only three or four times a year.

During these visits, the doctor will perform a careful interview and physical examination, with emphasis on possible symptoms related to the cancer and any residual side effects from your treatments. You will also have regular blood tests and other studies to monitor your condition. You will need lifelong follow-up because of possible problems that occur secondary to cancer treatment, such as the risk of new cancers or recurrence.

CANCER RECURRENCE—Cancer may recur in the same part of your body where it was found originally (a local recurrence), or it may reappear in a more distant part of your body (a metastasis). In either case, a new treatment plan must be developed. Diagnostic tests will be repeated to determine the extent of the cancer recurrence. The type of treatment that is selected for the recurring cancer will depend on the specific type of cancer, on its extensiveness, and on what previous therapy you received. Some recurrent cancers can still be cured, although the chance for cure is usually lower than it is for the first incidence of cancer.

Advanced and incurable cancer may exist at the time of diagnosis, or it may occur after many years of cancer treatment and follow-up care. In either case, the usual goal of treatment for this phase of cancer is symptom relief. Some patients, however, may want to participate in clinical trials of new experimental treatments (see page 11 for an explanation of *clinical trials*).

TYPES OF TREATMENTS

Traditionally, cancer has been treated initially with surgery, radiation, chemotherapy, or a combination of the three. In addition, hormonal therapies play a major role in the management of some hormonally responsive cancers, such as breast and prostate cancer. Now, newer classes of biological, immunological, and/or molecularly targeted therapies are being incorporated into standard treatments.

Surgery can be performed under local or general anesthesia, and may be limited to a small biopsy or be extensive. Some cancers, such as colorectal and lung cancers, are treated with surgery and may be cured by the surgical procedure alone. Many times, surgery is combined with radiation and/or chemotherapy to limit the extent of the surgery and to improve the chance for cure. This approach is called *combined modality therapy.*

Radiation therapy is the treatment of cancer with high-energy radiation. These treatments usually are given to defined or limited parts of the body. Radiation therapy alone, without major surgery, can cure some cancers, such as cancer of the cervix and larynx. More often, it is used to reduce the size of a cancer before surgery or to destroy any remaining cancer cells after surgery. Radiation therapy also helps many patients with advanced cancer by shrinking local areas of the cancer that are causing pain or other symptoms.

Chemotherapy is a general term for treatment with drugs. These medications usually are given by injection or infusion into a vein, but also can be given by injection into the muscle or skin, or can be taken by mouth. Chemotherapy treatment may be used alone to cure a number of cancers—for example, Hodgkin's disease, non-Hodgkin's lymphoma, and testicular cancer—but more often it is used in combination with radiation and surgery.

Chemotherapy treatments have the advantage of traveling in the bloodstream to almost all parts of the body, and thus are able to eradicate cancer cells that are out of reach of the scalpel or radiation beam. Chemotherapy is also used to provide long-term control for some cancers and to relieve symptoms in patients with advanced cancer.

Hormonal therapies are commonly used to treat cancers whose growth is regulated by hormones. For example, most prostate cancers thrive in the presence of male hormones such as testosterone, so that much of the therapy of prostate cancer focuses on depriving the cancer cells of this hormone. This can be achieved through medications that decrease the body's own production of testosterone or through medications that oppose the effects of testosterone on the cancer cell (antiandrogens).

Similarly, in breast cancer treatments, a wide array of medications oppose the effects of estrogen on the growth of breast cancer cells. The most commonly used hormonal treatment for breast cancer is the drug tamoxifen. Other drugs in widespread use are arimidex and megestrol acetate. As with chemotherapy, hormonal therapies are often used in the early treatment of breast and prostate cancers following surgery and radiation treatments.

Molecularly targeted therapies represent a major advance in cancer therapy. Chemotherapy and radiation therapy often damage healthy cells while they kill and damage cancer cells. In contrast, targeted therapies can be less toxic because they confine most of the damage to cancer cells. Hopefully, when used alone or in combination with other therapies, targeted therapies will improve cancer control and cure.

The first breakthrough drug in this group is trastuzumab (Herceptin), which prolongs the survival of advanced breast cancer patients when it is added to chemotherapy. It is now being tested in earlier phases of breast cancer treatment. Other examples of targeted therapy include Rituximab, which is a monoclonal antibody therapy used for treatment of some lymphomas.

Adjuvant therapy is given after the cancer goes into remission and the primary treatment is completed. The purpose of adjuvant therapy is to treat any stray cancer cells that cannot be detected by the usual tests. Adjuvant therapy may delay recurrence and prolong survival.

Neoadjuvant therapy is chemotherapy or hormone therapy given to shrink tumors before the cancer is removed.

High-dose chemotherapy with rescue (bone marrow transplantation [BMT] or peripheral stem cell therapy) is a treatment where patients are given extremely high doses of chemotherapy (often including radiation therapy) to eliminate the cancer cells that are in the body. The theory behind this treatment is that the higher the dose of chemotherapy or radiation, the more cancer cells that will be killed. Unfortunately, these high doses of treatment can harm normal tissues in the body, such as the cells of the bone marrow that make white cells, red cells, and platelets, as well as the cells that line the gastrointestinal tract. The treatment ordinarily would cause death because it damages the bone marrow—the blood-producing organ. Through the use of bone marrow transplantation, however, the patient is "rescued" by the transplanted stem cells, which find their way to the patient's marrow and take over production of blood cells.

BMT involves removal, under general anesthesia, of about one-half liter of bone marrow from a healthy donor who is genetically identical or extremely well-matched to the recipient (allogenic transplantation) or from the patient him/herself (autologous transplantation). Alternatively, stem cells from the bone marrow may be obtained by stimulating the marrow to release them into the blood circulation, and then obtained from the donor's blood. The donated cells are then processed and return to the patient by vein after the patient has received high-dose chemotherapy and radiation treatments. High-dose chemotherapy and radiation has many side effects and is performed only at specialized centers. BMT and stem cell transplantation have become standard treatment for some cancers, such as acute leukemia and lymphoma.

Modification of the immunologic system is a type of therapy used to boost the body's own natural defenses against cancer. Until recently, most of these results have met with limited success. Innovative technologies have permitted the large-scale production of new agents, broadly classified as *biologic response modifiers,* which are derived from the body's own natural products. Interferon, interleukin-2, and tumor necrosis factor are a few substances that are undergoing active study. Some of these agents already have found a place in cancer treatment, such as in patients with melanoma and renal cell carcinoma.

CLINICAL TRIALS

For most cancers, the majority of physicians and researchers have agreed on a "standard treatment approach"—the way in which cancer should be treated based on years of systematic study and research. However, doctors may have different opinions about how to treat some cancers because several equally effective treatments may be available. Under these circumstances, seeking a second opinion is helpful to learn about all your treatment options. See Chapter 17 for how to find information about the standard treatments for cancer.

Clinical trials involve research with new experimental treatments and with new ways of using standard treatments. Most trials are conducted at cancer treatment centers affiliated with universities, but many community cancer specialists can participate as well. In general, these trials test the effectiveness of a new treatment, usually in comparison with the best available standard treatment. If a treatment has not been accepted as one of the standard treatments, it is called *experimental* or *investigational.*

Because of the experimental nature of the treatment, you will be monitored very carefully for benefits and side effects. You must give your informed consent to participate in such research before any treatment is administered (see pages 43–45 for an explanation of informed consent). Unfortunately, very few patients treated in the United States today are given the opportunity to participate in clinical trials, a situation the National Cancer Institute is trying to improve. If you are considering receiving treatment in a clinical trial, ask your doctor ten questions suggested by the Coalition of National Cancer Cooperative Groups:

1. Why would this trial be important to me? What is it trying to prove?
2. What are my potential benefits and risks compared to other treatment options?
3. What are the eligibility requirements?
4. Who will monitor my care and safety, and review the trial?
5. What are the trial's tests and treatments? Will I be hospitalized? If so, how often and for how long?
6. How do the possible side effects of the new treatment option compare with those of the standard treatment option, and how will they affect my life?
7. What support will be available for me and my caregivers during the trial? Can I talk to other people in the trial?
8. Will my insurance company, Medicaid, or managed care plan cover these costs? Who will help me answer coverage questions?
9. What are my out-of-pocket costs and responsibilities?
10. What is the long-term follow-up care?

To find a trial, ask your doctor if she or he enrolls patients in a trial that may help you. If your doctor is unaware of a trial, contact the National Cancer Institute at (800)-4-CANCER or **www.cancer.gov.**

You may want to participate in a clinical trial for several reasons. It may give you the chance to receive treatment that is more effective or less toxic than the standard treatment. You also may be able to get access to a new drug that is not generally available. In addition, your participation in this research may help future cancer patients by testing new types of cancer treatment.

The process of cancer development is a long one. A single cell may take many years to transform from a healthy cell into a precancer and then a cancer. Therefore, researchers believe that blocking or preventing early steps in the transformation process can prevent the development of cancer. Researchers are studying *chemoprevention,* the use of various agents, such as drugs, vitamins, and micronutrients, to prevent several types of cancer.

The Breast Cancer Prevention Trial (BCPT), which tested the antiestrogen drug tamoxifen, was the first major trial to test chemoprevention. Over 13,000 women at high risk for breast cancer participated in this trial, which began in 1992 and was closed early in 1998 because it found a 50 percent reduction in the risk of developing breast cancer in those who took tamoxifen. Now, tamoxifen has become a standard treatment option for women with strong family histories of breast cancer or with precancerous changes in the breast that put them at risk for developing cancer. Chemoprevention and vaccines may be important for cancer survivors to prevent second cancers, as well as for close family members of cancer survivors who may be at high risk for developing the same cancer.

Symptoms and Side Effects

Pain

Pain is the most feared aspect of cancer, even though not every cancer patient experiences pain. Most people equate cancer with pain; yet, many are often surprised to find that their cancer was not painful at the time of diagnosis. Pain is, however, commonly associated with advanced cancer and with some treatments. Two types of pain are associated with cancer and its treatment: acute pain and chronic pain.

- *Acute Pain*—This pain—of sudden onset and relatively short duration— is generally related to the cancer pressing on adjacent tissues or to stretching the organ in which the cancer is located. With successful cancer treatment, usually all of the pain disappears. If the cancer remains and continues to grow in the same place, the pain often becomes chronic (constant and permanent).
- *Chronic pain* sometimes develops as a result of treatment. This usually occurs in a part of the body where surgery and radiation have been used together, leading to the development of scar tissue that entraps and injures the adjacent nerves.

Although treatment to alleviate pain may be a simple matter, survivors are sometimes reluctant to admit they are experiencing pain because they erroneously believe that

- pain associated with cancer is to be expected;
- pain is unimportant when life is at stake;

- pain is a sign that the illness is progressing;
- pain medication is addictive;
- people become immune to pain medication if they start taking drugs in early stages of pain.

A reluctance to admit you have pain can result in uncontrolled and unnecessary discomfort that interferes with daily life. You are the best judge of your own pain. You should not hesitate to give your doctor a detailed description of your pain symptoms. If pain becomes an ongoing problem for you, keep a pain diary to chart when the pain began and what helped to relieve it. You need not accept pain as a "necessary evil" in cancer treatment.

The general principle underlying the use of pain relievers is to get the pain under control and prevent it from returning. This can be accomplished by giving scheduled pain treatment whether or not you are in pain, and giving small additional doses of pain medication between the scheduled doses should the pain become worse. Giving pain medication on a regular schedule leads to more effective pain relief and to a lower total dosage of medication than if it is given only when the pain is severe. Ninety percent of all cancer patients can have their pain effectively controlled if they take their medications appropriately. Addiction is extremely rare unless the individual has a history of substance abuse. Efforts to control pain should be made at all phases of the disease, but it is especially important that pain be controlled in the advanced cancer patient. Different treatments are used to control pain from different sources.

Medication is the most common form of pain treatment. Nonprescription analgesics, such as aspirin, acetaminophen, and ibuprofen are effective in relieving mild pain. If your pain is moderate to severe, your doctor may prescribe a narcotic for you to take orally. For extremely intense pain, you may be given narcotics by injection, sometimes continuously using a portable infusion pump.

Radiation or surgery to anesthetize pain fibers may be used to control pain that is localized in one area, such as in a bone. Radiation and surgery also may be used to shrink tumors that are causing pain.

Skin stimulation excites nerve endings in the skin and may lessen or block the recognition of pain. Different types of skin stimulation include massage, pressure, vibration, heat, cold, menthol preparations, and transcutaneous electric nerve stimulations (TENS).

The relaxation techniques discussed in Chapter 6 may help eliminate or alleviate pain.

Biofeedback, acupuncture, and hypnosis are sometimes used in combination with more traditional pain relief.

Pain clinic—You may find other solutions at a pain clinic. Ask your doctor, nurse, or social worker about pain clinics in your community.

You have a right to seek adequate pain control. "Understanding Cancer Pain" is an excellent booklet that describes cancer pain management. It is available from the National Cancer Institute at (800)-4-CANCER or **www.cancer.gov.**

FATIGUE

Fatigue is one of the most common physical problems reported by cancer patients. Fatigue can occur as a specific symptom of the cancer, especially in persons with advanced cancer. Fatigue, which leaves a patient tired for weeks or months, also results from radiation and chemotherapy. For some patients, energy never returns to pretreatment levels. A few points to consider are:

- Fatigue is a warning sign that the body needs more rest; the best response is to heed the warning.
- Pace your activities according to your energy level, especially during and soon after treatment.
- If possible, exercise routinely to maintain stamina.
- Unless your physician prescribes against it, drink plenty of fluids—at least eight glasses of water per day.

NUTRITION AND WEIGHT MAINTENANCE

Cancer survivors experience nutritional and weight problems for a variety of reasons. Cancers occurring in the abdomen can cause problems when they invade or compress digestive organs, such as the stomach. Some patients experience nausea and vomiting, while others feel too bloated to eat. However, most dietary problems experienced by survivors are caused, in part, by cancer treatment.

Although most problems involve weight and appetite loss, some patients, especially those receiving adjuvant therapy for breast cancer, may suffer from too much weight gain, possibly because of decreased physical activity, increased food intake, and/or onset of menopause. Because weight gain and a high-fat diet may be risk factors for breast cancer recurrence, these women usually are encouraged to maintain their weight or lose weight if they are overweight.

On the following pages are the seven most common nutritional problems, their causes, and suggestions for relief.

Of the seven most common nutritional problems, nausea and vomiting, which are caused by chemotherapy and radiation, can be the most physically exhausting. Chemotherapy-associated nausea and vomiting usually begin about four to six hours after an intravenous injection or within an hour after taking some oral medications. The intensity of these side effects varies with the drug. Many drugs cause no or minimal nausea, while others cause fairly severe nausea followed by frequent vomiting.

PROBLEMS RELATED TO NUTRITION AND EATING

PROBLEM	CAUSE	WHAT WILL HELP
LOSS OF APPETITE	May be caused by illness, anticancer drugs, loss of sleep, depression, or fatigue.	• Light exercise to increase appetite. • A glass of beer or wine before meals (with doctor's OK). • Plan meals with favorite foods; small, appetizing meals in pleasant surroundings. • Speak with a doctor or registered dietitian for suggestions. • Keep nutritious snacks around: offer a snack before bedtime (ice cream with ginger ale, a milk shake, or yogurt). • Use seasonings like basil, oregano, tarragon, and lemon.
WEIGHT LOSS	Maintenance of normal weight is indicative of sufficient calories. Weight loss may be part of the disease process or the result of anorexia.	• Keep a record of foods eaten each day. • Offer between-meal snacks high in calories and protein (for example, add ¼ cup nonfat dry milk to 8 oz. whole milk; add this milk to sauces, soups, and gravies). • Use cream, not milk, in cereals. Extra calories may be added with a dietary supplement.
NAUSEA & VOMITING	May be a result of anticancer drugs or a consequence of the cancer itself.	• Small, frequent meals with no liquid during meals. Drink liquids one hour before meals to prevent large volume of fluid in the stomach. • Overly sweet foods may cause discomfort. • Greasy, fried foods can cause nausea; try foods like toast and crackers (especially in the morning). • May need to try several antinausea medications to find the one that works. Check with a doctor and keep a record of when symptoms start and how long they last.
TASTE	Anticancer drugs may change the way food tastes; for example, sweet	• For overly sweet taste, force fluids. Serve protein at room temperature. Some foods may taste better with salt or sugar. Marinate meats in sweet wine or fruit juices. Salt may

{continued}

PROBLEM	CAUSE	WHAT WILL HELP
	foods taste too sweet. Radiation to the head and neck area can cause a metallic taste.	need to be restricted if heart disease also exists.
HALITOSIS	Can occur with anti-cancer drugs and is caused by breakdown of cells that line the gastrointestinal tract.	• Use frequent mouthwashes (except when there are sores in mouth) and antacids (check with doctor). Sucking on hard candy can be helpful.
STOMATITIS (Inflamma-tion of the mouth)	Both anticancer drugs and some-times the illness itself can leave a person subject to mouth sores and "furry tongue" indicative of fungal overgrowth	• A soft, bland diet or favorite foods blenderized. Avoid spicy, hot, or acid foods (orange juice) and coarse vege-tables or fruit. Cold drinks are soothing. • Use a straw for easier drinking. • Remove dentures except when needed for chewing. • Mouth care three times a day after meals. • Salt water gargles if mouth sores occur. • Call doctor if sores do not get better after three days. • Soft-bristle brush if mouth sores occur. • Doctor may order topical anesthesia. • Do not use mouthwash that contains alcohol.
DRY MOUTH	Radiation to the head and neck area. Pain medication.	• Sips of water frequently. • Lubricate lips. • Artificial saliva may help. • Lemon drops may stimulate saliva.

Note: Each patient is an individual and may or may not have any of these symptoms. No problem is too insignificant to deserve an answer. Call your doctor if you are concerned.

Source: *Caring for the Person with Cancer at Home: A Family Caregiver's Manual.* American Cancer Society, 1985.

To prevent or decrease nausea and vomiting, your doctor may give you several medications, usually by vein. In addition, you may be given pills to take at home, usually for the first 24 to 48 hours after treatment. The preventive medications sometimes cause drowsiness as a side effect, so you may need someone to drive you home from your treatment. You may be hospitalized because the treatment and preventive medications are so complex that you may need to have more frequent nursing care. If the preventive treatments do not work, tell your doctor or nurse immediately so alternative approaches can be tried.

With effective prevention of post-chemotherapy nausea and vomiting, fewer patients develop "anticipatory nausea and vomiting." This is a problem in which you are conditioned, like the dogs in Pavlov's experiments, to associate many of the aspects of your treatment with the nausea and vomiting that occur after treatment. Patients who have anticipatory nausea and vomiting usually start to feel anxious and nauseated the day before their treatment, with increasing symptoms as they approach the doctor's office. They often will have nausea as they enter the chemotherapy treatment room or have a needle inserted into their vein. These responses are not effectively treated with anti-nausea medications. Instead, behavioral treatments that involve relaxation or self-hypnosis are usually helpful to decondition the response.

Hair Loss

Hair loss can result from head and neck radiation and from certain types of chemotherapy. Chemotherapy and radiation result in atrophy of the hair follicle. Your hair becomes weak and brittle, and either breaks off at the surface of the scalp or falls out of the follicle. The amount of hair loss depends on the type, dose, and length of the treatment you receive. Before you begin treatment, ask your doctor whether you are likely to experience some hair loss.

You may lose hair not only from your scalp but also from other parts of your body, such as eyebrows and arms. Most hair loss is temporary. Your hair may return as before or regrow in a different texture and color.

You can take several steps to minimize hair loss:
- Cut your hair in an easy-to-manage style before treatment begins.
- Avoid excessive shampooing, rinse thoroughly, and gently pat your hair dry.
- Avoid heat, such as hair dryers and hot curlers.
- Avoid excess tugging on your hair by brushing only when necessary, by using a wide-tooth comb, and by avoiding hair clips and elastic bands.

You can take several steps to prepare for expected hair loss:
- Choose a wig prior to losing your hair so that you can match it to your natural hair color and texture. Some insurance policies cover the cost of a wig.
- If you do not want to wear a wig, consider a hat, a scarf, or a turban.
- If you do not wish to cover your head, you may want to shave off any remaining hair for a neater appearance. However, keep your head protected from

a strong sun to prevent sunburn, and keep it covered in the winter to prevent heat loss.

• At home, consider wearing a hairnet to minimize shedding on your clothes or bedding.

LOW BLOOD COUNTS

The majority of patients receiving chemotherapy, and some receiving radiation, will experience low blood counts. This is because treatment often slows the growth of cells in the bone marrow, which produces red cells, white cells, and platelets. White cells are needed to fight infections. When the white cell count falls below a certain level, it is unsafe to give additional treatments because they would continue to slow the production of white cells. If you are receiving chemotherapy or radiation therapy and develop a fever, you should call your doctor immediately. A fever might be the first sign of a low white blood cell count (also called *neutropenia*) and an associated infection.

If your blood cell counts are too low, your treatments will usually be postponed for several days until the counts improve. If your counts are extremely low, your doctor might prescribe a white cell growth factor (G-CSF or GM-CSF), which is given by injection daily. These growth factors stimulate the bone marrow to make new white cells that will travel into the circulation and prevent an infection. If you develop severe neutropenia with chemotherapy, or if your doctor thinks you will be at high risk for this condition, you may be given the growth factor preventatively to avoid a low white cell count. This preventive approach is particularly common when the doses of chemotherapy are very high, which can severely lower white cell counts. These growth factors can help prevent life-threatening infections in cancer patients.

New medications are available to help reverse anemia (low red blood cell counts) and thrombocytopenia (low platelet counts). The medication used to counteract anemia is called Epogen, which is given by injection either once or twice a week. This medication increases the red cell count significantly, decreases the need for transfusions, and improves the fatigue associated with anemia. Thrombocytopenia can be a serious problem for some patients, leading to easy bruising and bleeding. A number of new products are available to stimulate the growth of platelets in the bone marrow. Some people, however, may still require platelet transfusions to avoid serious complications of bleeding.

SKIN CHANGES

Skin problems in the treatment area can result from both radiation and chemotherapy. Changes can range from a minor reddening to blistering and peeling. Itchy skin, called *pruritus,* is a common side effect of some cancers and treatment.

Your doctor may prescribe antihistamines or cortico-steroid creams for itching. Additionally, you can take several steps to heal dry, itchy, or burned skin.

- Avoid sunlight exposure, which can cause additional burning.
- Lubricate your skin with a water-based, rather than oil-based, moisturizer.
- Drink at least eight glasses of water or other fluids each day.
- Protect your skin from extreme temperatures and wind. Keep indoor temperatures cool.
- Bathe in cool or lukewarm water: cornstarch, baking soda, oatmeal, or soybean powder added to the bath may be soothing.
- Wear loose fitting, lightweight clothing.

NEUROTOXICITY

Injury to the nerves (*neurotoxicity*) is a side effect of some treatments. Usually this is first noticed as a numbness or tingling in the hands or feet, and rarely as complete weakness in an extremity. Some drugs can cause hearing loss or ringing in the ears. If you are having any of these problems, you should immediately bring them to your doctor's attention so he or she can consider changing your medications.

LOSS OF CONCENTRATION

Many patients report difficulty concentrating, remembering, and thinking clearly while they are receiving cancer treatments. These effects are caused by several factors: direct effects of the chemotherapy and radiation treatments on the brain, side effects from the medications used to prevent nausea and vomiting, and the increased fatigue associated with the disease and its treatment.

It is important to eat and sleep well, to get enough rest, and to do the best you can to maintain your physical condition and stamina. Usually, the greatest loss of concentration will be associated with the treatments themselves (the day of treatment and the first few days thereafter) with return of concentration between treatments. Try to postpone activities that demand your concentration until after treatment.

RESPIRATORY PROBLEMS

Lung cancer patients and other cancer patients may experience shortness of breath that can be caused by the cancer itself; by chemotherapy, anemia, malnutrition; and by other factors. You can improve your breathing in a number of ways.

- Inhale through your nose and exhale slowly through your mouth with your lips pursed as if blowing out a candle. Use your abdominal muscles, rather than your chest muscles, to pull air in and push it out.
- Rest in a comfortable position when experiencing shortness of breath. For example, you will find it easier to sit up in bed than to lie down.
- Move around as much as possible to help your circulation. Even if you are confined to bed, you may be able to do simple arm or leg exercises. A res-

piratory therapist can suggest the best exercises for you.
- Aid circulation in your feet by not sitting in one position too long or by crossing your legs.
- Drink at least eight glasses of water a day to help mucous membranes clear your lungs of secretions.
- Cough deeply from within your chest to help clear your lungs.
- Use a humidifier to keep the air in your house from becoming too dry.

SEXUAL FUNCTIONING AND FERTILITY

A number of sexual problems are associated with cancer and its treatment. Sometimes these are related specifically to the type of cancer (for example, gynecological or urological cancers), but more often they are related to general problems such as fatigue and discomfort. Even in healthy people, fatigue leads to a loss of interest in sexual activity, which is a very normal response. In addition, certain treatments lead to specific physical problems that affect sexual function. See Chapter 4 for a discussion of the impact of cancer treatment on sexuality.

Cancer and its treatment can affect fertility and fetal development. If you are sexually active during cancer treatment, you should use contraceptives. Both radiation and chemotherapy can lead to malformations or injury to the developing fetus. Conception can occur even if you are receiving treatment. If you wish to have a child, speak with your doctor before trying to conceive. You may be advised to wait several years after your treatments to reduce the risk of a problem pregnancy.

A parallel concern is the risk of permanent sterility from chemotherapy or radiation treatments. Radiation will cause permanent sterility if the testes or ovaries receive direct radiation. For this reason, these organs are usually shielded with lead barriers. Sometimes the ovaries are relocated surgically so that they will not be in a radiation treatment field. When such protective measures are used, subsequent fertility is preserved. It is, however, more difficult to protect these organs from the effects of chemotherapy. Not all chemotherapy treatments cause a decrease in fertility, but some will.

If you have concerns about the effect of cancer treatments on your fertility, you should consider the following:
- Discuss your questions with your doctor before you begin treatment so that your treatment can be changed, if possible, to minimize effects on your fertility. Sometimes you will have a choice between two equally effective treatment programs, one of which has a high rate of infertility and another that does not.
- Men should consider preserving their sperm in a sperm bank prior to treatment. If your sperm have not been impaired by the cancer itself, sperm banking may increase your chances of having a child after treatment.

- Women cannot preserve their eggs in the same way that men can store sperm. The only way to save a woman's eggs is to fertilize them and store them as embryos. This can be a problem for a woman who does not have a partner or a suitable sperm donor at the time of diagnosis. In addition, the harvesting of eggs may require hormone administration as well as several menstrual cycles (in other words, time) to retrieve eggs for this use. Thus, the opportunities for the preservation of fertility in women are more limited.

MEDICAL PROBLEMS OF LONG-TERM SURVIVORS

Fortunately, an expanding community of long-term cancer survivors have gotten past the early and often complex initial phase of cancer treatment. If you are among them, you will find that as time passes, and you are further removed from the early phase of treatment, you will tend to distance yourself physically and psychologically from the professionals who were involved in your cancer treatment. Although this is natural, you should maintain some form of regular medical follow-up with a physician who knows the details of your previous cancer treatment and its potential long-term side effects.

For example, a patient who has had the spleen removed for staging of Hodgkin's disease is at a lifelong risk for serious infections. In these individuals, fever must be treated promptly with antibiotics. Many cancer survivors are at a risk of long-term organ toxicities, infection, and second malignancies as a result of previous treatment. Therefore, it is important for survivors to inform their current physicians about their past treatments so that appropriate monitoring can occur.

LONG-TERM AND LATE EFFECTS

Long-term effects are known or expected problems that may occur with some frequency in individuals who have received certain treatments: for example, the risk of infection after splenectomy or infertility after certain chemotherapy drugs. *Late effects,* in contrast, are secondary conditions that arise as a result of having received certain cancer treatments: for example, leukemia secondary to alkylating agent therapy or congestive heart failure many years after treatment with anthracycline chemotherapy.

Information about the long-term and late effects of treatment on important organs, such as the heart and lungs, is growing. Chemotherapy and radiation treatments received many years earlier can lead to premature aging of these vital organs. As the number of survivors increases, more information about these problems becomes available, and this information is used to modify the type and intensity of treatment for patients currently receiving treatment. Specific examples of some long-term and late effects of cancer treatment include the following.

HEART MUSCLE INJURY is associated most commonly with high total doses of the anthrocycline drugs (doxorubicin or daunorubicin). In addition, high-dose cyclophosphamide, such as used in transplant regimens, can contribute to chronic heart failure. When chest radiation is combined with these drugs, the risk of heart failure is possible at lower doses of the chemotherapy drugs. Although heart muscle imaging studies (MUGA scans) are useful for monitoring the acute effects of treatment on how well the heart is pumping, some recent studies have noted the onset of heart failure in cancer survivors many years after their last chemotherapy or radiation treatments. In these individuals, the heart failure was apparently stable and compensated for over many years, until their hearts were stressed by the added physical demands of new situations, such as vigorous exercise or pregnancy.

CORONARY ARTERY DISEASE—Some cancer survivors may experience premature coronary artery disease from past radiation therapy. This may put them at risk for heart attacks at an age much younger than the general population.

LUNG TISSUE INJURY is an expected long-term problem when the drug bleomycin is used. This drug may lead to lung scarring and to a certain degree of shortness of breath in some individuals, as well as an increased risk of lung failure during anesthesia. Other groups of drugs can also cause this problem (for example, alkylating agents, methotrexate, and nitrosoureas), and these can be a concern in long-term survivors of bone marrow transplantation. Some patients may experience a gradual increase in shortness of breath with exercise, which may be a sign of lung injury from past chemotherapy or radiation therapy.

KIDNEY DAMAGE can occur after treatment with several chemotherapy drugs (for example, cisplatin, methotrexate, and nitrosoureas). These agents can be associated with both acute and chronic toxicities. Rarely, some patients may require hemodialysis as a result of chronic injury to the kidneys.

NERVOUS SYSTEM INJURY, which is commonly associated with the vinca alkaloids and Taxol, may cause considerable disability—for example, pain or difficulty walking or using hands. Whole brain radiation, with or without chemotherapy, can cause progressive dementia and cognitive dysfunction in some long-term survivors. This is particularly a problem for brain tumor patients and for patients with small-cell lung cancer who have received prophylactic radiation therapy to the brain. In children with leukemia, a variety of abnormalities (problems with learning and concentration) have been associated with whole brain irradiation.

BLOOD AND IMMUNE SYSTEM PROBLEMS (low blood cell counts, anemia, increased susceptibility to infection) are common during and shortly after receiving chemotherapy and radiation treatments. In some instances, however, some survivors will have persistent abnormalities as a long-term effect of treatment. A damaged immune system is a long-term problem for patients with Hodgkin's disease, which may be related to the underlying disease as well as to the treatments that are used. Those patients who have received a splenectomy may also be at risk for serious bacterial infections.

MONITORING FOR RECURRENCE

All survivors should be regularly monitored for recurrence. You should discuss even minor symptoms with your doctor. To get the best follow-up care, have the detailed records of your cancer treatment forwarded to your current family physician, internist, or pediatrician. These records should be carefully reviewed by your doctor. Keep a set of records for yourself.

In addition to monitoring you for a recurrence of your initial cancer, your physician also should be aware that some forms of cancer treatment can lead to an increased risk of second malignancies. A few specific examples are described below.

ACUTE MYELOGENOUS LEUKEMIA—Acute myelogenous leukemia may occur as a result of intensive therapy with radiation and chemotherapy—initially used to cure cancer—or as a result of prolonged therapy with certain types of chemotherapeutic drugs (alkylating agents or nitrosoureas). In general, this form of treatment-related acute leukemia occurs because of serious damage to the cells in the bone marrow that are responsible for making new blood cells. This type of leukemia is difficult to cure.

The peak time of occurrence of secondary acute leukemia in patients with Hodgkin's disease is five to seven years after initial treatment. Thus, a slowly developing anemia in a Hodgkin's disease survivor should alert the doctor to the possibility of a secondary leukemia. Newer adjuvant treatments using high doses of adriamycin and cytloxan have noted an increased rate of leukemia.

SOLID TUMORS AND OTHER MALIGNANCIES—Cancer survivors who have been treated with chemotherapy or radiation therapy are also at risk for solid tumors and other malignancies. Non-Hodgkin's lymphomas have been reported as a late complication in patients treated for Hodgkin's disease or multiple myeloma. Patients treated with long-term cyclophosphamide are at risk for bladder cancer. Patients who have received radiation therapy for Hodgkin's disease have an increased risk of breast cancer, osteosarcoma, and lung carcinomas.

In these cases, the second cancer usually involves tissues that were heavily radiated as part of the original cancer treatment. In general, the risk of solid tumors begins to increase during the second decade of survival after Hodgkin's disease. As a result, young women who have received radiation to the chest as part of their treatment for Hodgkin's disease should be screened more carefully for breast cancer starting about ten years after treatment. Screening for breast cancer should include a clinical breast examination every six months and a mammogram annually. Experts are studying whether tamoxifen may help some of these women in the prevention of breast cancer.

Other Late Effects

Endocrine Problems—A variety of endocrine problems are a result of cancer treatment. Patients receiving radiation therapy to the head and neck region can develop an underactive thyroid gland. This is a particular risk in patients receiving chest and neck radiation therapy for Hodgkin's disease. You should ask your doctor to be sure to monitor your thyroid function if you have had this type of treatment.

Menopause may start earlier than expected in women who have received certain chemotherapeutic agents (for example, alkylating agents and procarbazine) or abdominal radiation therapy. The risk is age-related, with women older than age 30 at the time of treatment having the greatest risk of treatment-induced menopause. Early hormone replacement therapy may help some women reduce the risk of accelerated osteoporosis and premature heart disease.

Treatment-related gonadal failure or dysfunction can lead to infertility in both male and female cancer survivors. Infertility can be temporary, especially in men, and they may recover over time after therapy. Psychological counseling may be helpful if you have experienced this long-term result of therapy.

Radiation therapy can affect the muscles, bones, and joints, especially in children and young adults. The radiation can injure the growth plates of long bones and can lead to muscle atrophy. Short stature sometimes occurs as a result of radiation therapy, but it also can be secondary to growth hormone deficiency in some people who have had brain radiation. Finally, abdominal radiation in young girls can change the size and shape of the immature uterus, which may make pregnancy difficult.

Childhood Cancer Survivors

Childhood cancer survivors are an important and rapidly growing segment of the survivor population. One in 900 young adults between the ages of fifteen and thirty-five is a survivor of childhood cancer. One in 330 children will be diagnosed with cancer by the age of twenty. Experts are studying the special problems of childhood cancer survivors.

Some children experience slower growth because of their treatment, especially radiation to growing bones. This can lead to some long-term physical limitations and changes in body image. Children who received radiation to the brain may experience learning and behavioral problems. Most childhood survivors have normal fertility and healthy children. Some survivors, however, are unable to have children.

Treatment programs are being designed to minimize these long-term problems. For more information about special issues for childhood cancers, see the Resources on page 325.

CANCER PREVENTION AND EARLY DETECTION

Although cancer survival rates are improving every year, the ideal goal is to decrease the occurrence of cancer through prevention. While screening and early detection of cancer will improve survival once cancer is diagnosed, preventing the development of cancer will provide an even greater impact on mortality rates. Cancer prevention is in its infancy, however, because only some of the causes of cancer are known. In addition, because complex behavioral and lifestyle changes often are required to lower the risk of cancer, prevention of cancer is very challenging. Increasingly, we are seeing the evaluation of medications in clinical trials to prevent the development of cancer in high-risk populations, and these may hold some promise as an alternative strategy. What are some of the approaches that can lead to a reduction in cancer incidence and mortality?

ELIMINATING THE USE OF TOBACCO

Tobacco kills approximately 25 percent of those who use it. Approximately 500,000 Americans and three million people worldwide die each year from tobacco-induced diseases, including cancer of the lung, head and neck, esophagus, bladder, and pancreas. Roughly half of the cancer deaths each year in the United States are causally related to tobacco use. Many Americans have heeded the warnings of the medical profession and decreased their use of cigarettes, pipes, cigars, and chewing tobacco. Between 1965, when the federal government first required a health warning on packages of cigarettes, and 1999, the smoking rate among adults in the United States decreased from 42 percent to 24 percent. In several states, increased tobacco taxes have encouraged further decreases in tobacco use. While adults have decreased their consumption, unfortunately adolescents are smoking more. Strong antismoking laws also have contributed to making this habit appear less socially acceptable.

EATING A WELL-BALANCED DIET

Americans have begun to change their diets significantly to reduce the risk of cancer and heart disease. Morning ham and eggs have given way to oat bran muffins, while fast-food chains promote salad bars and chicken sandwiches. Although scientists do not agree on the impact that diet has on cancer, they do agree that dietary changes can affect the chances of getting certain types of cancer. For example, high-fat diets increase the risk of colon, breast, and uterine cancer. High-fiber diets decrease the risk of colon cancer. The micronutrients found in many fruits and vegetables have been shown to have anticancer properties. Their high rates of consumption are associated with lower rates of cancer in various populations throughout the world.

A well-balanced diet, low in fat and high in fresh fruits and vegetables, is the most prudent cancer prevention diet. People who do not overeat and who maintain a balanced diet do not need extra vitamins and other supplements, which can be harmful in large quantities. Beware of dietary supplements that claim to prevent cancer. No diet can prevent cancer; it can only affect the risk of some types of cancer. For more information on diet and cancer, contact the Cancer Information Service at (800)-4-CANCER or **www.cancer.gov.**

AVOIDING EXCESSIVE RADIATION

Cosmetic and pharmaceutical manufacturers are selling a wide variety of sunscreens in response to the evidence that overexposure to the sun is the major cause of skin cancers. During the 1990s, a dark suntan began to lose its value as a status symbol as many Americans avoided the sun during midday and protected their skin with clothing and sunscreen.

Radon is another source of radiation to be avoided. A natural, odorless, radioactive gas, radon in high concentrations increases the risk of lung cancer; radon is found in the ground and can become trapped in buildings with inadequate ventilation. A simple, inexpensive test can measure the amount of radon in a building. Many people in areas with high levels of radon, such as parts of Pennsylvania, New Jersey, and New York, have improved their ventilation systems to decrease the radon levels in their homes and offices.

DECREASING ALCOHOL CONSUMPTION

Alcohol consumption increases the risk of oral cancers, especially when combined with tobacco use. Heavy drinking also increases the risk of liver cancer through the development of cirrhosis. In addition, regular daily alcohol consumption increases the risk of breast cancer.

SEXUALLY TRANSMITTED DISEASES AND CANCER

Cervical cancer and penile cancer are both associated with an infectious agent, the human papillomavirus (HPV). Given that the infection is transmitted sexually, men and women can take several steps to prevent the development of these cancers:
- avoid sexual activity as a young adolescent;
- avoid having multiple sexual partners;
- practice good hygiene;
- use barrier contraceptives, such as condoms or diaphragms;
- avoid intercourse with individuals who have numerous sexual partners.

REPORTING WARNING SIGNS TO YOUR DOCTOR

Although early diagnosis does not decrease the risk of getting cancer, it can dramatically improve the effectiveness of your treatment.

- Report to your doctor any symptoms or warning signals of cancer as defined by the American Cancer Society:

    Change in bowel or bladder habits.

    A sore that does not heal.

    Unusual bleeding or discharge.

    Thickening or lump in breast or elsewhere.

    Indigestion or difficulty in swallowing.

    Obvious change in wart or mole.

    Nagging cough or hoarseness.

- Conduct monthly self-examinations of your skin, breasts (women), and testicles (men). The American Cancer Society and National Cancer Institute have booklets that describe how to perform a self-exam.

- See your doctor for routine physicals that include a screening for breast, cervical, and colon cancer.

Chapter Two

Working with Your Doctor and Hospital

Becoming a Wise Consumer

by Natalie Davis Spingarn
and Nancy H. Chasen, J.D.

W E ARE ALL CONSUMERS—users of goods and services. In no other area of life do we know as little about our choices as in the field of health care. Yet to be effective members of our health care team, we must become informed consumers. You must gather a lot of information to make sound choices about your caregivers, hospitals, and treatment.

This chapter provides a road map to help you find the right doctor and then to communicate with him or her to your best advantage—both inside and outside of a managed care setting. This chapter also offers suggestions to select the most appropriate hospital for your needs, as well as important tips for protecting your personal privacy.

GATHERING INFORMATION AND CHOOSING A DOCTOR

A HISTORICAL PERSPECTIVE

We investigate prospective schools and colleges carefully before enrolling, asking detailed questions about facilities and faculty. Whether we buy a big item like a house or car or a smaller one like a computer, we often shop around for weeks, even months, comparing quality and price to see which is the best buy.

When it comes to purchasing health care, however, cancer survivors used to follow their doctor's advice without question and without exploring other options. But in recent years a revolution in attitudes and a growing candor about medical matters, including preventive health care, have transformed patients from passive to active participants in their care. Civil rights, women's rights, consumers' rights, and human rights have helped to empower survivors. Now many feel that they should have a hand in choosing their treatment to improve their quality of life. The growing wealth of consumer health-related information has given survivors the means to become informed participants in their own health care.

When you become a cancer survivor today, you become a consumer in a vast medical marketplace, which you typically enter with little or no experience or training, but where you must play an active role. The many recent advances in research and technology complicate the survivor's job with a mind-boggling array of treatment choices. The choices you make affect the quality of your life as well as your finances. Before you select your doctor, learn which providers are covered by your insurance plan. See Chapter 12 for information on health insurance for cancer survivors.

LEARNING ABOUT YOUR TREATMENT

Learn about your diagnosis and the different treatment options available to you so that you can understand and participate in crafting a treatment plan. A vast quantity of information is available on the Internet, from government and private organizations, and from survivors willing to share their experiences. Chapter 17 explains how to find this information.

Do not be surprised if you suffer from information overload. This can be an overwhelming and confusing time, especially at first. After all, you are learning about a disease that is complicated to understand and that has its own vocabulary.

THE PRIMARY DOCTOR: ORCHESTRATING YOUR CARE

Cancer survivors need a primary care doctor—an oncologist—to orchestrate their care. Your primary care doctor will become a significant part of your life, not only during treatment, but perhaps for years of follow-up care.

The "best doctor" means more than the doctor with the best education, although training is important. The "best doctors" practice in fine hospitals, use excellent radiologists and other specialists, refer patients to clinical trials, run efficient patient-centered offices with caring staff, and communicate in a way that leaves you feeling good about yourself and your treatment.

In a managed care setting, you may be limited to doctors within the network who meet these criteria, or your plan may permit you to see a doctor outside of the system if you pay a larger share of the cost. Older patients will find that some doctors will not take new Medicare patients.

No "ONE SIZE FITS ALL"—The quality of your cancer experience depends, in part, on whether you find a doctor who is sensitive to your needs and your concerns, one who understands you as a person as well as a patient with a disease, and one who has the personality and clinical skills that allow you to be comfortable in a lengthy medical relationship.

Do not use a "one size fits all" formula in your search. Patients differ greatly in their preferences and needs. You may not want to conduct in-depth discussions with your doctors about your disease and treatment. You may not want detailed statistics about your chances for long-term survival. You may assume that the doctor knows best and be more comfortable leaving the tough medical decisions to him or her, which is your privilege. Many survivors, particularly older ones, share such views. Others feel better when they are involved actively in making decisions and gathering information about cancer care.

IDENTIFYING CANDIDATES–Begin by identifying a few candidates from among your previous doctors, from your health plan, and from your friends and family. You can call the local medical society, the chief resident or experienced nurses at the hospital, or local peer-support groups of seasoned survivors for suggestions. Be cautious: Doctors and other medical professionals willingly tell you good news about each other, but they seldom level with you about the bad news.

If you live near a comprehensive cancer center, check the center's Web site. These sites typically include detailed information about each center's staff physicians, including their areas of expertise, publications, and practical information such as addresses and phone numbers. Chapter 17 lists comprehensive cancer centers and their Web sites, as well as information to help you find a doctor.

Consider the following in making your choice:

Basic Credentials—Though credentials are not everything, they are still important. Note the doctor's basic credentials, including education, teaching affiliations, and whether he or she is board-certified in a specialty.

Board Certification—Find out whether the doctor is the type of medical specialist you need (for example, medical oncologist, radiation oncologist, general surgeon). Note that some are self-proclaimed specialists who have not satisfied the requirements for certification established by the professional board that supervises that field.

Certification means that doctors have passed rigorous peer-administered written and oral examinations in their field and satisfied residency training requirements. Some physicians are *double boarded,* meaning they are certified in more than one field. A few specialty boards require recertification after a certain number of years. Initials starting with an "F" (like F.A.C.P.) after a doctor's name mean that he or she has been honored by election to a specialty college fellowship.

Experience—Length of experience is always important, but medical oncology is a relatively new subspecialty of internal medicine, certified as such only since 1973. So when you consider older doctors who may lack this formal credential, check carefully on other factors, such as reputation among support group members, publications, teaching affiliations, and whether they enroll and/or follow patients in clinical trials (or have colleagues who do so).

Hospital Affiliation—Learn which hospitals the doctor is affiliated with, and which ones he or she prefers and why. Also determine where arrangements will be made for you to have radiation therapy, chemotherapy, or any other outpatient treatment.

Style of Practice—How do the doctors you are considering practice? If they practice independently, do they work closely with other physicians? If they are with a group or in a university setting, do they see you each time you have an appointment, or are you seen by an assortment of associates (and if so, who are these associates and what is the level of their education and training)?

"Chairside Manner"—In the old days, people talked about a physician's "bedside manner." Now, when doctors rarely come to see you in bed, and you are seen in an office chair more often than a hospital bed, it is appropriate to check out the "chairside manner" of a doctor. Do prospective doctors seem warm and concerned with you as a person? Talking with you, do they sit down or glance at a wristwatch while they hover at the door? Do you feel so rushed that your questions have gone unanswered? If called away in an emergency, do they arrange a time to answer your questions?

Office Procedures—When are the doctors usually in the office (days and hours of the day)? Can they be reached evenings or weekends? Who "covers" for them when they are away or not available by phone? How long, on the average, do patients have to wait to see them? Are your prospective caregivers part of that rare breed who still make house calls? How do they want you to proceed in the event of an emergency?

Who manages the office, answers the phones, and deals with the billing? What are the office policies toward the confidentiality of the information you choose to share with them? (See page 47 for a discussion of your privacy rights.)

Office Atmosphere—Note the manner in which the doctor's staff conducts business. Are they warm and patient with you and with others—on the phone as well as in person? Do they seem efficient and willing to answer your questions, even if your questions concern such mundane things as your next appointment? Check out the appearance of the office. Is it comfortable and cheerful, or dark, drab, and cluttered? In one major city, patients left a practice because chemotherapy was administered in a small, dark, messy room crowded with black chemotherapy chairs. As one such survivor put it: "That depressing place makes me feel like death warmed over; why make things worse than they have to be?"

Quality of Staff—The nurses and other paraprofessionals who work with a doctor may draw your blood and administer your chemotherapy. Find out how many of them are RNs (registered nurses), and how many have been tested and awarded the OCN (oncology certified nurse) credential. Consider the importance of experience, just as you did in choosing the doctor.

SPECIFIC TIPS–To see if you feel comfortable with a doctor, you will have to visit his or her office. Even then it is sometimes difficult in the first interview to determine whether you have chosen wisely; sometimes it takes months to find out.

Here are a few suggestions about what to watch for and how to proceed at the beginning of your professional relationship:

- Some doctors encourage you to take notes during important visits—and even to tape conversations—so you will remember the details of a diagnosis or answers to your questions about treatment. Ask about office policy in this regard.

- To test a doctor's ability to relate to you, you might show him or her the *American Cancer Society's Survivor's Bill of Rights* (reprinted on pages 53 and 54). Ask how he or she feels about statement number one, specifying that those involved in cancer care, for example, should be "sensitive to the cancer survivor's lifestyle choices and need for self-esteem and dignity" and should take symptoms seriously and not dismiss aches and pains. Any marked disagreement about such statements should serve as a warning that you may not have chosen the right doctor.

- If you have other compelling reasons to stay in treatment with a particular doctor—including, for example, the limits placed on your freedom of choice by a managed care plan—discuss them frankly with him or her.

- If your test results, biopsies, and other indicators of the success of your treatment (including how you feel) do not please you at any time, get a second or even third opinion. Some health plans cover and may require second opinions, while others may require your primary care doctor's approval of such opinions. Even if you decide to stay with a particular doctor, a second opinion approving your treatment may make you more comfortable and reinforce your trust.

- If all this does not work, if you feel your doctor does not have the necessary skills, or if you simply cannot feel comfortable with him or her, consider looking for a new doctor. The process will be much the same as the search for your first doctor, except that you have gained experience, know more about what you are looking for, and know what questions to ask.

COMMUNICATIONS—THE TWO-WAY STREET

To work successfully with your doctor, you must be able to talk frankly. As a survivor, you need an anchor, a coordinator, and an interpreter of information with whom you can conduct a comfortable dialogue—a dialogue that may continue for years.

Modern medical care can be highly technical, complex, and difficult to understand. Moreover, it is delivered by a team of specialists, including surgeons, radiologists, and a multitude of nurses and technicians. Psychiatrists, gastroenterologists, gynecologists, neurologists, and others may be consulted. Communicating with these specialists, and getting the benefit of their shared views, is an integral part of survivorship.

BARRIERS TO COMMUNICATION

Communication between the doctor and patient is a two-way street. Good communication can improve the quality of your cancer journey. The primary responsibility for it rests with the doctor. Your doctor needs accurate information from you to provide appropriate cancer care. Yet sometimes patients fail to tell their doctors crucial information.

Why is this so? Although talking with a doctor sounds easy, many survivors report that it is not. Survivors want to know more about their treatment options. They may not know what, when, or how much medicine to take. They may be anxious to learn whether new pains are serious or are unimportant side effects of old treatments. Certain attitudes and fears restrain survivors from talking with their doctors, including:

AWE OF THE DOCTOR—Many survivors stand in awe of their doctors, in whose hands their comfort and even their lives rest. They want these doctors to make them better, to like them, and not to consider them pests or hypochondriacs.

LACK OF SELF-CONFIDENCE—Survivors too often fear to ask the questions that lurk in their minds, afraid that the doctor will consider these questions "stupid" or "dumb." They worry: Doesn't this busy physician have more important things to do than answer my questions? The answer is "NO!"

DIFFICULTY REMEMBERING—No matter who they are, or how extensive their experience or impressive their education, survivors can grow anxious discussing life-and-death matters with their doctors. Hearing new words and new concepts, they can suffer "information overload." They can have trouble focusing, absorbing abstract ideas, and remembering all but certain emotionally charged "buzz words"—like *cure* or *disability*. Survivors commonly return home from an important medical interview and find they are unable to tell family or friends exactly what the doctor said.

"IATROGENIC" BEWILDERMENT—*Iatrogenic* means "induced by a physician." Some doctors make it difficult for you to understand them by using complex, technical language instead of plain English (for example, *alopecia* rather than "hair loss"). They may act as though they have no time for you, failing to sit down during your interview, or even hovering near the door. An NCCS survey explains in *Words That Heal, Words That Harm* (available from the National Coalition for Cancer Survivorship) that the doctor who told his patient "You're a walking time bomb," and another who observed that certain treatment was "only palliative," were using negative and harmful words that left patients shaken. Some doctors may simply seem insensitive to hints or cues you give as to how you would like to be treated.

Suggestions for Effective and Meaningful Communication

Some survivors argue that medical competence is more important to patients than communication skills. As one lawyer put it, she would rather see a "bleeding bastard" who would cure her than a less competent, "sweet-talking" physician. To provide you quality cancer care, however, your doctor must get sufficient information from you and explain important concepts to you.

The following are suggestions for how to communicate effectively with your doctor and other caregivers:

Speak Frankly with Your Doctor—Your doctor cannot read your mind. Describe your symptoms—not only the obvious aches and pains, but other signs you have observed, such as trouble falling asleep at night, unhealthy eating habits, or overindulgence in alcoholic beverages. Keep a notebook of your symptoms when you experience them and of questions when you think of them so you can bring a written list to your doctor. You can then record your doctor's answers directly next to your questions in your notebook. Include questions about office procedures and confidentiality policies. For example, ask, "Who has access to my medical records? Will you charge me for photocopying my medical records?"

Bring a Family Member or Friend—If you have trouble asserting yourself, bring a family member or friend to speak for you. If several people are involved, be sure your doctor understands who they are and to what extent your doctor can discuss your situation with them.

Tape Important Conversations—Because most people have trouble absorbing new information when they are upset, some doctors ask patients to tape important conversations so they can listen to the tape again later in the quiet of their homes. That way, they can review medical explanations and instructions in calmer, more rational moments.

Insist on Privacy During Important Interviews—Under no circumstances should such an interview take place in a busy hallway, where anyone passing by can hear it. Preferably, consultations should be conducted with you and your physician seated and facing each other in a private room with the door closed.

Tell Your Doctor How Much Information You Want and Need to Know—Doctors used to tell patients nothing about cancer, not even that they had it. Now they tend to tell everything, including statistical chances for survival. Patients have different "coping styles"; for some it is frightening to know these things, for others it is frightening not to know. If your doctor is overloading you with facts and statistics that you do not want, simply say so; or offer a hint or cue as to how you feel. Try something like, "My father's already gotten the statistics about my tumor from PDQ" or simply "You know best." Sometimes body language—such as turning away and looking down—can help indicate you have had enough. If you want to know more about your disease, its treatment, and possible outcome, say so.

Ask for Explanations of Long, Puzzling Medical Terms–Never be embarrassed if you do not understand a word like "metastasis" or "sarcoma." Insist on a translation into plain English. Ask your doctor to show you a diagram or picture of the organs he or she is describing so you can understand where they are in your body and their relation to one another. Your doctor will probably respect your need to have your situation described in a way that makes sense to you.

Do Not Forget That Doctors Are People, Too–Medical professionals respond to you just as you respond to them: pleasantness is usually met with pleasantness, and courtesy with courtesy. Express your appreciation when your doctor sits down to talk with you—either at the side of your bed in the hospital or in an office chair—and gives you complete attention during your limited time together.

If the doctor is called away from a consultation for an emergency, you should be told when he or she will return. If you are not told, or if the doctor looks at his or her wristwatch in the middle of an important conversation, or takes non-emergency telephone calls, speak up. Say you realize that he or she is a busy person, but you would like to know when you will be able to finish your talk because you still have unanswered questions.

Do Not Present Yourself to Your Doctor As a Disease, but As a Person Living with a Disease–One survivor reported that she made it a rule to tell her doctor one thing about her life on each visit: that she had been to London, or had seen a ball game, or taken a poetry course. In this way, the doctor learned more about her and could look at her and treat her as a whole person. Another reported that she traveled frequently, but was anxious about going too far from sophisticated medical care. The physician prepared a special medicine kit for her to take when she went to underdeveloped countries.

Be Sure That You Understand Your Treatment Plan before You Leave the Doctor–Be sure you understand which tests and medicines have been prescribed, and how long and when you will be taking them. Ask the doctor to repeat whatever you are not sure of, including the benefits and risks involved in your treatment. Find out where and when you can call him or her in case a new problem occurs. Do not be embarrassed about taking too much of your doctor's time, although you should use your time together wisely. Informed patients are more cooperative patients, and doctors report that good communication with patients saves them time in the long run.

IF YOU FIND YOURSELF UNABLE TO COMMUNICATE WITH YOUR DOCTOR, TRY TO FIND ANOTHER ONE—If you feel hurried as you talk, or if you feel that your doctor is not listening to your questions or giving you clear answers, discuss your concerns with your doctor. You may be surprised at the results.

Consider the advice of a support group or a cancer counselor to see how other patients have handled such problems and how you and your doctor may communicate better. As doctors themselves will tell you, if all this fails, consider changing physicians. Although this may be difficult for some—for patients in managed care or Medicare, or in rural areas—keep trying. With persistence, you can probably find new caregivers.

THE HOSPITAL: A WORLD UNTO ITSELF

Cancer survivors do not spend much of their health care time in the hospital, mainly because hospital stays are expensive and outpatient care is used whenever possible. But most survivors do spend some time as inpatients, particularly at the beginning of treatment. This is usually a significant experience that may set the tone for how you view your care in the future.

EVALUATING HOSPITALS

Patients are often unprepared for the hospital experience. You may have been in the hospital briefly to have an appendectomy (a nuisance) or a baby (a joy) or to visit a sick grandmother (a duty). Unless you are an unusually sophisticated consumer of medical services, you probably did not shop carefully for a hospital. In the fee-for-service system, your doctor usually stipulated one of the hospitals where he or she had privileges. If you were covered by a managed care plan, your choice of hospitals may have been limited.

No matter where physicians and particularly surgeons practice, one of the first questions you should ask them is, "With what hospital, or hospitals are you—or your managed care plans—affiliated?" Managed care plans vary widely. Some are restricted to one or two local hospitals; others include services at comprehensive cancer centers in distant cities.

When you have the names of these hospitals, check them out. The public library is a good starting resource. Check the Internet for the hospitals' Web sites. The advice of seasoned survivors, nurses, and other health professionals may be more impartial than that of the local medical society or hospital association.

Gourmet cooking and cable television are both very nice but should not be the determining factors in evaluating a hospital. What you are seeking is an excellent workplace for your health team—a humane haven in a difficult period of your life. The following is a checklist to use as you consider specific hospitals.

TYPE OF HOSPITAL—Cancer care is offered in many different settings, from major cancer centers to small community hospitals. A comprehensive cancer center— one that is designated by the National Cancer Institute—is likely to offer high-quality, modern medical care. Researchers at these institutions have been involved in many of the most important medical advances.

Comprehensive cancer centers offer a wide variety of services, from counseling and rehabilitation to home-care supervision. If you belong to a managed care plan, find out if it offers a point-of-service option covering the full services of a cancer center. If not, you can still go to one, at least for a consultation, if you are able to pay for it out of your own pocket.

In addition to these comprehensive centers, clinical cancer centers around the country are funded in part by the National Cancer Institute to carry out research and training programs, as well as patient care. Be aware, however, that some for-profit hospitals call themselves cancer centers or even comprehensive cancer centers.

But if they are free-standing (not affiliated with medical schools) and do not have research or teaching obligations, they probably are not designated as cancer centers by the federal government. See pages 313–321 or call (800)-4-CANCER (the NCI's cancer information service) for a list of NCI-designated comprehensive and clinical cancer centers.

Other important questions to ask when evaluating hospitals include—

- Is this a teaching hospital, and is its cancer program affiliated with a medical school?
- Does a medical school use the hospital for internship and residency programs?

The advantages of medical school affiliation—the availability of doctor-faculty members, round-the-clock medical attention, a broad variety of services, and a greater likelihood of state-of-the-art oncology—usually outweigh the disadvantages (for example, being treated as a teaching case, which means being poked and prodded, especially when the medical team makes its early morning teaching rounds).

ACCREDITATION & RANKINGS—Many community hospitals provide cancer care. The American College of Surgeons Commission on Cancer has established standards for cancer programs and accredits over 1,400 hospitals that have met its standards. You can find at **http://web.facs.org/cpm/default.htm** hospitals in your community that have voluntarily sought accreditation as a cancer program.

If you are considering a community hospital that is not a federally designated cancer center and is not affiliated, either directly or indirectly, with a medical school, be sure your hospital is accredited. The Joint Commission on Accreditation of Healthcare Organizations (JCAHO), a professionally sponsored group employing physicians, nurses, health-care administrators, and other experts, holds hospitals to some one thousand staffing, safety, and quality-of-practitioner-care standards. You can learn whether a hospital is accredited either by calling the Illinois-based JCAHO's customer service line at (630) 792-5800, or online at **www.jcaho.org**. You can also learn about various hospital services from the *American Hospital Association Guide to the Health Care Field,* an annual hospital survey published every fall and available in most public libraries.

You are also likely to find helpful information in articles that rank medical institutions. Some large-city magazines periodically carry articles rating local hospitals. Such lists include information from various sources, both objective and subjective. *U.S. News and World Report* has published a national listing of top hospitals every year since 1990, ranking hospitals within various specialties. The most recent list can be found online at **www.usnews.com** (click on Rankings) where you can search under the "Cancer" specialty and narrow your search to the hospitals in a particular geographic region. Clicking on any hospital's name will take you directly to that institution's Web site.

CONVENIENCE—Going to a hospital close to home, where your friends and family can visit you easily, offers many advantages. But if that hospital cannot provide you with the quality of care you need, you should consider another one, even if it is some distance away. A sensible compromise is a consultation at the closest comprehensive cancer center. Often the experts there can make the diagnosis, map out your treatment plan, and consult with your local doctors and hospital as they carry it out. If you cannot travel to a cancer center far from home for family or financial reasons, you may find the care you need in your own community (see Services below).

SIZE AND SOURCE OF FUNDING—When considering the size of a hospital, bigger is not always better. Some large hospitals (500 or more beds) are very good, some are not so good, and some are poor. The same is true of medium-sized (100–500 beds) and small (fewer than 100 beds) hospitals. Although bigger hospitals may seem more bureaucratic and impersonal, they may have more cancer treatment resources, such as expensive high-technology equipment. Moreover, staff members often are more experienced, since they see a wide variety of cases.

As for the source of a hospital's funding, public hospitals (like veterans hospitals, county hospitals, and some urban hospitals) may suffer from a poor image and may not provide certain amenities. But amenities are less important than quality care. If it is affiliated with a good teaching hospital, attracting interns and residents eager to care for a variety of patients, and if it is well organized to deliver care, a public hospital may provide outstanding service.

SERVICES—It is difficult to assess the services of a given hospital until you have experienced them. But you can check on the quality and variety of services a hospital has to offer through your doctor, the hospital's administrative offices, and through other survivors who have used them. If you are having surgery, for example, you might ask your surgeon for details regarding the hospital's recovery room or intensive care unit. Ask about the reputation of its pathology laboratory and blood bank.

Some community hospitals do not serve enough cancer patients to have a special cancer unit. They may, however, offer treatment in local alliances, through which you can get scans in one hospital and radiation in another. Such an arrangement may suit your needs. Be sure you have answers to the following questions:

- Where will you receive care?
- Will the hospital have the high-tech equipment necessary to treat you after surgery? For example, are radiation therapy and scanning equipment available? If not, where will you receive such therapies when they are necessary?
- What is the reputation of the hospital's other services, such as respiratory and physical therapy, social work services, or posttreatment program?
- Most meaningful perhaps, what is the reputation of the hospital's nursing staff and of the non-R.N. staff who are performing nursing functions? Whether the people taking hands-on care of you are called "nursing aides" or "patient care associates" or something else, their number and the quality of their work, including their sensitivity to your needs, will affect your health and your well-being.

THE HOSPITAL EXPERIENCE–The quality and length of your hospital stay will be determined, in part, by your health insurance plan. Your insurer may determine whether you receive cancer treatment as an inpatient or outpatient, in a private room or semiprivate room, and for how many days.

Most hospitals have a preadmission process for nonemergency admissions to collect insurance, medical, and other information about you. You may go through a battery of tests before you are admitted, from which you may first learn the atmosphere of the institution. You can be passed from hand-to-hand efficiently and cheerfully and treated as a human being instead of as a body hosting a disease. Or you may face a seemingly disorganized, loud, and crowded environment.

Once you are admitted, you will become a part of the special hospital culture. Different caregivers will draw blood, perform tests, and care for you in different ways. Others can answer your questions about daily routine, such as visiting hours, meal times, and where to keep your personal items.

The hospital is a world unto itself, a world to experience and to master. This world brings both good and bad news. The good news is that you can feel hopeful, even ennobled, by the marvelous care the modern hospital can offer through many well-trained, devoted, and talented professionals and paraprofessionals. Your caregivers now are more likely to look at you as a whole person, rather than as a lung or breast or set of bones.

The bad news is that a few impersonal staff members wedded to sometimes mindless institutional routines can make you feel dehumanized. For example, they may wake you up to give you a sleeping pill or ask you why you let yourself get cancer. More crucial, even the best hospitals with excellent reputations occasionally make mistakes. Though these mistakes are seldom fatal, survivors should remain alert to the possibilities.

The tragic death in 1994 of *Boston Globe* health columnist Betsy Lehman made this painfully clear. Though this 39-year-old mother of two had chosen one of the country's preeminent cancer centers for bone marrow transplant treatment, and though she repeatedly complained of increasing pain and had a gut feeling that something had gone dreadfully wrong, Ms. Lehman was administered a fourfold chemotherapy dosage, four days in a row. Her resulting death, and the cardiac crippling of a fellow patient in the same hospital program, focused national attention on the issue of hospital errors.

A series of public and private investigations resulted in increased awareness that more hospitals must take steps to oversee quality treatment, including installing computerized techniques for ensuring dosage ceilings, clarifying guidelines for highly toxic drugs, better supervision of junior staff, and the design of unambiguous physician order forms. Essential as such improvements are, they will prove ineffective unless they are supplemented by sensitive professional education and on-the-job training in doctor-patient communication.

DEALING WITH HOSPITAL LIFE

Seasoned survivors have found that their attitude—the way they respond to the hospital culture—can improve their hospital experience. The following suggestions may help you deal with hospital life.

BE ASSERTIVE—If your common sense tells you something is wrong, learn to act, not aggressively or rudely, but assertively. If someone wakes you up for no good reason or jabs at your veins until your arm is speckled black and blue, ask politely but firmly for an explanation and a remedy. If you cannot speak up for yourself, ask your spouse, a relative, or a friend to speak up for you.

KNOW YOU CANNOT PERFORM THE IMPOSSIBLE—Be equally assertive in dealing with new and sometimes misguided staff efforts to help you avoid hospital errors. Someone may suggest that you should check your own drug dosages and other aspects of your care. If you wish to do this, and feel well enough to try, fine. If not, and particularly if you are alone with no one to speak up for you, respectfully make clear that you are unable to perform what is really your caregiver's job.

EMPATHIZE WITH OTHERS—Make an effort to treat hospital staff and fellow patients as you would like to be treated. They will likely respond to your respectful and polite attitude in kind.

DO NOT TAKE YOURSELF TOO SERIOUSLY—Even as you take your situation seriously, try to keep your sense of humor. When you can laugh, joke, and empathize with others, you will find your experience to be a little more pleasant.

STAY ALERT. SPEAK OUT. ASK QUESTIONS—Many people are fearful of hospital authority. An extreme example is the patient who is given a pill she feels sure is wrong, but does not ask questions because she fears doctors and nurses will consider her uncooperative, pushy, or ignorant. You and your caregivers will benefit if you tell them what bothers you and what information you need to feel more comfortable.

IF YOU MUST, COMPLAIN—When you have exhausted your assertiveness and you are still not satisfied, by all means, complain. Complain to your doctor, to the nursing supervisor on your floor, to the chief nurse, to the hospital administrator, or to the hospital patient representative. Present the facts calmly and clearly, but demand attention to your concerns.

GOING HOME AND REENTERING SOCIETY

Some patients enjoy the often abbreviated postsurgery part of hospital life. Free of the cares of job and household, they savor their visitors, the plants they bring, the ministrations of the staff, and the companionship of other patients—particularly when the prognosis is good. Others find their hospital stay more stressful than the time spent at home immediately after their release.

Everyone looks forward to going home. Hospitals usually help you plan to assure that your reentry into the real world of self-care and many responsibilities is accomplished smoothly. In the discharge planning process, a nurse, social worker, or some other designated professional works with you to make sure you have the appropriate help and are in other ways prepared to convalesce at home. (See Chapter 3 for a discussion of the roles of these helping professionals.)

KNOWING AND UNDERSTANDING YOUR RIGHTS—INFORMED CONSENT, CONFIDENTIALITY, AND PATIENT RECORDS

PATIENT'S BILL OF RIGHTS

Congress may eventually pass a federal Patient's Bill of Rights that would, for example, curb or eliminate the most common abuses in managed care plans. These problems include restricting access to specialists, prohibiting doctors from discussing treatment options, and overruling the doctor's judgment on how long cancer patients need to stay in the hospital. Much remains to be done to ensure such rights as a matter of law.

In the meantime, many hospitals have their own Patient's Bill of Rights that govern hospital-patient relationships in those institutions. These statements typically list the rights and responsibilities of patients, such as the right to be treated with respect and compassion, to receive information about your diagnosis and treatment from your attending physicians, and to receive an itemized bill. A few are more treatment-oriented, such as the Johns Hopkins Breast Center's Breast Cancer Patient's Bill of Rights, which includes the right to be "evaluated by a multidisciplinary team of health care professionals dedicated to the diagnosis and treatment of women with breast cancer".

INFORMED CONSENT: YOUR RIGHT TO CHOOSE AND REFUSE TREATMENT

Your right to accept or refuse medical treatment both complicates good doctor-patient communication and makes it essential. Informed consent, the process by which patients agree to treatment, is more than a legal exercise. It offers an opportunity to learn about your medical options.

Doctors who take time to fully explain the consent form you must sign before you receive a specific treatment are at the same time explaining the treatment's benefits, side effects, and possible alternatives. Although state laws vary as to what treatments and procedures require your specific consent, they typically include chemotherapy, surgery, internal examinations such as a colonoscopy, and dye injections for a scan.

RESPONSIBILITIES—*The doctor*—Your doctor does not have to tell you everything about a proposed procedure, but must give you enough information to allow you to make an informed decision about whether you want to undergo it. You must be told the nature and purpose of the procedure, the risk and consequence of the procedure, the medically acceptable alternatives to the procedure, and the risks of not having the procedure. Your written consent is valid only if you have been given adequate information to make an informed decision.

The patient—If your doctor does not volunteer information about a procedure, ask for it. If you do not understand what you are told, ask for a clear explanation before you sign a form consenting to treatment.

Carefully read the informed consent form itself. When you sign it, you state two important things that help avoid future misunderstandings: that you are an "informed" patient and that you give your consent to be treated.

THE PATIENT'S RIGHTS—If you do not agree with every statement on the consent form, you can make changes. For example, if the form states that you agree to have your operation videotaped for use by medical schools, and you do not want to be videotaped, just draw a line through that sentence and put your initials next to your changes.

By signing a consent form, you give your doctor permission to treat you and acknowledge that you understand that a particular result cannot be guaranteed. You do not give up your ability to sue your doctor for malpractice should he or she fail to follow professional standards and cause you harm. Informed consent is not a waiver of the doctor's liability if he or she acts negligently or improperly. (See pages 283–286 for a discussion of medical malpractice.)

WHEN YOUR CONSENT IS NOT NEEDED–Your doctor does not have to obtain your consent if—
- emergency treatment is needed to save your life or to prevent permanent harm;
- you have given your consent to one type of surgery, and during that surgery, a serious unanticipated condition arises (for example, you gave your consent to have cancerous lymph nodes removed, and during surgery, your doctor finds involvement in another organ and therefore removes it, too);
- you waive your right to consent to each treatment and agree to let your doctor make decisions about your care without consulting you;
- you suffer from a progressive illness and, having previously given informed consent to an anticipated course of treatment, are no longer capable of making decisions.

THE RIGHT TO REFUSE TREATMENT–A competent adult has the right to refuse medical treatment, even if the result may be death. Although these rights are limited by concerns such as danger to the public if treatment is withheld in case of AIDS or potential harm to the fetus of a pregnant woman with cancer, these limits vary from state to state.

In the case of incompetent patients, states increasingly respect the patient's previously expressed wishes. In the absence of clear direction, credible surrogates may be permitted to refuse treatment on the patient's behalf. See pages 277–281 for a discussion of your right to refuse treatment and to prepare advance health directives.

CHILDREN AND INFORMED CONSENT–Under most circumstances, parents have the right to make treatment decisions for their children, although they cannot typically refuse life-saving care for their children. Most states give children the right to choose their own medical treatment at the age of 18, with two exceptions:
- Minors deemed mature and emancipated (married or self-supporting and living away from home) usually are permitted to make their own medical decisions.
- If a parent's refusal to consent to treatment may cause avoidable harm to the child, a court may decide that the child is suffering from neglect and appoint a guardian to make medical decisions for the child.

CONFIDENTIALITY

We used to take for granted that our doctors, sworn under the Oath of Hippocrates not to "nose abroad" or divulge their patients' "holy secrets," would keep the information we shared to themselves. In those simpler days, medical record keeping was a comparatively simple business, with doctors filing facts about your health on 3 × 5 cards, and maintaining them—unmolested—from the patients' birth through their death.

You can no longer take the sanctity of your medical records for granted. Some of what you tell your doctors, including sensitive and highly personal information about your emotional as well as physical health, may no longer be held in confidence.

Most doctors object as strongly as do survivors to this erosion of doctor-patient confidentiality. But your doctor has little control over the increasing complexity of the medical marketplace, reliance on third-party insurers to pay medical expenses, and electronic movement of personal information.

ACCESS TO YOUR MEDICAL RECORDS BY OTHERS–During the course of your cancer treatment, you are likely to be treated by many doctors in several different settings. To coordinate your care, treat you successfully, and be paid, your doctor will probably share information about you with other doctors, nurses, office staff, and insurers.

The Risks—In a managed care setting or in a private physician's office, your medical record may be seen by various caregivers, even though it contains sensitive information such as "patient appears depressed" or "patient reports husband suffers sexual dysfunction." The same is true at hospitals, laboratories, and at the pharmacy that maintains your prescription records.

Your routine signature authorizing your doctor to disclose health information to your insurers triggers a more far-reaching risk. This signature allows access to your entire medical file, including personal information that may not be relevant to a particular claim. But the time-honored bonds of confidentiality that apply to the doctor-patient relationship do not extend to "third party payers" under the law. So insurance companies can, and frequently do, transfer or even sell such information to other data banks. In some circumstances, your records flow to data banks maintained by institutions like health maintenance organizations, hospital networks, drug companies, or medical information clearinghouses, which collect information from member insurance companies and distribute it to similar companies.

If you want to be sure your treatment is covered, refusing to authorize your doctor to open your records to insurers is not a realistic option. You probably can, however, cross out particularly offensive phrases in release forms without dire consequences. For example, one seasoned survivor routinely crossed out "now and forever" from the sentence defining the time frame of her releases.

The Benefits—Ready access to your complete medical history can be a lifesaver if you are traveling, relocating, or changing doctors. Well-organized, computerized medical records can eliminate mistakes resulting from a doctor's sloppy handwriting and can avoid the need to retest when x-rays are mislaid or blood counts lost. One metastatic breast cancer survivor reports that she would have preferred submitting her medical data to a host of computers to the experience of searching with hospital authorities one Fourth of July weekend for her spinal x-rays (they had slipped behind a file cabinet).

Still, you should be alert to the fact that your medical records travel routinely along computerized highways at incredible speeds. Your medical information can flow, not only to insurers, but to employers through whom most Americans get their health care paid for.

PRIVACY AND YOUR MEDICAL RECORDS

Putting sensitive information in the hands of the wrong person, or even in the hands of the right person who unknowingly misuses it, can stigmatize you. It can result in your losing a job, failing to qualify for insurance, keeping you out of school or university, or adversely affecting your credit rating. Yet, our laws have long fallen short of fully addressing the perils of record keeping in an age of massive computerized data banks and third-party payers.

After years of discussion, the federal government issued privacy regulations in 2003 under the Health Insurance Portability and Accountability Act (HIPAA). Patients now enjoy the right to: 1) inspect and obtain copies of their medical records and request corrections of errors and mistakes; 2) receive a notice from doctors and other health care providers regarding their rights under the regulations; and 3) request that their doctors take reasonable steps to keep their communications confidential.

Health providers must get your written permission before they can share your records with employers or with insurance companies who consider you for life or disability insurance coverage. They also must receive your written permission before they can share information about you with marketers who sell products, such as wigs, of potential interest to cancer patients. You also must authorize the release of information about you for medical research. In the case of clinical trials, the consent form and HIPAA authorization form might be combined. Finally, health providers and insurers will no longer share information about adult patients with their family members unless the patient has given written permission to do so. You may refuse to give your permission to share your information for any of these purposes.

Doctors and hospitals are not required to obtain patient consent to use and release confidential health information for the purposes of treatment, payment, or health care operations. Some providers may, however, ask you for permission to disclose your records for these purposes, too, just to be on the safe side. Read these disclosure forms carefully. If you are uncomfortable with or do not understand them, discuss them with your health care provider. He or she may be willing, although not required, to give your records more protection.

In the wake of these new rules, you may also notice certain privacy-related changes in your doctor's office. For example, some no longer use public sign-in sheets and do not place patient charts or lab orders where other patients can see them. Some no longer call out the names of patients in the waiting room. If you feel that your privacy is being compromised by certain office procedures, tell your doctor or his or her staff.

If you have a complaint about the privacy practices of a health care provider, contact:

Office of Civil Rights
Department of Health and Human Services
http://www.hhs.gov/ocr/hipaa
866-627-7748

Although state laws vary widely, some may offer more protection than federal law. To find out if you have more rights under your state law than under federal law, call your state attorney general's office or your local Office of Consumer Protection. You can get a summary of state and federal health privacy laws from:

The Health Privacy Project
1120 19th Street, NW
8th Floor
Washington, DC 20036
(202) 721-5632
www.healthprivacy.org

Getting Your Own Medical Records

You have several good reasons for wanting a copy of your own medical records. Having these records on hand may make it easier to seek a second opinion, to change health care providers, to ensure that the records are accurate, or simply to be more informed about your prognosis and health care program. Ready access to records is particularly important in an emergency, if your doctor's practice closes, or if you move to a new community. Given that others may have seen these records, you may want to know what they have seen. You may also want to know what information has been sent to the Medical Information Bureau (MIB), a vast database where insurance companies exchange medical information about people who have applied for health insurance. See more information on the MIB on page 228.

Once you have seen your records, you may want to change this information in some way, perhaps to correct inaccuracies or to add comments about your feelings about your illness or treatment. This kind of information is likely to improve communication with your doctor and provide important information to other providers who see these records as your treatment progresses.

Fortunately, the new federal privacy regulations (see page 47) give you the right to get copies of your own medical records from virtually all hospitals and doctors and to amend them if you find mistakes. You may be required to make your requests in writing and to pay "reasonable, cost-based fees" for copying and postage. Providers must give you these records within 30 days, or, if they cannot, they must tell you in writing the reason for the delay and produce the records within the next 30 days.

These rules have some exceptions. Providers can, but are not required to, withhold psychotherapy notes and records that may compromise another person's privacy, such as notes from group therapy sessions. Laboratories do not have to give you any information, although lab results are likely to be available from your doctor anyway. Additionally, you will probably have to wait until research is complete before you can get information gathered as part of a clinical trial.

A few doctors and hospitals, typically sole practitioners in small towns or small rural hospitals, are not covered by these regulations. Ask for your records anyway, and if you are unsuccessful under federal law, you may have rights under state law. About one-half of the states have laws permitting some access to medical records, although these laws vary greatly. Access to your records under state law may depend on the type of records you want to see, whether certain exclusions apply, whether you want to copy or just see your records, and whether you need a court order or merely a doctor's consent.

For a description of state laws, see *Medical Records: Getting Yours* (1995), available from:

Public Citizen's Health Research Group
1600 20th Street, NW
Washington, DC 20009
(202) 588-1000
www.citizen.org/hrg

This consumer-friendly guide includes samples of a physician's office record, a hospital's clinical record, a hospital's progress notes, a physician's order sheets, a daily nursing care sheet, and a pathology report, with helpful information about how to interpret them.

NEW CHALLENGES TO CONFIDENTIALITY

CONFIDENTIALITY AND THE INTERNET—Computers have become indispensable tools for researching medical conditions, identifying and evaluating doctors and medical centers, and, for some, communicating with health professionals by electronic mail. But as helpful as these electronic resources are, they are not risk-free. According to the Privacy Rights Clearinghouse, "Virtually no online activities or services . . . guarantee an absolute right of privacy." Cyberspace is virtually unregulated, leaving the Internet, at least for now, a classic "buyer beware" environment.

The risks to your privacy vary with the type of activity you undertake. Do not expect communications to be private if you choose to post messages on electronic bulletin boards or participate in medical chat rooms. Though ethically questionable, anyone who finds information about you on these public forums can legally share what they have learned with anyone else. These postings can also find their way electronically into other databases, where they can be retrieved indefinitely by many people with whom you never intended to share personal information or opinions.

Federal law, however, provides some privacy protection to your e-mail. The Electronic Communications Privacy Act (ECPA) prohibits almost everyone—except your employer and law enforcement authorities—from reading or disclosing the content of your electronic communications. Your e-mail, however, can be disclosed to others if your recipients keep these messages on shared or insecure computers, or because you or the recipients inadvertently send messages to an erroneous address, or worse, to an unintended list. The instant you hit the "send now" button, you cannot stop the inevitable delivery of the mail.

Surfing the Internet in search of useful medical information also carries some risks to privacy. Internet service providers and operators of many sites collect information about your "browsing patterns"—for example, where you have stopped on the information highway and how you have used the sites you have visited. Many sites leave data bits called "cookies" on your computer so they will remember you and your identifying characteristics when you return.

The Center for Democracy and Technology (CDT) also maintains an excellent Web site on Internet privacy, including a list and discussion of the "Top Ten Ways to Protect Privacy Online." You can find this information at **http://www.cdt.org/ privacy/guide/basic/topten.html.** CDT suggests, for example, that you clear your computer's memory cache after browsing (particularly if you are using a computer at work) and that you reject unnecessary cookies. You can set your browser's preferences either to reject all cookies or to ask you before accepting any new ones. The Center also suggests that you check to see whether sites disclose their privacy policies or whether they display a privacy seal of approval from a group such as TRUSTe, WebTrust, or the Better Business Bureau.

Just as you use extra caution before entering credit card or other financial information online, exercise special care before you enter sensitive medical information. Do not provide private medical information unless you are confident that you are on a secure page, that is, a page that transfers information only in encrypted form. Sites that offer security typically tell you when you are on a secure page. This secure status is often indicated by a graphic of a closed lock.

CONFIDENTIALITY, COMPUTERS, AND THE WORKPLACE—You may find it most convenient to surf the Web for medical information and to communicate with your doctors by phone or e-mail at work, but be aware that doing so can seriously compromise your privacy. If you want to protect details of your medical situation from your employer, research and exchange medical information someplace other than your office.

Employers have a legal right to listen to or read virtually all communications that take place in the office, and they may do so without telling you. Your employer can legally read your e-mails, listen to your voice mail messages, and access your office computer to determine what is stored on it and which Internet sites you have visited. They are required by federal law to hang up when they realize they are monitoring personal calls, but, as a practical matter, the damage may already have been done by the time they become aware that you are discussing personal information. Even deleting e-mail and voice mail messages does not necessarily protect them from prying eyes since all of these can be retrieved even after they have been "erased."

Sometimes employer rights are limited by written office policies or union contracts, but in the absence of such agreements, courts have typically sided with the employer's right to monitor information flow in the workplace. So, forewarned is forearmed. If you must make medically related calls at work, consider doing so on a pay phone or personal cell phone. Consider getting a separate e-mail account for your personal use so you do not have to go through the officer server. Some accounts permit you to check your e-mail online without downloading it to your company's computer. And if you must do medical research on your office computer, decline or delete cookies and clear the cache, as discussed above.

For a more detailed discussion of these workplace issues, see the Privacy Rights Clearinghouse fact sheet, "Employee Monitoring: Is There Privacy in the Workplace?" at **http://www.privacyrights.org**.

CONFIDENTIALITY AND GENETIC INFORMATION—Just as the Internet has opened a world of both information and privacy risk for cancer survivors and their families, so too has the leading-edge field of modern genetics. This exciting frontier of science gives caregivers the potential for improving your health through more precise diagnostic tools, new medications, screening, and counseling about how to avoid or ease a disease. But at the same time, genetic information poses an ominous threat to privacy.

Calling genetic information your "future diary," one leading medical ethicist, Professor George Annas of Boston University, has warned that access to it "gives others potential power over the personal life of the individual." He warns that when the day comes that a blood test might reveal the extent of your chance of developing an inheritable cancer (some are inheritable, others not)—or your child's risk of getting the cancer you already have—that information will become part of your medical record. These records travel far beyond your doctor's office and open the way to stigmatization and discrimination. Genetic testing expands the scope for invasion of privacy from your definite past to your possible future.

This development is so dramatic, and the prospects for abuse so disturbing, that several states have enacted laws preventing disclosure of genetic information without your permission. As of late 2003, Congress had not passed a federal law prohibiting insurers from denying health insurance on the basis of genetic information. The Americans with Disabilities Act may protect some survivors from employment discrimination because they have a genetic marker for cancer. See Chapter 14 for discussion of the Americans with Disabilities Act.

In most circumstances, though, state law will determine whether your employer or insurer can discriminate against you because of a genetic marker for cancer. If your insurer asks you for a blood test to conduct DNA-based testing, or if you suspect that you have been discriminated against because of genetic testing, check with your state insurance department or state attorney general's office to see if your rights have been violated. You also can learn more about laws that prohibit genetic discrimination from:

The National Partnership for Women and Families
1875 Connecticut Avenue, NW
Suite 650
Washington, DC 20009
(202) 986-2600
www.nationalpartnership.org

The National Partnership publishes an excellent booklet on the laws that govern genetic discrimination and provides links to the National Human Genome Research Institute, a project of the National Institutes of Health that lists state laws that regulate how employers and insurers must handle genetic information.

CONFIDENTIALITY AND SUPPORT GROUPS–The burgeoning of support groups, important and meaningful as they are, also raises privacy concerns. Whether such groups are professionally or peer-led, participants often grow close and share a great deal of personal information. A 1993 study published in *Hospital and Community Psychiatry* showed that over half of the group leaders responding to a survey reported experience with group members breaking confidentiality—although almost all of them (87 percent) said they had briefed their groups on confidentiality principles.

But no matter how sensitive group members are to privacy concerns, difficult situations can arise. Consider the dilemmas arising from these examples cited during an expert panel discussion titled "Eavesdropping on Your Cancer" at the National Coalition for Cancer Survivorship's Eighth Annual Assembly in Seattle (1993).

A survivor absent from a group session called another member to fill her in on what she had missed. When this conversation got back to the group, an active participant felt her confidentiality had been violated.

A survivor who shared the fact that she had been a longtime member of Alcoholics Anonymous became very upset months later when a fellow member raised her AA connection in front of new members.

A couple participating in a group suffered when, at a session that the woman did not attend, her husband asked the group to keep secret the fact that he had sent for a book advising how to end one's life, and that he intended to follow its approach when the time came. The woman later told the group (when her husband was absent) that she knew he had sent for the book but that he would not discuss it. Constrained by his request, the group simply encouraged her to keep trying. When the husband's lung cancer accelerated and he did commit suicide without discussing his decision with his family, the group, its social work leader, and his physician all agonized as to whether they should have spoken up, even against his wishes.

The doctor-patient privilege is almost always lost when information is discussed in front of other people. That means that each member of the group must trust the others to protect their privacy. While nothing is foolproof, and ambiguous situations may arise, groups should establish an understanding at the outset—perhaps even in writing—that information discussed in the support group is confidential and that no one can discuss what anyone says outside of the room.

THE CANCER SURVIVORS' BILL OF RIGHTS

WRITTEN FOR THE AMERICAN CANCER SOCIETY BY NATALIE DAVIS SPINGARN

1. Survivors have the right to assurance of lifelong medical care, as needed. The physicians and other professionals involved in their care should continue their constant efforts to be:

    Sensitive to the cancer survivor's lifestyle choices and their need for self-esteem and dignity;

{continued}

THE CANCER SURVIVORS' BILL OF RIGHTS *(CONTINUED)*

Careful, no matter how long they have survived, to have symptoms taken seriously, and not have aches and pains dismissed, for fear of recurrence is a normal part of survivorship;

Informative and open, providing survivors with as much or as little candid medical information as they wish, and encouraging their informed participation in their own care;

Knowledgeable about counseling resources, and willing to refer survivors and their families as appropriate for emotional support and therapy which will improve the quality of individual lives.

2. In their personal lives, survivors, like other Americans, have the right to the pursuit of happiness. This means they have the right:

To talk with their families and friends about their cancer experience if they wish, but to refuse to discuss it if that is their choice and not to be expected to be more upbeat or less blue than anyone else;

To be free of the stigma of cancer as a "dread disease" in all social situations;

To be free of blame for having gotten the disease and guilt of having survived it.

3. In the workplace, survivors have the right to equal job opportunities. This means they have the right:

To aspire to jobs worthy of their skills, and for which they are trained and experienced, and thus

To be hired, promoted, and accepted on return to work, according to their individual abilities and qualifications, and not according to "cancer" or "disability" stereotypes.

To privacy about their medical histories.

4. Since health insurance coverage is an overriding survivors' concern, every effort should be made to assure all survivors adequate health insurance, whether public or private. This means:

For employers, that survivors have the right to be included in group health coverage, which is usually less expensive, provides better benefits, and covers the employee regardless of health history;

For physicians, counselors, and other professionals concerned, that they keep themselves and their survivor-clients informed and up-to-date on available group or individual health policy options, noting, for example, what major expenses like hospital costs and medical tests outside the hospital are covered and what amount must be paid before coverage (deductibles).

Chapter Three

You and Your Health Care Team

Working Together

by Elizabeth J. Clark, Ph.D., M.S.W., M.P.H.

Quality care means providing patients with appropriate services in a technically competent manner, with good communication, shared decision making, and cultural sensitivity.

—The National Institute of Medicine's 1999 report on
Ensuring Quality Cancer Care

EFORE YOU WERE DIAGNOSED with cancer, you may have had infrequent contact with health care professionals. Perhaps you saw your family doctor or primary care physician every year for a checkup or if you had the flu or some injury. If a woman, you probably had a gynecologist whom you saw each year for a checkup, breast exam, and Pap smear to rule out cervical cancer. Many of us take good care of our health but do not know much about special problems unless we, or someone in our family, develop a certain condition.

For example, many of us have a vague understanding about diabetes because someone we know lives with the disease. We might understand something about insulin injections or diet management because we have learned those facts from interacting with the friend or family member with diabetes.

In a similar fashion we may have a basic understanding of hypertension (high blood pressure) because an older relative or coworker has it. We know that they need to limit their salt intake and to exercise and manage stress. We may not understand how blood pressure is controlled or what the readings mean or the types of treatment regimens available for persons with high blood pressure.

Each of us also knows friends or family members who have been diagnosed with cancer. That does not make us experts about the disease of cancer or its treatment. In fact, with a cancer diagnosis, comparing the cancer you have with others' cancer is unwise. Cancer is not just one disease, but many. In fact, there are over 100 different kinds of cancer—each with its own characteristics, treatment plans, and outcomes. *Like any other disease, cancer can be treated, controlled, and cured. It is not an automatic death sentence.* You can learn to live with cancer just as people learn to live with diabetes, asthma, high blood pressure, and heart disease.

When you are diagnosed with cancer, you need to become as expert as possible about the type of cancer you have. Comparisons with other people or other types of cancer are not useful, and, in fact, can cause you needless stress and fear. Becoming an expert seems almost impossible at first. Often, you cannot even pronounce or spell the formal name of your cancer or its treatment regimen. You will need to learn the language of cancer. It will seem like a foreign language, but it eventually becomes familiar.

The other major task is learning about all the different types of health care specialists who will work with you to treat and control your disease. For quite a while your life seems to focus only on medical appointments. Everything else is secondary to getting your cancer under control.

YOUR HEALTH CARE TEAM

A team approach to treating cancer is the ideal and the norm. Because cancer is such a complex disease, many specialists are needed to ensure that you receive expert care; that your medical, social, psychological, and spiritual needs are met; and that you maintain the highest quality of life possible after your cancer diagnosis. Because of the complexity of cancer, the National Cancer Institute recommends that a "multidisciplinary" team including physicians, nurses, social workers, pharmacists, dietitians, and rehabilitative specialists manage your disease. Clergy may also be added to your health care team.

As the cancer survivor, you are an important and essential part of your own team. You have equal status and equal responsibility. Without your input, your team does not know how to best proceed with your treatment and care. They need to know your wishes, concerns, and suggestions. Sometimes it is difficult to take on this role when you are sick and overwhelmed and feel that you lack adequate knowledge to fully participate. Sometimes it seems easier to be a passive participant by letting others decide your treatment.

Yet only you can know what your needs are. Only you can help the medical team know how much treatment you can tolerate, what side effects you are willing to live with, or if you are experiencing pain. Decisions about cancer treatment are too important to leave solely to your health care team. Your quality of life and your life itself may depend on your being an active part of your own team.

Who else will be a part of your health care team? The heart of your team will be your doctors and nurses.

ONCOLOGY DOCTORS

To begin with, your family doctor will probably refer you to a cancer specialist—an oncologist. Oncologists specialize in diagnosing and treating cancer. Because cancer is such a complex disease, oncologists also have specialty areas. For example, a surgical oncologist is a doctor who specializes in cancer surgery. A medical oncologist is a specialist who treats cancer with drugs (chemotherapy). A radiation oncologist (sometimes also called a radiation therapist) uses radiation to treat cancer.

Depending on the kind of cancer you have, you may see all three types of oncologists or only one of the oncology specialists. You may see other doctors who combine the word "oncologist" with some other term. For example, if you are a woman with ovarian cancer, you may be referred to a gynecological oncologist. If you are a man with prostate cancer, you may see a urologic oncologist, who is a urologist specializing in treating cancer specific to the urinary tract and organs.

You may wonder why you need to see so many different doctors and how you will keep them all straight. How will you know that they are experts or if your insurance will pay for them?

Chapter 2 provides guidelines for choosing your doctors, making sure they are covered in your health care plan, and checking their credentials. Chapter 1 also discusses ways to assure good communication with your medical specialists. Another useful reference is a booklet called *Teamwork: The Cancer Patient's Guide to Talking with Your Doctor.* This publication is available from the National Coalition for Cancer Survivorship (NCCS). You may reach NCCS by calling 1-888-650-9127 or online at **www.canceradvocacy.org.**

For your part, keep a record of all the doctors you see. List the dates you saw them, their office addresses and phone numbers, and any other information that you think is relevant. If you do not understand their specialty or what they do, ask them directly. This is all a part of becoming an expert about your own care.

ONCOLOGY NURSES

Another important member of your health care team is the nurse. During your cancer treatment you will spend much time with nurses. Professional nurses have a wide range of skills including administering medicines, assessing and treating side effects, and teaching you about your disease and how to live with it. They also are excellent resources for patient education materials and for finding community support services.

Like physicians, nurses also specialize in various areas of practice. An oncology nurse usually has the initials "O.C.N." after her or his name. This means "oncology certified nurse," which indicates a registered professional nurse who has met numerous requirements and who has successfully completed a certification exam in cancer management.

If your illness requires hospitalization during your treatment, you may be admitted to a unit that specializes in cancer care. This unit will be staffed primarily by oncology nurses who are expert at caring for persons with cancer. They are knowledgeable and committed, and will provide excellent and competent care while you are an inpatient.

Once you are discharged, you will probably see an oncology nurse at the office of your cancer specialist. They often are the persons who administer your chemotherapy and do other aspects of your physical exam during your office visit.

They will get to know you and your family, and will try to see you at each treatment. The nurse can help you manage your symptoms and side effects between appointments. He or she can mobilize your health care team when you or your family needs them. When you call your doctor's office with a question, often the oncology nurse will provide an answer. Oncology nurses are a wonderful resource, and many cancer survivors report that the nurses are a patient's strongest allies.

Oncology nurses can address many of your concerns, and some people find them easier to talk with than their physicians. They usually have a little more time to spend with you and can answer many of your questions. You should be comfortable asking any question of your oncology nurse. Some of the most difficult questions seem to center around sexual issues—for example, when can you resume sexual relations, or how will the treatment affect your sexual desire or fertility (Chapter 4 covers these topics). Oncology nurses are quite comfortable answering personal questions, and if they do not have the answer that moment, they can get it for you.

Oncology nurses are also knowledgeable about existing community resources including support groups and tangible services, such as where to find wigs and head coverings or how to find transportation for medical appointments. They also will be able to assist you with a referral to a social worker, psychologist, or psychiatrist when appropriate. The services of an oncology nurse are covered as part of your physician's bill for treatment. You will not be billed separately for seeing the oncology nurse.

Oncology Social Workers

Like oncology nurses, oncology social workers are professionals who have advanced training and expertise in cancer. Oncology social workers are professional counselors who have a broad understanding of the complex issues and needs facing cancer survivors and their families. They are particularly concerned about quality-of-life issues and seeing that the concrete needs, as well as the emotional needs, of cancer survivors are met.

Oncology social workers provide a variety of counseling services. They may work with the individual alone, with the family, or with a support group. They use many interventions to help individuals and their families adjust to the diagnosis and treatment of cancer. The choice of intervention depends upon the problems identified by the cancer survivor, the family, and the health care team. Frequently these problems are related to making difficult treatment decisions, feeling overwhelmed or out of control, and living with limitations required by the illness. They also have excellent family counseling skills and can help when family members have problems communicating.

Social workers are the largest providers of mental health services in this country. There are over half a million professionally trained social workers, and, frequently, in rural areas social workers are the only mental health professional available. Social workers with advanced clinical skills also provide psychotherapy and address serious emotional issues such as clinical depression. Other oncology social workers who have gained expertise in sexual therapy focus on sexuality and fertility, especially issues around sexual functioning and maintenance of intimate relationships, which are important aspects of quality of life.

Social workers also are experts in helping you find needed community services and practical assistance with home care, transportation, childcare, financial problems, and other concerns that frequently arise during cancer treatment, including your eligibility for services. Oncology social workers can help with employment or insurance discrimination issues. They can make telephone calls, write letters, and follow up with schools, employers, or agencies to see that you receive needed services and consideration.

Most hospitals have social workers on staff who are available when you are an inpatient or an outpatient. You can ask your doctor or nurse to arrange for you to meet with a social worker, or you can call the hospital Social Work Department yourself. Most hospitals do not charge for these services.

Most doctors' offices do not have a social worker on staff, and you may need to ask your doctor or oncology nurse for a referral. You can also find information about oncology social workers by calling your local unit of the American Cancer Society or the Leukemia and Lymphoma Society.

The names of clinical social workers in your area can be obtained by checking the *Register of Clinical Social Workers* on the Web site of the National Association of Social Workers at **www.socialworkers.org**. This registry is published every two years and contains over 7,000 qualified and credentialed social workers who are independent providers of mental health services. Included in the listing are social workers' names, addresses, telephone numbers, and areas of expertise, and whether the social worker speaks a language in addition to English.

Social workers are licensed by state boards, and with the proper credentials they can receive third-party payments for their services from Medicare and from managed care companies. Other oncology social workers offer their services on a sliding-scale fee according to what the individual requesting services can afford to pay.

CASE MANAGERS

Sometime during your treatment, you may be assigned a case manager to help plan, coordinate, and monitor your cancer care. Most hospitals have Case Management Departments (some of these were previously Discharge Planning Departments) that will help you coordinate your post-hospital care and make referrals to appropriate community agencies. Your insurance company or managed care company may also use this method.

Social workers and nurses are the professionals who most often fulfill this function. The goals of case management are to limit the problems that arise from a lack of coordination of services and to ensure that you receive needed services on a timely basis.

PSYCHIATRISTS AND PSYCHOLOGISTS

Psychiatrists and psychologists also provide mental health services. Psychiatrists are medical doctors who specialize in emotional disorders and mental illness. They provide psychotherapy and can prescribe medications as needed. A cancer diagnosis can create feelings of acute distress and sadness as you try to adjust to the diagnosis and incorporate it into your life. Chapter 6 goes into more detail about the emotional impact of cancer and how you can manage it.

Research has shown that cancer survivors are no more depressed than persons with other serious illnesses, but sometimes the feelings of sadness and stress are intense, and sharing these concerns with family members and friends may not alleviate them. If this continues for long periods and interferes with your daily activities, a psychiatrist may be able to help. Psychiatrists can prescribe medication for problems such as depression, severe anxiety, and sleeplessness. Some psychiatrists also are trained in hypnosis and relaxation techniques that can help manage and reduce anxiety.

You may ask your family doctor or oncologist for a referral to see a psychiatrist. It is particularly helpful to see one who has experience in counseling cancer survivors. You can also find a referral to a psychiatrist by calling the psychiatry department of your local hospital or by calling the local medical society. Psychiatric help is covered by most private insurance, but you will need to determine how many visits or sessions will be covered and whether the entire fee will be paid or if you will have to pay for part of it.

Psychologists are also professional therapists. They usually have completed a doctoral degree in psychology and use the title *doctor.* They are doctors in psychology, not medical doctors, so they cannot prescribe medications. Psychologists usually have specialty areas. Some psychologists work only with adults or only with children. Some specialize in marital or couples counseling or family counseling. Others may specialize in areas such as eating disorders or alcohol and drug treatment. Still others focus on stress management or post-traumatic stress disorders. They use a variety of behavioral techniques including biofeedback, hypnosis, imagery, and meditation. They also are expert at administering psychological tests.

Some psychologists specialize in oncology, and they are frequently linked to major cancer centers. Ask your oncologist or oncology nurse if they can recommend a psychologist in your community. You can also contact the American Psychological Association's help center to assist you in finding a psychologist in your area. To reach the help center, call 1-800-964-2000. The operator will use your zip code to locate and connect you with a referral system in your area.

Psychologists must be licensed to practice psychotherapy. You should learn the individual's credentials and ask about cost and insurance coverage before going to your first appointment.

Sometimes cancer survivors assume that seeing a therapist is a sign of weakness or an indication that in addition to having cancer, they are now "going crazy." This is not true. Going to a therapist simply means that you are having difficulty dealing with a very stressful period in your life and need some assistance to manage better. Seeking help for emotional problems is like seeking help with physical problems. When needed, psychiatrists and psychologists can be important members of your health care team.

PHARMACISTS

Sometimes cancer survivors overlook an important resource for their health care team. Pharmacists provide essential input into your care. While you are an inpatient, hospital pharmacists review and prepare your drug therapy, often mixing your chemotherapy. They also review your complete drug regimen to guard against drug interactions or drug and food interactions. Like other health care professionals, some pharmacists specialize in cancer care and may participate in clinical trials and other research.

Community pharmacists are vital to good care. They, too, watch out for drug interactions, and they are the professionals who call your doctors if any question arises about your prescriptions. Frequently you see more than one doctor and you may receive prescriptions from each. Your pharmacist will make certain that you are not taking duplicates of one kind of medicine and will check to see that the combined dosages of different drugs are not dangerous. Pharmacists are an excellent source of information and are willing to answer any questions to help you understand how to best take your medicines. They also can contact your doctor if you cannot remember something about a prescription. Get to know your community pharmacist. For the best protection against drug interactions, use only one pharmacy whenever possible.

HOME HEALTH PROFESSIONALS

Many health services are available to you at home. These include visits from a professional nurse, a private-duty nurse, or a home health aide. Your doctor can request that a nurse come to your home to take blood, supervise dressing changes, or monitor intravenous lines. Nurses may come on a daily basis or less frequently. They will work with you and your caregivers to help you deal with problems related to your illness and treatment. Many people now have chemotherapy administered at home, which works especially well if you have difficulty traveling to the doctor's office. The cost of the nurse's visit is covered by insurance after approval of the visit is obtained from your doctor. Be sure to determine that your insurance covers the services your doctor orders.

Sometimes cancer survivors need help with tasks that are not considered skilled nursing tasks. You may then need a referral for a home health aide. Home health aides provide care at home for brief visits to help with bathing and light household chores such as cooking meals, changing linens, or doing laundry for the patient. Their services may be available at night as well as during the day. This care is sometimes reimbursed by Medicaid, depending on state rules, and sometimes by Medicare if a nurse supervises the care. Rarely are the services of home health aides covered by private insurance. Many agencies have sliding-scale fees based on your income, and you should not be embarrassed to ask about these.

You and your family also can request a private-duty nurse to stay at your home for longer periods of time, such as for eight hours of care at night or during the day when your family members are at work. This care arrangement can provide many advantages by allowing you to stay at home rather than in the hospital, or it may help to better manage pain or side effects. It also may help your family become more comfortable in managing your care at home. Fees for private-duty nurses are quite high, and Medicare or Medicaid does not cover them, and only seldom are they covered by private insurance. Be sure to check your health care policy carefully before hiring a private-duty nurse.

Your doctor, nurse, or social worker will know about resources for nursing care and home health care in your community and can refer you to a reputable agency. The yellow pages of your phone book also contain home care listings. You should check the credentials of the agency and of the staff who will be providing care.

Home health care services can ease the burden of care for you and your family. Sometimes, just a few hours of outside help a week is all that is needed for family and friends to be able to coordinate their efforts to provide care.

REHABILITATION SPECIALISTS

You may experience physical changes resulting from your cancer and its treatment. You may have had surgery, or you may need some assistance in regaining your physical health and strength. Rehabilitation specialists may best address these concerns. A doctor who specializes in rehabilitation medicine is called a physiatrist. Other rehabilitation specialists include physical therapists, occupational therapists, speech and hearing therapists, and rehabilitation counselors. Their services are offered in hospitals and outpatient settings, and in your home.

Many cancer survivors are not familiar with how rehabilitation specialists can help them. They may be familiar with some of the services because they had an elderly relative who needed assistance after a stroke, or they may know of someone who was in an accident and needed help in learning to walk with crutches or had to find other ways to do routine chores.

Physical therapy can strengthen a body part or function weakened by cancer. It can also keep your muscles strong if you are bedridden for several weeks or longer. For example, physical therapy is used to help you regain strength after major surgery. Frequently, you will see a physical therapist while you are an inpatient. Physical therapy also is used after a mastectomy and/or lymph node dissection to reduce swelling and to help the cancer survivor regain movement of the arm.

Occupational therapy helps cancer survivors adjust to needed changes in daily routines that are required because of surgery or treatment or the need for a prosthesis. This can include helping you learn new ways of getting dressed, cooking, or moving around the house so that you can continue with your normal activities even when your physical activity is limited.

Speech and hearing therapy are essential for cancer survivors who need to learn different ways to communicate after head or neck surgery or after undergoing a laryngectomy (removal of the voice box). Many assistive devices can help cancer survivors resume normal life activities, including their occupations.

Rehabilitation counseling addresses concerns and problems related to physical changes and limitations brought about by cancer or cancer treatment. Changes in body image or body functioning, whether temporary or permanent, can be especially distressing for cancer survivors. Rehabilitation counselors have training and experience in helping cancer survivors emotionally adjust to these changes so that they may maintain their quality of life.

When needed, most doctors will refer you for rehabilitation services. If you are not told about them, ask your doctor or nurse what is available to help you adjust to your new limitations. Be certain that your insurance company will pay for the needed services.

Some agencies offer free rehabilitation programs. The best known of these is the American Cancer Society's "Reach to Recovery" program for breast cancer survivors. The American Cancer Society also offers programs for cancer survivors with ostomies or laryngectomies. Other community agencies offer various programs. Ask your nurse or social worker for suggestions.

Ostomy Therapists

Ostomy nurses are formally known as enterostomal ("entero" means intestine; "stoma" means opening) therapists or ET nurses. These are registered professional nurses specially trained to help persons adapt to surgeries that result in ostomies (colostomy or ileostomy for elimination of stool or a urostomy for elimination of urine). These nurses recognize that good information about stoma care can make a huge difference in a person's quality of life. Besides teaching and counseling patients about ostomy care, ET nurses also help with sexual difficulties resulting from ostomy surgery.

Many hospitals do not have an ET nurse on staff. Some ET nurses work for home care groups like the Visiting Nurse Association or in a rehabilitation clinic. Some are employed by ostomy supply companies, or they may be in private practice. Many ET nurses work not only with people with ostomies, but also with patients who have draining wounds, bedsores, incontinence, or impotence. If you have an ostomy, either temporary or permanent, ask your physician for a referral to an enterostomal therapist.

DIETITIANS

Professionals who deal with nutritional and dietary concerns are called registered dietitians. Some dietitians specialize in oncology and work to help relieve nutritional problems that result from cancer and its treatment. Many persons with cancer experience a significant weight loss prior to having their cancer diagnosed. When treatment such as chemotherapy is added, the weight loss may become even more severe. Cancer treatment also can result in weight gain. Other survivors find that their eating habits and preferences for certain foods change dramatically, especially if their taste buds are affected by treatment. Therefore, a referral to a dietitian early in your treatment process may be helpful.

A dietitian can help you minimize weight change by recommending a diet that meets your needs for calories, vitamins, and protein. The dietitian can suggest food substitutes if your tastes change because of treatment or if you are unable to tolerate some foods. The dietitian also can provide recipes written specifically for people who are undergoing cancer treatment. Another important role for the dietitian is explaining to your family why your appetite has changed or why you cannot tolerate or swallow some foods. Family members often spend a lot of time worrying about feeding you and may feel like failures if they are unable to coax you to eat. They may be unaware of the barriers to eating that cancer survivors face during treatment. A dietitian can help family members feel more comfortable with their concerns, too.

Most hospitals have registered dietitians on staff, and you can request to see one before discharge. If you are looking for one on your own, be sure you find someone who is reliable and not someone who promotes dietary cures for cancer. As with the other professionals, ask about training, credentials, and experience in working with cancer survivors, and the dietitian's fees for service. Most dietitians will have at least a bachelor's degree; many will have a master's degree. Although anyone can call themselves a *nutritionist,* a *registered dietitian* must meet certain standards.

Your insurance should cover your consultation with a dietitian in the hospital. Ask your doctor, nurse, or social worker about community-based programs that offer free educational sessions.

CREATIVE ARTS THERAPISTS

A variety of professionals use creative arts in their counseling and support work. Some modalities, such as art therapy and music therapy, have been around for decades, have degree programs and professional certifications, and have been used to provide interventions for numerous areas including cancer-related problems and concerns. Other modalities, such as poetry therapy, drama therapy, visual arts, and photography, have only recently been used to help people adapt to cancer.

Each of these specialty areas can be further broken down. For example, art therapy may include mask making as a creative way to help persons with cancer express fears and emotions and to gain personal insight into their coping patterns. Poetry therapy may involve expressing emotions through writing poetry, or established poetry may be used as a starting point for analysis into the human condition and living with adversity.

Bibliotherapy, the use of literature for better understanding of situations and insight into the meaning of life, can be a powerful therapeutic technique. Similarly, keeping a journal about your feelings related to your cancer experience can be a positive action when learning to live with cancer. Other people make quilts or paint murals in a group format or make something symbolic from art materials.

These therapies frequently form the basis of support groups. Cancer survivors self-select into them according to their interests and talents. Chapter 8 discusses ways to find and use peer support, including support groups.

Insurance coverage for these therapies is rare unless the therapist using the technique also has credentials in an insurance-covered therapeutic modality such as psychology. If offered as part of a hospital or community support group, these services may be free or may charge a small weekly fee to cover materials.

CLERGY

Spiritual well-being is an important part of most persons' overall quality of life. In times of serious illness, questions often arise about the meaning of life. You may wonder why you developed cancer or why that happened at this particular time in your life. You may wonder if you can, or should, find spiritual meaning in your illness. Depending on your religious or spiritual inclinations, you may want to discuss these questions and concerns with a member of the clergy.

A compassionate member of the clergy who is trained to provide support during a cancer crisis can be a valuable asset for you and your loved ones. Prayer can be useful as a means of providing hope and comfort, and spiritual counseling can help you through a difficult and stressful time.

Almost every hospital has a pastoral care department, and while an inpatient, you can request to see a chaplain or pastoral counselor of your own faith. If you have no regular religious affiliation in the community, you can contact your local Council of Churches for a referral. Clergy also are important resources for learning about local organizations and agencies that provide services you may need.

TELEHEALTH SPECIALISTS

The concept of telemedicine has been around for decades. It was first used in 1948 to transmit radiological images by telephone. In the 1970s, federally funded projects linked health care professionals at large medical centers with patients in remote areas of Alaska and Canada by using videoconferencing. Today the use of modern information technology to deliver health and mental health services is referred to as "telehealth."

For some cancer survivors, a lack of transportation or physical problems such as weakness, nausea, or pain may make it difficult to travel to a mental health counselor's office on a regular basis. One alternative may be telephone counseling or counseling by Web site, which is called "online counseling."

One nationwide resource for telephone counseling for cancer survivors is CancerCare, Inc., located in New York City. Professional social workers at CancerCare, Inc., provide counseling by telephone for the emotional aspects of cancer. They also provide referrals to community resources, including local support groups in your community.

In addition, CancerCare, Inc., offers weekly teleconferences on a variety of topics. The conferences usually begin with an expert's talk followed by a question-and-answer period. CancerCare, Inc.'s, free counseling line can be reached at 1-800-813-HOPE (4673).

Online counseling is a rapidly growing area of mental health services. This may involve e-mail where clients e-mail a counselor who responds either by traditional e-mail or in real time through interactive e-mail messages. Interactive counseling chat rooms are online discussions moderated by a counselor. Some experts feel that this type of counseling may be more comfortable for some people than face-to-face counseling. Teleconference counseling sessions, in which the counselor and the clients can see and hear each other, also exist, but both the counselor and the client need interactive video hookups.

As might be expected, the field of telecounseling is basically unregulated, and fees vary tremendously and are usually billed directly to your credit card. Insurance reimbursement is not readily available for electronic counseling. Chapter 17 discusses ways to make sure your telephone and Web resources are reliable.

MAINTAINING QUALITY OF LIFE

One of the major goals of your health care team is helping you and your family members maintain the highest possible quality of life after a cancer diagnosis.

We know from research that quality of life is a broad concept that includes physical, psychological, emotional, social, and spiritual components. Some researchers also include sexual and financial components. Many experts can help you with challenges to any of these quality-of-life areas. You play an important part in your own health care. You need to tell team members what is troubling you and if you are having a problem; you should not be afraid to *just talk* about your concerns, nor should you be embarrassed to ask for help or services. You must be your own best advocate so you can live life fully after cancer.

Chapter Four

Sexuality and Fertility

by Debra Thaler-DeMers, R.N., O.C.N.

*T*HE EXPERIENCE OF LIVING with cancer affects everything in your life. While a survivor's immediate focus may be on finding successful treatment, a cancer diagnosis has physical, emotional, spiritual, economic, legal, sexual, interpersonal, and reproductive effects. Of these issues, health care providers rarely discuss sexuality and fertility unless prodded by the cancer survivor. Many cancer survivors experience changes in their level of sexual desire, their ability to enjoy their usual sexual activities, and their fertility. These are frequent side effects of either the disease itself or its treatment.

Your sexuality and fertility are an important part of your overall treatment for your cancer. If your doctor or oncology nurse does not raise these topics with you, ask them about fertility and sexuality *before* you begin treatment. They may be uncomfortable talking about it. Few medical schools or nursing schools teach how to talk to patients about intimate or personal matters. Recognizing a health care provider's discomfort can help move the conversation along. You might start the conversation by saying, "I'm not entirely comfortable bringing up the subject of sexuality, but it is important for me to know how my cancer and my treatment may affect my sexual function and my fertility." If your health care providers are too uncomfortable talking about it, or are not well informed about treatments to preserve sexual function and fertility, ask them to refer you to someone who can help you. Find a physician, a psychologist who specializes in this area, a nurse with expertise in this area, an oncology social worker, a licensed sex therapist, or some other member of the health care team who is both comfortable talking about the subject and well informed about how your treatment may affect your interest and ability to engage in sexual activity.

Some cancers naturally lead survivors to think about issues of sexuality and fertility. These include cancers of the breast, prostate, ovary, uterus, vagina, cervix, penis, and testes. Any type of cancer, however, can impact sexuality, and many types of cancer treatment can temporarily or permanently affect sexuality and/or fertility.

After they are first diagnosed, most cancer survivors focus on choosing an appropriate treatment plan and beginning treatment as soon as possible. Although their doctors may discuss the side effects of treatment, survivors are overwhelmed with a lot of new, complex information. Their concerns about sexuality, intimacy, and fertility may be deferred until treatment has started. To provide quality cancer care, however, health care providers must tell newly diagnosed survivors how their treatment may affect their sexuality and fertility before they make a final treatment decision. Consider these examples:

Bob has been diagnosed with prostate cancer and has been given several options for treatment. These include surgery, radiation implants, radiation therapy, chemotherapy, and hormone therapy. He is told that any of these treatments may cause impotence. Bob tells his doctor that he wants to have the best chance at being cured, but also would like to preserve his ability to engage in sexual activity. His doctor then tells him that among the types of surgery that can be performed, some are less likely than others to cause impotence. They also talk about penile implants and other ways that impotence can be treated if this occurs as a result of his treatment.

Jim, a college student, has been diagnosed with testicular cancer and will have surgery and chemotherapy. He competes in sports and is worried about how his teammates will react to the change in his appearance after surgery. He is also concerned about the impact his cancer will have on his social life. Because body image is important to him, he should know *before* the surgery that he can have a prosthetic testicle implanted at the same time the tumor is removed. Prosthetic testicles are available in different sizes and are made of different materials. If he is not told about this prior to surgery and finds out about it later, he will have to undergo another surgical procedure to have the prosthesis inserted. In addition, he may wonder why his health care team did not make this information available to him.

Before you have chemotherapy, consider storing sperm for future use (sperm banking). Once treatment begins, the chemotherapy may cause a significant change in fertility. While you can bank sperm after you have started treatment, the quantity and quality of sperm harvested may not be the same as sperm harvested prior to treatment. Sperm banking should be offered to men of all ages and should be discussed with teenagers, adolescents, and the parents of young children as well. Recent advances in reproductive medicine make it possible for men to father children despite a low sperm count at the time of diagnosis.

Susan has been diagnosed with lymphoma. She has decided to have high-dose chemotherapy and a stem cell transplant. She is told that the chemotherapy will probably cause her to become infertile after treatment. She is also told to use birth control during treatment because the chemotherapy has the potential to harm any child conceived during treatment. Susan has read about the possible side effects of chemotherapy. She asks her health care team about harvesting ovarian tissue to preserve her future fertility options. The team is not familiar with this technique, so she asks for a referral to a reproductive endocrinologist prior to starting her chemotherapy.

Susan is an example of a survivor who has read about potential side effects of treatment and learned about her options to minimize the impact of those side effects on her life. She is well informed, but she also is assertive about communicating her wishes to the health care team. When she discovers that they are not familiar with the information she has obtained, she asks to talk to a specialist who can help her explore her options for preserving her fertility.

This chapter describes the sexuality and fertility issues cancer survivors may face. Every year, new medical discoveries bring better surgical techniques, new medicines, and more cancer treatment choices that minimize harmful side effects. Quality of life has become an important consideration in choosing cancer treatment. If sexuality and fertility are important to you, tell your health care team *before* you begin treatment.

SEXUALITY

Sexuality is more than just the physical acts related to sexual activity. Your sexuality comprises how you see yourself both as an individual and in relation to others. It includes how you feel about your body, the need for touch, interest in sexual activity, communicating your sexual needs to a partner, and the ability to enjoy sexual activity. Sexuality is a complex interaction of many factors, including the desire for emotional intimacy. For some people, the ability to have children affects their sexuality.

A cancer diagnosis can affect sexuality in many ways. From the moment of diagnosis, you may have physical, emotional, psychological, and spiritual life changes. These changes can begin before you choose your treatment; any one of them can affect your sexuality and desire for intimate contact with others.

"Sexual response" is the term Masters and Johnson used to describe the changes that occur from the time of sexual arousal (becoming excited) to the period of resting after sexual activity. Every person has a unique response; your response may be different from that described in this or any other book. Use the basic physical changes described here as a guide. If you are experiencing difficulty in achieving any of the stages described, or if you have any physical discomfort during sexual activity, discuss it with your physician. Physical, chemical, or psychological changes that cause sexual problems can be addressed by the health care team.

Many people who experience discomfort, a discharge, or bleeding during their first attempts at sexual activity during cancer treatment assume that they can no longer enjoy sexual activity. This is *not* true. Different positions, various types of lubrication, more attention to foreplay, improved communication between partners, or referral to a certified sex therapist can help cancer survivors deal with problems encountered during sexual activity. See Chapter 17 for how to locate a sex therapist. A lack of desire for sexual activity is often caused by medications or by the fatigue associated with cancer treatment. Sometimes a change in medication or planning intimate moments following a rest period can help.

Sexual response begins in the mind—the brain, to be exact. Something triggers a physical response. It can be an erotic thought, something you see that excites you, a smell, a touch, or something that you read. It may be one thing or a combination of things. The brain then releases chemicals that begin a series of physical changes.

Blood begins to build up in certain parts of the body—notably in the shaft of the penis, the clitoris, vulva, and vagina. The breasts enlarge and the nipples can become erect. Women secrete fluid that lubricates the vagina. The penis becomes erect, the scrotum thickens, and the testes enlarge, become bluish in color, and rise closer to the body. The heart beats faster, the rate of breathing increases, and blood pressure increases. Some people become flushed or feel tense or anxious. Muscles become tense and may have involuntary spasms. Nothing that happens during this phase of the sexual response cycle should be painful.

If you continue with sexual activity, these sensations will heighten until they culminate in orgasm. Muscle contractions in the pelvic area cause men to ejaculate. Orgasm provides a sense of release and well-being. Muscle spasms can occur as the tension in muscles is released. This is followed by a period of recovery for the body, which varies in time depending on the individual. Heart rate, breathing, blood pressure, and muscle tension all return to normal levels.

Communication with your partner is essential during sexual activity. If you experience pain, let your partner know immediately and try to isolate what triggered it. You may need to change position, use more lubricant, support yourself with pillows, or make other changes in your sexual activity to make it a pleasurable experience for both you and your partner.

Many parts of the body must work together for the sexual response to take place. Messages travel from the brain to muscles and blood vessels through the nervous system. Nerves help control the muscles as they become tense or relax. Blood must flow to the genital area to prepare the sex organs for intercourse. Hormones must be released at certain times during the process for these body changes to take place. The heart beats faster. The lungs need to take in more oxygen to help the body during this time of increased physical activity. A change resulting from illness, surgery, radiation, chemotherapy, or biologic therapy may alter the body's sexual response. Emotional stress or depression can block sexual arousal.

SEXUALITY ISSUES COMMON TO MEN AND WOMEN

You may need to take some precautions if your cancer affects your blood cell counts. Low red blood cell volume (anemia) can cause shortness of breath, limited endurance, and fatigue, which can affect your sexual activity. A low platelet count (thrombocytopenia) can make sexual intercourse dangerous. Platelets are one of the factors that help your body form blood clots. If you have a very low platelet count, you will bruise easily and bleed longer than normal if you cut yourself. Low platelets can also cause spontaneous bleeding because of dry mucous membranes. You might notice this as a nosebleed or bleeding from dry, cracked lips. Check with your physician or oncology nurse to see if it is safe to engage in sexual activity when your platelet count is low.

A high white count, such as from leukemia, can also pose a risk for sexual activity. The high number of white cells crowd the blood vessels and can increase blood pressure. This can become a problem because sexual arousal also causes an increase in blood pressure and an increase in heart rate. If you have a very high white cell count, you should check with your physician to be sure it is safe for you to engage in sexual activity. When your white blood cell count is very low, you are at increased risk for infection, so you should not engage in certain types of sexual activity. You and your partner should use good personal hygiene when your white cell count is low to minimize the possibility of infection.

Any cancer that affects your ability to breathe, or that causes you to get short of breath with physical activity, can affect sexual activity. Low red blood cell counts can make you feel short of breath with activity. If you are using supplemental oxygen, be sure that you have enough oxygen in the tank and that the oxygen tubing is long enough to allow you to move freely during sexual activity. You may find it easier to breathe if you are not lying flat on your back. Try positions that involve either sitting upright or standing. This will help your diaphragm expand, allowing you to take in more oxygen with each breath. Tell your partner if you are getting short of breath. Take a rest or slow the pace of your activity until you no longer feel short of breath.

If you have a colostomy, ileostomy, nephrostomy, or ileal conduit, you may want to empty the pouch before any anticipated sexual activity. If you are concerned about odor, you can place substances in the pouch to eliminate unpleasant odors. Be sure any clamps are securely fastened.

If you routinely need pain medication or if you are taking pain medication on an "as needed" basis after surgery, you may want to take a dose of pain medication about 20 minutes before any sexual activity. People normally become tense when they experience pain. This causes muscles to contract and may make the pain worse. If you take the pain medication before your pain level becomes unbearable, you can break this cycle and need less medication to control your pain. Generous use of pillows for positioning can help alleviate pain caused by cancer or recent surgery. If you are having nausea from your treatment, take your prescribed antinausea medication about 20 minutes before any sexual activity, because movement can sometimes make the sensation of nausea worse.

If you have multiple myeloma, take extra precautions. Multiple myeloma causes your bones to break very easily, sometimes without any obvious reason. Choose positions for sexual activity that provide support and comfort. Make generous use of pillows or rolled towels or blankets for support. Tell your partner immediately if you experience pain at any time during sexual activity. Make sure you can move that part of your body without pain. If it turns red or swells, or if the pain does not subside, call your doctor right away.

Anyone engaging in sexual activity, whether they have cancer or not, should take precautions against sexually transmitted diseases. When you have sex with someone, you are essentially taking the same risk as if you were having sex with every sexual partner your partner has ever had. Some sexually transmitted diseases have no symptoms, so it is possible to have a disease without knowing it. Anyone undergoing treatment for cancer, and people with lymphoma or leukemia in particular, are at risk for herpes and genital warts, which are spread by skin-to-skin contact. Parasites can be passed between partners through anal intercourse or anal-oral contact. Hepatitis and HIV are spread through many kinds of sexual contact. Any exchange of body fluids risks transmission of a disease.

The best protection from sexually transmitted diseases is to use a latex condom and water-based lubricants, such as KY jelly. Condoms should be used with any contact between a penis and a mouth, a penis and the genital area, or a penis and an anus. If you are a man performing oral sex on a woman, you should place a dental dam or plastic wrap over the woman's vulva to prevent infection. Using flavored condoms or topping the condom with chocolate or whipped cream can diminish the taste of the barrier.

In addition to protection from sexually transmitted diseases, anyone undergoing cancer treatment should protect themselves from becoming pregnant or causing a pregnancy. Many types of cancer treatment can cause harm to a developing fetus. Wait for a period of time after completing cancer treatment before attempting to conceive a child.

Having cancer is only one part of who you are. While you go through treatment, your attention can be so focused on getting well that you forget about all the things you did and enjoyed before your diagnosis. Give yourself permission to take a vacation from the cancer experience and enjoy yourself. The sexual response cycle begins in your mind, which is also the source of memories of things that made you feel happy, relaxed, and safe. Think about the things that gave you pleasure before you had cancer and can continue to after your diagnosis. What was your favorite music? What was your favorite restaurant? Who did you enjoy being with? What did you enjoy doing? Thinking about things that brought you joy can help you focus on things other than your illness, such as your interest in sexuality and intimacy.

INTIMACY

Intimacy involves sharing oneself with another person in far more ways than through sexual intercourse. Holding hands, touching, hugging, and caring deeply about another person, and sharing feelings, hopes, dreams, fears, emotions, and religious values are all aspects of an intimate relationship.

If you are involved in a relationship when you are diagnosed, your partner may have concerns to discuss with you and your doctor. For example, some people incorrectly believe that cancer is contagious. It is not. You cannot get cancer from kissing, hugging, or from most forms of sexual contact. Confusion may arise if you have an active infection with a virus associated with the development of cancer. For example, if you have cervical cancer caused by human papillomavirus (HPV), the concern is transmitting the *virus* that causes genital warts that lead to cervical cancer. If you have an active case of genital warts, using a condom during intercourse will protect your partner from the virus. Similarly, the virus that causes AIDS (HIV) can also be spread through sexual contact. While AIDS is not a form of cancer, people with AIDS can develop certain forms of cancer such as Kaposi's sarcoma, central nervous system (CNS) lymphoma, and non-Hodgkin's lymphoma. Practicing safe sex will protect you and your partner from getting or passing on viruses that may lead to cancer.

Talk with your partner about your fears, worries, or beliefs about how cancer will affect your relationship. Sharing these thoughts and feelings will strengthen your relationship. For example:

> Beverly believed that all kinds of cancer were extremely painful. Even though John's cancer had been diagnosed from a painless lump in his testicle, and he had never experienced pain except for the first week after his surgery, Beverly was afraid to touch him or to have any sexual activity. She believed that sexual arousal would cause him severe pain. When John tried to interest Beverly in sexual activity she avoided him, truly believing she was doing this to protect him. John felt rejected. He wondered if Beverly was no longer attracted to him because he had testicular cancer. Their relationship began to suffer until John finally decided to ask Beverly why she no longer wanted to be sexually intimate with him. When Beverly was able to say, "I'm afraid I'll hurt you," it was a great relief to both of them. They were able to talk about their feelings and agreed that if anything they did was painful for John, he would let Beverly know right away. He was also sure to tell her when something she did felt good. This helped Beverly to relax and begin to enjoy their physical relationship again.

See Chapter 7 for suggestions on how to communicate with family members.

DATING

If you are not involved in a relationship at the time of diagnosis, you may become involved with someone during or after treatment. Think about when you will share the fact that you have had cancer. When and how to disclose your cancer history is a personal decision that should consider the needs and desires of each person in the relationship. The way you approach the subject of your cancer diagnosis is important. If you are defensive or confrontational, you may frighten your partner.

You might want to tell your partner up front—before or during the first date. This way, if she or he has any concerns about having a relationship with someone who has cancer, you will learn about it early in the relationship. If you decide to tell your partner about your cancer early in the relationship, be sure to let her or him know to what extent you want to discuss it. One person might want to put the whole thing in the past and never talk about it again. Another person may think the experience is important in shaping who they have become as a person and want to talk about the impact cancer has had on his or her life. If you do become involved in a relationship, you will want to share your cancer history at some point so your partner understands the effect your cancer history has on your health and life perspective.

Cancer, through the drama of television specials, movies, and feature articles, has a reputation as a painful, traumatic, and fatal disease. An unfortunate, but normal response to hearing the word "cancer" is to be afraid and to believe that the person with cancer is going to die in a short period of time. If you are entering a new relationship, you might consider waiting until you and your partner have had a chance to get to know one another and feel comfortable with each other before discussing your cancer experience in depth. Once you have established good communication skills and feel comfortable being with and talking with each other, it may be easier to share feelings about the cancer experience.

INTIMACY IN A HOSPITAL

The fact that you are hospitalized will not prevent you from having erotic or loving thoughts about your partner. You should feel free to invite your partner to share your bed for hugging, cuddling, or just to be physically close to each other. If you feel that you want to engage in more intimate activities and if your partner is available and willing, you can be intimate while you are in the hospital—provided you take a few simple precautions.

Talk to your nurse about having some private time with your partner. Post a "Do Not Disturb" sign on the door, and make sure all members of the staff know not to interrupt you to check your temperature and blood pressure or give you medications. Make sure you are not scheduled for a test or procedure that requires you to leave your room during your planned private time. You might ask your nurse to inform other staff who may enter your room that you and your partner have requested some private time together. If you need to take some pain or nausea medication before any sexual activity, ask your nurse to give it to you at least 30 minutes ahead of time. If you receive medication according to a set schedule, plan your activity for the time between doses. Consider putting something in front of the door that will make a noise if someone should try to enter without knocking first, but do not block the door in a way that will prevent the medical staff from entering should you need immediate help.

If you want to use lubricant, your nurse can provide you with a tube of KY jelly. Your partner may have to obtain condoms or other methods of birth control for you. The nurse or a nursing assistant may be able to provide you with extra pillows to provide comfort and support. Make sure you know where the nurse and emergency call lights are. Put them close to you and show your partner how to use them. This way, if you become short of breath or experience any other problems, someone can come to help you immediately.

Not all people who work in a hospital are comfortable with sexual intimacy. If you find that your nurse or nursing assistant is not willing to help you arrange for some intimate time with your partner, ask the charge nurse or unit manager for someone who is at ease with this issue to be assigned your care. A simple change in staff assignments can help everyone feel more comfortable.

If you do not have a partner, or your partner is not available, you may still have erotic thoughts and desire some form of sexual activity. If you take steps to ensure your privacy and safety, you can masturbate in the hospital setting.

BIRTH CONTROL

Birth control is important during cancer treatment. Even if the treatment has the potential to cause infertility, you can become pregnant or impregnate your partner during treatment. Some chemotherapy drugs can have a harmful effect on a developing fetus. Radiation therapy can cause chromosomal changes in sperm and egg cells. To avoid the possibility of birth defects, discuss with your physicians how long you should delay attempts to conceive a child after treatment is completed to give your body time to replace any damaged cells and to be sure you have recovered from any side effects of treatment. Women with tumors that are hormone dependent should not use birth control pills containing estrogen. Women with leukemia are often given medication to suppress their menstrual cycle during treatment. If you are taking medication to suppress your menstrual cycle, or if you are not having a regular menstrual cycle during treatment, you should still use an effective method of birth control. Ask your physician to recommend a type of birth control that will not interfere with your treatment.

Special Issues for Women

When thinking about sexuality, the types of cancer that typically come to mind are those involving the parts of the body associated with sexual activity—the breast, vulva, vagina, uterus, and ovaries. Surgery that alters the function or appearance of these organs can inhibit sexual feelings by changing how you see and value your physical appearance. Other cancers that may cause a change in body image are cancers of the colon, rectum, bladder, head and neck, larynx, and skin. In many cases, reconstructive surgery can lessen the impact of changes to those body parts.

The most commonly reported sexual problems women face after cancer treatment are little or no interest in sexual intimacy, pain during sexual intercourse, inability to achieve orgasm, and problems with lubrication. Many women report a change in their relationship with their partner, which they attribute to concerns about their health or feelings of inadequacy related to their physical appearance.

A lack of interest in sexuality can be caused by many things. Depression may cause a lack of interest in any social interaction. Depression can be related to the diagnosis itself, medications used to treat the cancer, changes in body image resulting from tumors or surgery, changes in your role in the family, changes in finance, or many other factors related to cancer treatment. See Chapter 10 for a discussion of cancer-related depression, which can affect survivors of all ages.

Fatigue is the most common side effect reported by cancer survivors. It can be related to the disease itself, the treatment for the disease, or the side effects of treatment. When you are too tired to even think about sex, you may still desire intimacy. If anything, your need for intimacy may be increased. See Chapter 1 for discussion of cancer-related fatigue.

When you are tired, pace your daily activities to accommodate sexual relations. During those sexual encounters, pace yourself so that you do not become exhausted. Tell your partner if you feel that you need to rest or slow down. Slow, relaxing, intimate contact can be the best solution.

Sexual desire is affected by hormones. Women need both estrogen and testosterone. The levels of these hormones can be affected by surgery or other cancer treatments. A lack of estrogen can cause vaginal dryness. If your cancer is estrogen dependent, talk with your doctor about the local application of estrogen. This can be in the form of a cream, vaginal pill, suppository, or through an estradiol ring inserted into the vagina to provide vaginal lubrication without allowing estrogen into your body's circulatory system. If your cancer is not estrogen dependent your doctor may prescribe hormone replacement therapy. This is a controversial subject because long-term hormonal replacement has advantages and disadvantages. Long-term estrogen replacement therapy may reduce the risk of colorectal cancer and hip and other bone fractures, but it also may increase the risk of breast cancer, stroke, heart attack, and blood clots. One of the rationales for hormone replacement therapy has been to reduce the incidence of osteoporosis in women who are no longer producing estrogen. Newer medications without estrogen can help prevent osteoporosis. When you talk to your doctor about hormone replacement, ask about medications to prevent osteoporosis. The risks and benefits of each option must be evaluated for each individual.

Women with estrogen-dependent tumors who are lacking sufficient levels of testosterone may be able to take supplemental testosterone in the form of injections or pills. You should ask your physician about the risks and benefits of testosterone replacement therapy.

Vaginal dryness can be caused by many types of cancer treatment. In addition to hormonal treatments, several excellent lubricants are available. Generous amounts of water-based lubricant should be applied to the labia, vagina, and penis to ease penetration, prevent pain, and minimize the risk of injury to the vaginal wall. Application of sufficient lubricant can be incorporated into sexual foreplay so that it becomes a source of pleasure for both partners.

Sildenafil (Viagra) has been prescribed to women to treat diminished sexual arousal. In women, sildenafil increases relaxation of the smooth muscles of the vagina and clitoris, and increases blood flow to the genital area. Other medications, such as phentolamine and L-arginine, have been used in clinical trials with promising results to treat women with diminished sexual arousal. Ask your doctor for the most current information about medications to increase sexual arousal.

Painful intercourse may be related to surgical changes, chemotherapy-induced harm to the nervous system, or psychological factors. A fear of pain during intercourse will cause an involuntary tensing of the genital muscles. This reaction makes penetration difficult, causing pain, which in turn increases fear and anxiety, causing involuntary muscle tension, which only makes the situation worse. Many survivors were used to certain sexual activities prior to their diagnosis. If they experience pain when they attempt their usual sexual activities during treatment, they can become conditioned to feel fear and anxiety with subsequent sexual activity. Many then give up on sexual activity. If your usual pattern of sexual activity is no longer comfortable, you may need to change positions, add lubrication, or practice muscle relaxation exercises before attempting the same type of sexual activity. You can also use this as an opportunity to learn about other sexual positions and techniques that you might enjoy. See chapter 17 for resources to help you learn about different types of sexual activity.

Pain from nerve damage, a side effect of some types of chemotherapy, has been reported in the vulva. This can be treated with corticosteroid cream, testosterone cream, or a topical anesthetic gel. The anesthetic gel may cause a feeling of numbness for both partners. If this is not a pleasant sensation for your partner, be sure he communicates this to you. Use of a condom will prevent direct contact between the skin of the penis and the anesthetic gel.

A hysterectomy may cause the vagina to become shorter, which may lead to painful intercourse in certain positions. If you experience pain during intercourse, ask your partner to try a different position so that you are more comfortable. You might want to try positions where the woman is on top, or you are side by side, so that you can have some control of the angle and depth of penetration. Generous use of lubrication will also help minimize discomfort.

Surgery and radiation can cause the vagina to become narrower and less elastic. This is called vaginal stenosis. Women who are at risk for vaginal stenosis should be instructed in the use of vaginal dilators. These are made in various sizes and are inserted into the vagina to ensure that it remains open. You start with a very narrow, well-lubricated dilator and gradually increase the size of the dilator used until a normal vaginal opening is achieved. You must continue to use dilators for the rest of your life to maintain an open vaginal canal. Even if you do not continue sexual activity, your vagina must remain open for future physical examinations by your physician.

Cancer affecting the vulva may require surgery to remove the tumor and surrounding tissue. Recent advances in surgical technique allow for a localized tumor of the vulva to be removed in a way that preserves a woman's ability to achieve orgasm.

Most survivors treated for advanced ovarian cancer with surgery to remove the ovaries, uterus, vagina, bladder, and rectum do not continue sexual activity. Extensive surgery creates changes in body image, such as having a stoma or pouch for emptying the bladder or bowel. This surgery is often followed by chemotherapy, and survivors may be dealing with too many physical issues to feel any interest in sexual activity. However, when you recover from the surgery and any subsequent treatment, your desire for sexual activity may return. Preserve your options for future sexual activity at the time of your original surgery by telling your surgeon about your interest in future sexual activity and asking your surgeon about the most current information on reconstructive techniques. For example, a surgeon can reconstruct the vagina using a loop of the bowel or muscle from the inner thigh or other suitable tissue.

Any type of surgery has the potential to interrupt nerve pathways. If the nerve pathways involved in the sexual response cycle are damaged or destroyed, survivors may need to learn new ways to enjoy sexual activity. For example, if tissue from your clitoris has been removed, you can learn where other sensitive tissue remains by experimenting with different types of touch. You can use your hands to explore different sensations on the remaining tissue. You can also experiment with vibrators once the surgical site has healed sufficiently. Try using lubricants as you massage the area. You can also try other sensations, such as those created by a piece of silk or a feather. While you try to stimulate nerve endings, remember that sexual response begins in the mind. You can enhance the process by employing fantasy as well as touch. Above all, give yourself time to become reacquainted with your body and its responses to different physical and mental stimuli.

SPECIAL ISSUES FOR MEN

Ask your physician about all possible treatments for your tumor, as well as their side effects, before deciding on a course of treatment. Tell your doctor whether the ability to maintain sexual function is important to you.

One of the things many men worry about after having cancer is that they will be unable to have or maintain an erection. This is called *erectile dysfunction,* or ED, and is now discussed in television and print advertisements, which indicates how common it is among men. Sildenafil, or Viagra, is widely prescribed to treat some forms of erectile dysfunction.

The ability to have an erection depends on several things. Because the sexual response cycle begins in the brain, a thought, an image, an odor, a touch, or a kiss may cause sexual arousal, which then causes the brain to release certain chemicals that begin a cascade of events, potentially culminating in sexual intercourse. Many things can interfere with this series of events. A common problem among men is "performance anxiety," which means worrying about whether you are able to have an erection may make it difficult or impossible for you to have an erection. To determine whether a problem producing an erection is physical or mental, notice whether you have erections in your sleep. Many men awake in the morning with an erection. Others have erections during sleep, but do not wake up until after it has subsided. To test whether you had an erection while you were asleep, put a loose paper band around your penis at night. If the band is ripped in the morning, you had an erection. Be sure the paper is something that rips easily. If it is too tight it can cause permanent damage to your penis.

If you find that you have erections while you sleep, but still cannot have erections when you desire, you may need to look at mental or emotional barriers to enjoying sexual activity. A professional counselor can help you overcome these barriers.

Changes in hormones may interfere with the sexual response cycle. If your body is not making sufficient amounts of certain hormones, or if your treatment intentionally inactivates the hormones because they are feeding the tumor, the sexual response cycle must be started in another way.

If the nerve pathway from the brain to the penis has been interrupted at any point, the message from the brain to initiate sexual response never arrives and an erection may not occur. Nerve-sparing surgical procedures, particularly for prostate cancer, are more successful in preserving the nerves that help a man achieve and maintain an erection. Ask your surgeon what the success rate is for maintaining sexual function with this type of surgery. Surgical techniques are constantly being refined, so be sure that the information you get is current. If the nerve pathway has been interrupted because of damage to the spinal cord, other methods, such as touching the face, nipples, scrotum, and inner thigh can stimulate erogenous feelings and trigger a sexual response.

Good blood flow is necessary for the penis to enlarge and become erect. Medical conditions other than cancer, such as diabetes and high blood pressure, can impair circulation to the penis. Be sure your physician is aware of all your health conditions when you talk to him or her about any erectile problems you experience. Some chemotherapy drugs can cause changes in your blood pressure. Your physician can prescribe medication to control your blood pressure. For some people, however, blood pressure medications can interfere with their sexual function. Tell your physician if you notice changes in sexual function when medications are added or changed during your cancer treatment.

Several forms of medication can treat erectile dysfunction. Some are taken in pill form; others are rubbed on the penis to relax blood vessels, or inserted or injected into the penis to cause an erection. Probably the most well known treatment is Viagra, or sildenafil. In men, Viagra relaxes muscles so that blood can flow into the penis. If you have leukemia, multiple myeloma, or cardiac problems, you should not take Viagra. Because Viagra changes the effect of some other medications, the doctor who prescribes it must be aware of all medicines, including over-the-counter and herbal medicines, that you are taking. If you are not able to take Viagra, other treatments may help you have and maintain an erection. If you have a problem with the blood supply to the penis, ask you doctor to order a study, such as a Doppler ultrasound study, venogram, or arteriogram, to identify the problem. A blockage or other type of problem may be surgically corrected.

An erection can also be obtained by using a device that will create a partial vacuum around the penis. This pulls blood into the penis. An elastic ring fits over the base of the penis and traps the blood so that the erection can be maintained.

Surgery can also be performed to place a device inside your body that will allow you to have an erection when you want one. This is called a *penile implant* or *penile prosthesis*. A prosthesis is either a replacement part for some part that is missing or something that will help a part of you to work better, such as a hearing aid. A penile prosthesis is surgically implanted; it is possible that no one will be able to tell you have one. One type of penile implant, a *semi-rigid* implant, makes the penis hard and somewhat erect all of the time. This will allow you to have sexual intercourse. A fully erect penis is not necessary for penetration and intercourse. The disadvantage is that the penis will always look semi-erect and may be seen through tight clothing. Another type of penile implant allows you to have an erection by pressing on a small pump. The pump moves fluid into one or more tubes implanted in the penis. The fluid serves the same purpose as the blood that would normally flow into the penis when you are aroused, and causes the penis to become hard and erect. The erection stays until the fluid is released.

Erectile dysfunction is a specialized area of medical treatment. If your physician does not know about the most recent research and techniques to treat erectile dysfunction, ask for a referral to a physician who specializes in treating this problem.

Ejaculation is the release of fluid from the penis during sexual activity. Most men (and women) think that ejaculation should happen at the same time they reach orgasm, or at the time of greatest pleasure sensation during sexual activity. This happens in the movies and romance novels, and sometimes in real life—but not always. Many men reach orgasm just before or after ejaculation. After the fluid is released, the penis returns to its normal, relaxed state. Sometimes, though, the time between orgasm and the release of fluid is too long or the fluid is released before the man has satisfied himself or his partner.

Cancer surgery may remove some of the body parts that produce semen or help cause semen and sperm to move into the penis. If your prostate and seminal vesicles are removed, of if nerves that control the movement of semen and sperm into your penis are damaged, you can have an orgasm with little or no fluid being released from the penis. The absence of fluid will not affect your ability to have an orgasm. If you are concerned about fertility, you can retrieve sperm without ejaculation (see pages 88–89).

In some cases, semen is being produced, but rather than moving into the penis, it moves backward into the bladder. This condition is called *retrograde ejaculation.* Normally, an opening between the bladder and the prostate connects to the *ureter,* the tube through which both urine and semen pass down the penis and are pushed out of the body. When the sexual response cycle begins, the opening closes so that urine stays in the bladder and semen travels down the penis. If the muscles or nerves that control this opening are damaged, it could stay open during sexual activity. Semen and sperm would move into the bladder instead of down the penis. The sensation of ejaculation will not be affected, but no fluid will be released. The semen and sperm will eventually be washed out of the bladder with the urine, which may look cloudy. If this occurs, talk to your physician. The condition is not harmful, but your physician can help you decide if you want to try to have it corrected.

Cancer of the penis is rare, but it does occur. If the entire penis has been removed because of an invasive cancer, the surgeon will create an opening for urine that is located behind the testicles and in front of the anus. You will have to sit down to urinate. Removal of all or part of the penis does not physically affect your ability to become sexually aroused, achieve orgasm, or ejaculate because you still have sensation in the area. Take the time to explore sensations in the genital area as well as other areas of the body. The nipples, inner thigh, ears, neck, and face are very sensitive to stimulation. Try different types of touch—from a light touch using the fingers, a piece of silk, or a feather to deeper, massaging type of touch until you discover techniques that work for you and your partner. If you ejaculate, semen will be released through the same opening as urine.

Colorectal cancer involving a tumor that is located low in the colon, near the rectum, or in the rectum itself may require a surgical procedure to remove the tumor and close the rectal opening. The surgeon will create a colostomy for elimination of feces. Homosexual men who have enjoyed anal intercourse prior to this surgery will no longer be able to engage in this activity. Explore with your partner other methods of sexual activity to enhance your relationship.

If you have a testicle removed to treat testicular cancer, you can get a testicular prosthesis. These can be custom made so that you can select both the size and the material from which the prosthesis is made. In many cases, the prosthesis can be inserted at the same time the malignant testicle is removed. Some men are not bothered by removal of a testicle and may not want a prosthesis. Removal of a single testicle should not affect your ability to produce sperm or to have children. Lymph node surgery to determine whether testicular cancer has spread may damage the nerves that control ejaculation. If these nerves are damaged, you may not experience a release of fluid when you ejaculate, but you can still experience the sensations that accompany sexual activity and ejaculation. If you wish to have children, you will have to use another method to retrieve sperm and cause fertilization (see pages 88–89). You may want to bank your sperm before having surgery or any other treatment for testicular cancer.

FERTILITY

Fertility is a concern for childhood cancer survivors and those diagnosed during their childbearing years. In some cultures, a woman's fertility is extremely important for marriage. Reproductive technology is becoming more sophisticated at the same time that cancer treatment is being refined to minimize harming fertility. Unfortunately, many insurance companies do not cover the cost of harvesting and storing sperm, ovarian tissue, or embryos. In vitro fertilization (fertilization of an egg by a sperm in a laboratory followed by implantation in the uterus) can be quite expensive. See chapter 12 for a discussion of how to obtain insurance coverage. Additionally, while many oncologists know about sperm banking, many are not aware of the latest reproductive technologies. Every year doctors make new advances in reproductive technology. If possible, talk with a reproductive specialist to learn the latest options in preserving fertility so you can make decisions *before* you get cancer treatment. Tell your health care team about your fertility concerns so they can consider your needs in proposing treatment options.

Certain chemotherapy drugs cause temporary or permanent infertility. In some cases, you can choose drugs that will have little effect on your fertility. In other cases, the choice of treatment itself may make a difference in preserving fertility. For example, women treated for Hodgkin's disease with total lymphoid irradiation had better fertility rates than those treated with combination chemotherapy or with both radiation and combination chemotherapy. In cancers such as Hodgkin's disease, where the survival rates are fairly high, you have more treatment choices with fewer side effects that do not affect long-term survival.

If you are going to freeze sperm, eggs, ovarian tissue, or embryos, you will need to decide who has control of the frozen tissue. Before the tissue is harvested, you should state, *in writing,* whether

- any of the tissue may be used at a later time for a medical experiment;
- a surviving spouse, significant other, or parent has the right to use the frozen tissue;
- the tissue may be donated to a specified infertility clinic for use by other infertile couples;
- the tissue may be destroyed at any time in the future and under what specific circumstances you would want the tissue to be destroyed; and
- one of the partners may use the frozen tissue should your current relationship end in divorce.

Special Issues for Women

Women with gynecologic cancers should discuss with their doctors preserving fertility at the same time they discuss treatment options. Combining more conservative surgical procedures with radiation and/or chemotherapy improves a woman's chance of preserving her fertility without adversely affecting her chances for long-term survival. Women with tumors that are estrogen receptor positive should learn about the risks of pregnancy after treatment is completed. Because pregnancy is accompanied by a surge in hormone levels, use birth control during cancer treatment, particularly when the tumor is "nourished" by hormones. Once you are in remission, weigh the risks and benefits of pregnancy, and the timing of any pregnancy, with your physician. Ask about the latest data about long-term follow-up of survivors who became pregnant after completing similar treatment. See Chapter 17 for information about long-term follow-up studies of cancer survivors.

Cancer treatment can cause chromosomal damage to ovarian and testicular tissue. Men make sperm on an "as needed" basis, so this is not as much an issue for men as it is for women. Women are born with all the eggs they will ever have during their lifetime. If you decide to have a child after completing treatment, consider genetic counseling and amniocentesis during your pregnancy. Your obstetrician should be someone who specializes in high-risk pregnancy and who is aware of all the treatments you received for your cancer.

While a man can produce sperm for cryopreservation (freezing) within a very short period of time, the process for harvesting eggs may take several weeks. If it is important to start cancer treatment immediately, you may not have enough time to harvest eggs prior to starting treatment.

In a normal cycle, one egg is released each month. In some cases, a woman will release two eggs, which is how fraternal twins are conceived. Hormones can be used to stimulate production of eggs for harvesting and freezing. This produces only a small number of eggs at a time. You have a better chance for successful pregnancy if the egg can be fertilized immediately and the embryo frozen for later implantation than if you freeze unfertilized eggs. If you do not have a partner with whom you want to have children at the time you are diagnosed, fertilizing an egg can be a problem. One possible solution would be to use a sperm donor—someone you know, or an anonymous donor from a sperm bank. If you use a known donor, make a written agreement concerning the legal rights of each parent regarding any child who is born.

Cancer treatment at a young age has been associated with the early onset of menopause. As a cancer survivor, you may have fewer childbearing years than someone who has not been treated for cancer.

Some adolescents and young women treated for Hodgkin's disease have had their ovaries moved outside the field of pelvic radiation to maximize their potential for preserving fertility. Discuss this option with your doctor if you are being treated with pelvic radiation.

In some cases, women whose cancer treatment has induced menopause may later recover ovarian function through the use of hormone replacement therapy. This may not be an option in some gynecologic cancers or in breast cancer. As discussed on pages 79–80, long-term use of hormone replacement therapy has many serious risks.

If you cannot preserve your fertility or harvest a viable egg for fertilization and implantation, other options are available. After completion of your cancer treatment, you may be able to obtain a donor egg, have it fertilized with your partner's sperm or with donor sperm, and have the embryo implanted in your uterus. As with the use of donor sperm, you should have a written agreement with the egg donor that contains your entire agreement regarding use of any frozen embryo, custody of any frozen embryo, and the parental rights and legal responsibilities of each party.

If you are not able to sustain a pregnancy on your own, consider a surrogate mother—a woman who agrees to have your fertilized embryo implanted in her uterus. At the end of the pregnancy, she agrees to give up any custodial rights to your biologic child. The embryo that is implanted may have been created from your egg and your partner's sperm or may have been created using either donor sperm, a donor egg, or both. Surrogate motherhood can be successful or can result in a lawsuit when the surrogate decides after the birth that she wants full or partial custody of the child. The surrogate can be a woman recruited by an infertility center or a surrogacy agency, or could be a member of your family.

You might also consider adopting a child after cancer treatment. Many attorneys and agencies specialize in arranging adoptions. Consider adopting a child who is older than an infant. Infant adoption may take years to arrange, and many older children need loving parents. International adoption has also become common in the United States. Most adoptions will involve questions about your health history. See pages 287–288 for an explanation of the role your cancer history may play in adoption. See Chapter 17 for resources to help you adopt a child.

Special Issues for Men

Some types of cancer affect the number and quality of sperm you produce. To fertilize an egg, the sperm must be able to move up the vagina toward the woman's egg (*motility*). To preserve your fertility options, collect and freeze your sperm before you begin any cancer treatment. Some insurance companies will pay for sperm banking as a part of your cancer treatment. For the company to pay for the collection and storage costs, your physician may need to write a letter to the insurance company stating that it is "medically necessary" to store your sperm.

If you have to pay for this procedure yourself, you will probably pay separate fees to analyze the sperm to see if the number and motility are sufficient to make sperm banking worthwhile, to process the sperm, and to store frozen sperm. When you decide you want to use the sperm, the sperm bank will return it to the physician or fertility clinic that you choose.

The procedure for collecting sperm is fairly simple and can be done in a medical setting, at the sperm bank, or in the privacy of your own home. Most sperm banks will provide you with a sperm collection kit. If you go to the sperm bank, a private room is used for sperm collection. The sample is collected by masturbation. A special type of "condom" is used to collect the sperm. If possible, collect three separate samples at least 24 hours apart so that the number of sperm in each sample will be as large as possible. In cases where time is a critical factor for starting cancer treatment, the samples can be collected with less time between each collection.

Anyone who has reached puberty can bank sperm. The fact that you are young, single, or may think that you do not ever want children should not prevent you from thinking about banking your sperm for future use. You should decide what you want done with the sperm if you decide later that you do not want to use it.

You have the option of having the sperm destroyed, donating it to an infertility clinic or a research facility, or donating it to a specific couple, such as a family member who is either infertile or who has agreed to have a child for you. If you are in a relationship, you should discuss these options with your partner. You should also decide what will happen to your sperm should the relationship end, either through divorce or the death of one of the partners.

Consult a fertility specialist if you have not banked sperm prior to your cancer treatment and find that you are having retrograde or dry ejaculation after treatment to determine whether you are producing sperm. If you are producing sperm, it may be possible to retrieve the sperm directly from the testicle or from that part of the body where the sperm has been diverted. The sperm that is retrieved can either be used immediately or frozen for future use.

A low or zero sperm count may not necessarily be related to your cancer diagnosis. If you never had a sperm count done prior to your diagnosis, you will not know what your sperm count was prior to your illness. You may have always had a low sperm count. The cancer diagnosis provided you with the opportunity to store your sperm to preserve your option for having children after your diagnosis. You may never need to use your stored sperm. Your cancer treatment may not permanently affect your ability to produce sperm.

With improved techniques, such as intracytoplasmic sperm injection (ICSI), a man need not have a large number of sperm, or highly mobile sperm, to have a child. This technique inserts a sperm directly into the cytoplasm of the egg. Technically, you need only one good sperm to create a baby. ICSI is particularly helpful if you have lymphoma, leukemia, or testicular cancer, because these cancers can lower sperm counts, so you may have a low sperm count before treatment begins.

The ability to produce sperm does not affect your ability to produce semen, the fluid that is ejaculated from the penis. Semen and sperm are made in two different parts of your body. The semen is a transportation system for the sperm to get out of your body.

The ability to produce active, healthy sperm in sufficient numbers to father a child does not physically affect your ability to achieve or maintain an erection. Some men have the mistaken belief that fertility is linked to sexual ability. If you are having trouble becoming sexually aroused or obtaining or maintaining an erection after learning that you are infertile, speak with your doctor or a urologist, fertility specialist, sex educator, or sex therapist.

If intimacy, sexual activity, or the ability to have children were important to you before your cancer diagnosis, you need not abandon them in your new life as a cancer survivor. Make sure your doctor and other members of your health care team know that these issues are important to you. If you have questions, do not hesitate to ask them. Many resources are available to help you. Do not focus on the losses in your life; use this time to learn new things about yourself and those people who are important to you. Be open to new ideas, different ways to approach problems, and to new experiences.

Chapter Five

Complementary and Alternative Medicines Therapy

by Georgia Decker, M.S.,
C.S.-A.N.P., A.O.C.N.®

A Short History of Medicine

2000 B.C.— "Here, eat this root."

A.D. 1000—"That root is heathen. Say this prayer."

A.D. 1850—"That prayer is superstition. Drink this potion."

A.D. 1940—"That potion is snake oil. Swallow this pill."

A.D. 1985—"That pill is ineffective. Take this antibiotic."

A.D. 2000—"That antibiotic doesn't work anymore. Here, eat this root."

—Author unknown

RESEARCH HAS DOCUMENTED an increase in the use of complementary and alternative medicine (CAM) therapies in recent years. In 1993 alternative therapies were defined by Dr. David Eisenberg and colleagues at Harvard as those that are not taught in medical schools and not usually available in American hospitals. This definition is no longer accurate, because many medical schools now include these therapies in their medical school programs. The terms now used to describe these therapies are controversial. Some feel that terms such as "unconventional" or "unproven" are judgmental, and prevent the communication and understanding needed between patient and practitioner. *Complementary and alternative medicine (CAM),* also known as *integrative medicine,* is the language currently used by the National Institutes of Health (NIH). Medical journals now include information about CAM therapies being researched.

Some authors say that a common reason for using these therapies is a patient's disappointment with conventional therapies. Others state that it is a perception of improved quality of life and an increased sense of control that appeals to patients. Patients want to be treated in a holistic way with what they consider to be natural or nontoxic remedies. These therapies may be used when conventional therapies fail, during conventional therapy, or when a patient seeks more control in his or her health care. From 1990 to 1997, the use of CAM therapies increased 25 percent, the use of herbal medicine increased 380 percent, and the use of high-dose vitamins increased 130 percent. Unfortunately, less than 40 percent of CAM therapies used were disclosed to a physician in 1990 and 1997. This low rate of disclosure is of concern to health care professionals. A survey conducted in 2000 of CAM therapy use by cancer patients participating in clinical trials revealed that most used at least one type of CAM therapy: spirituality (94 percent); imagery (86 percent); massage (80 percent); lifestyle, diet, nutrition (60 percent); relaxation (50 percent); herbal/botanical (20 percent); and high-dose vitamins (14 percent).

WHAT ARE COMPLEMENTARY AND ALTERNATIVE MEDICINE (THERAPIES)?

Complementary ≠ Alternative

The use of *complementary* and *alternative* as meaning the same thing has led to miscommunication and confusion. These terms are not interchangeable. They describe the intent with which a therapy is used, not the therapy itself.

TERMS USED TO DESCRIBE THERAPIES

(W)HOLISTIC	Considers the entire person, not just a diagnosis.
UNPROVEN	Has not been scientifically studied. Does not mean it has no value; the value has yet to be established.
DISPROVEN	Has been studied scientifically and has been shown to be of no use for a particular intention.
CONVENTIONAL	Therapy most often used by a particular culture or group of people.

A therapy is *alternative* when it is used in place of conventional therapy. An example is a patient using only herbs as a treatment for cancer. *Complementary therapies* are those used in addition to or to complement conventional therapy, such as the use of meditation in addition to medication to combat nausea. The more contemporary term *integrative* means combining conventional and unconventional therapies in a way that is safe and supervised, and with a result that is better than a result of either one used alone. What one person may consider conventional may not be conventional to another person. Culture, ethnicity, and previous experience affect what you consider conventional. It is very important that you communicate with your health care providers regarding any therapies that you are using.

Although the use of CAM therapies has grown in the United States and internationally, little is known about the safety and efficacy of many therapies, especially when used by a person receiving cancer therapy. The National Institutes of Health National Center for Complementary and Alternative Medicine (NIH-NCCAM) was created in 1998 to "facilitate the evaluation of alternative medical treatment modalities" to determine their effectiveness. The NIH-NCCAM does not provide referrals for CAM therapies or practitioners. It does conduct and support research and training, and provides information on CAM therapies to practitioners and the public (**www.nccam.nih.gov**).

NATIONAL INSTITUTES OF HEALTH
NATIONAL CENTER FOR COMPLEMENTARY AND
ALTERNATIVE MEDICINE (NIH-NCCAM):
CATEGORIES OF CAMs

CATEGORIES:

1. Alternative Systems of Medical Care
2. Mind-Body Medicine Modalities
3. Bioelectromagnetic Therapies
4. Manual Healing Methods
5. Pharmacological and Biological Therapies
6. Diet, Nutrition, and Lifestyle
7. Herbal Medicine

ALTERNATIVE SYSTEMS OF MEDICAL CARE

These systems stress prevention of "dis-ease" and promotion of health that includes personal responsibility and self-healing. These systems are a way of being and a way of living. They are not meant to be separated into individual modalities. Examples include traditional Chinese medicine (TCM), naturopathy, and Ayurvedic medicine.

MIND-BODY MEDICINE

Understanding that the mind influences the body is not new. These therapies are based on the connection of mind and body, and the potential for a person to influence healing. The therapies in this category are based on the belief that the mind and body are wholly integrated and that each has the ability to influence the other. Examples include meditation, guided imagery/visualization, relaxation, spirituality, and art therapies.

BIOELECTROMAGNETIC THERAPIES

The study of bioelectromagnetic therapies gained recognition when a German oncologist raised awareness of low-frequency electromagnetic currents in the earth. This theory (geopathic zones) was based upon the belief that energy is drawn from a person's body by low-frequency currents, resulting in disease. Electromagnetic field therapy theory is based upon making corrections in human energy fields and is a very controversial

{continued}

area of study. Examples include acupuncture, magnet therapy, and cymatics.

MANUAL HEALING METHODS

Manual healing methods involve touch. In conventional medicine, caregivers used to "touch" patients more than they do now. To receivers of manual healing methods, the benefits seem obvious; however, scientific proof is lacking for some. They appeal to us because we as human beings (in our culture) have a strong desire to touch and be touched. Examples include Reiki, chiropractic, reflexology, massage, and therapeutic touch/healing touch (a misnomer since actual touch may not be involved).

PHARMACOLOGICAL AND BIOLOGICAL THERAPIES

Some pharmacological and biological therapies claim to cure everything from obesity to cancer. Scientific proof is lacking for many of these therapies. Isadore Rosenfeld, M.D., describes these therapies as having "the lure of the cure." Examples include laetrile, shark cartilage, oxidative therapies, and antineoplastons.

DIET, NUTRITION, AND LIFESTYLE CHANGES

Much has been written about nutrition and its effect on health and disease. Many CAM diet programs promise "detoxification" and healing, and therefore nutrition and dietary changes are common choices as complementary therapies. The major appeal of nutritional therapies is that they can be started immediately. Controversies are related to the risk of malnutrition with restricted dietary programs, effects of antioxidants and/or vitamins during certain therapies, and the effects of dietary soy on breast cancer. Examples of CAM diet therapies include macrobiotics, the Gerson Program, and Kelley-Gonzalez.

HERBAL MEDICINE

The goal of herbal medicine is to assist the body to restore and maintain balance. The foundation of herbal medicine is based upon the Doctrine of Signatures. This doctrine states that a plant's

{continued}

NATIONAL INSTITUTES OF HEALTH
NATIONAL CENTER FOR COMPLEMENTARY AND
ALTERNATIVE MEDICINE (NIH-NCCAM):
CATEGORIES OF CAMS (CONTINUED)

HERBAL MEDICINE
(CONTINUED)

appearance or characteristics provide a clue to its medicinal value. This concept has not been scientifically established. Herbal remedies can be taken internally or applied to the skin and come in a variety of capsules, tinctures, poultices, creams, and compresses. Herbs may be used as a single agent or in combination.

ALTERNATIVE SYSTEMS OF MEDICAL PRACTICE

Homeopathy is a system of medicine that originated in 17th-century Germany. Homeopathy means treating "like with like." Practitioners believe the external signs of an illness are seen as the body's efforts to heal itself; the remedy they prescribe is tailored to support and enhance the body's own efforts. Western (conventional) medicine, referred to by homeopathic practitioners as "allopathy," suppresses symptoms with an antidote of superior force. In homeopathy, remedies are *minute* dilutions of a natural substance that would cause the same symptoms if taken in a higher dose. For example, nausea would be treated with a substance that causes nausea but is given in a minute dilution. The smallest dose is believed to increase the body's healing potential without causing side effects. Today, many homeopathic remedies for common illness have become standardized and are available over-the-counter in health food stores and drugstores.

COMMON HOMEOPATHIC REMEDIES*
(SOMETIMES CALLED A HOMEOPATHIC FIRST AID KIT)

Arnica: for shock after trauma, burns, bruising, nosebleeds, and strained muscles
Apis: for bee stings, edema, arthritis, and allergic reactions in eyes, throat, and mouth
Nux Vomica: for motion sickness and nausea, headache, and digestive problems
Silica: for migraines, and recurrent colds and infections
Tabacum: for motion sickness, nausea, vomiting, faintness, and anxiety

*When taken with medications, the action of these remedies may be altered.

Ayurvedic medicine comes from the traditional healing system of India. The primary belief is that human beings are a part of nature and are controlled by the same principles as nature. The goal of Ayurveda is to bring people into harmony with their surroundings. In Ayurvedic medicine, everyone is believed to be born with varying amounts of the three types of vital energy called *doshas*: 1) Vatta (symbolized by air and space—constantly moving); 2) Pitta (symbolized by fire—volatile and competitive); and 3) Kapha (symbolized by earth and water—solid and tranquil). Ayurveda, though, considers each person to be unique.

In Ayurvedic medicine, illness is related to imbalances in the doshas, and all aspects of one's life are affected by these imbalances. Health requires balance among all three doshas. Practitioners are expected to accurately identify each person's makeup, diagnose any imbalance(s), and then provide treatment. Detoxification, diet, herbs, exercise, and mind-body techniques contribute to a system that is a way of life, not an intermittent or occasional treatment option.

Naturopathy began in the late 19th century in Germany. It is a system of medicine that focuses on increasing the body's ability to heal. Naturopaths use herbal medicine, massage, nutrition, and other techniques to promote the elimination of toxins and improve health. Naturopaths combine modern diagnostic techniques with natural therapies.

MIND-BODY MEDICINE

Important caution: The symptoms of mental illness may worsen with some of these modalities. Therefore, choosing a therapist who is skilled in these therapies, as well as knowledgeable about physical and mental illnesses, is very important.

Relaxation and *meditation* are techniques that include a variety of modalities, including breath therapy, hypnotherapy, imagery and visualization, meditation, and yoga. Some authors include Tai Chi in this category. Although they vary in methodology, all require a quiet, stress-free environment. Patients have reported positive outcomes, including increased happiness and self-confidence.

Imagery and *visualization* may be referred to as guided imagery, creative imagery, or visualization therapy. These techniques incorporate the use of images or symbols and focus the mind on bodily functions. Imagery and visualization have been used successfully to decrease stress, pain, and heart rate. Recent studies have shown that these therapies may stimulate the immune system. Although imagery is used as a self-help technique, initial practice should be under the guidance of a therapist who is skilled in this technique, as well as knowledgeable about medical and psychiatric conditions. See chapter 6 for descriptions of mind-body exercises.

Music therapy is the intentional use of music or sound—writing music or listening to music to impact health. Practitioners of sound therapy, a subset of music therapy, believe the use of sound waves can restore body harmony. They may work with individuals or groups. Music therapy has been used in mental health care, stress management, and pain management. Choose a qualified music therapist to lessen the chance of having an unexpected problem.

BIOELECTROMAGNETIC THERAPIES

Acupuncture is an expression of electromagnetic pathways of body energy flow. The Meridian System, the primary map of the body used by acupuncturists, describes energy channels flowing throughout the body. Acupuncturists use 12 principal meridians and 365 points (*acupoints*). When acupuncture needles are placed at an acupoint, you may feel a slight ache, dull pain, or tingling sensation that lasts a few seconds. Once the needle is in place, you should feel no discomfort. In fact, some patients report a sensation of warmth. An acupoint may be stimulated in a number of ways. For example, crystals can be used instead of needles. Acupuncture is most widely used for a specific purpose, such as pain management or immune-system balancing. However, patients are treated as a whole with an understanding that signs and symptoms are interrelated. Acupuncture has been scientifically proven to decrease pain and is included in pain management guidelines.

Magnet therapy is based on the theory that the body consists of various energy processes that generate their own magnetic field and that the manipulation of these fields has therapeutic potential. Magnet energy as a cause of and potential cure for disease has been a topic of fascination for health care professionals for many years. Two types of magnets can be used. Electromagnets conduct electrical currents through wire. Permanent magnets create a magnetic field when the electrons in the atoms of the magnet are in motion. Magnets are said to have been used successfully in the treatment of peripheral neuropathies and pain syndromes. Research in this therapy is increasing.

HERBAL MEDICINE

The United States Food and Drug Administration (FDA) lists approximately 250 herbs as GRAS (generally recognized as safe). Only six herbs (aloe, capsicum, cascara, psyllium, senna, and witch hazel) received FDA approval before the passage of the Dietary Supplement Health and Education Act of 1994. Under this law, herbs in the United States are now classified and sold as nutritional supplements and no longer require FDA approval. The active ingredient content of these products is not controlled or standardized. A constant concern is the purity of the product. A 1998 study conducted by the California Department of Health found that some herbal products are contaminated with heavy metals as well as other substances. In 1997, an estimated 15 million adults took prescription medications concurrently with herbal remedies and/or high-dose vitamins. These individuals are at risk for potential adverse drug-herb or drug-supplement interactions.

Medicinal herbs can interact with pharmaceuticals. Herbs should be discontinued if any unpleasant side effects occur. *When in doubt, do without.* Most herbs have specific indications and therefore should not be taken in particular situations.

More information about potential interactions between herbs and drugs is available from the Food and Drug Administration at **www.fda.org** (click on "Medwatch").

PHARMACOLOGICAL AND BIOLOGICAL THERAPIES

Oxidative therapies are based upon the belief that cancer and viruses cannot exist in an oxygen-rich environment. Oxygen is essential to life; some people believe that oxygen deficiency is a component of illness. Oxidative therapies are believed to improve oxygen concentration and thus fight illness, including cancer. Hydrogen peroxide infusions and ozone are examples of oxidative therapies. Although research is being conducted regarding these therapies, they remain controversial.

Colostrum has been used to treat diarrhea, to improve gastrointestinal health, and to boost the immune system. Colostrum, the first milk new mothers secrete after giving birth, is a rich natural source of nutrients, antibodies, and growth factors for a newborn. Several studies show that bovine colostrum concentrates are highly successful in improving gastrointestinal health and in treating certain kinds of diarrhea. Product purity is a major concern. Potential side effects include mild gastrointestinal upset, mild nausea, and flatulence.

Laetrile (also known as amygdalin, Vitamin B_{17})—Amygdalin is a cyanide-containing substance that was once believed to be, *but has since been disproven as,* an effective cancer therapy. Laetrile is a concentrated form of amygdalin. It is usually administered intravenously, but also has been injected into an artery immediately above the tumor site. It may also be taken orally. There are documented reports of accidental poisoning with laetrile tablets. Potential side effects include weakness, dizziness, nausea, vomiting, diarrhea, and fever.

Shark cartilage and bovine cartilage are believed to inhibit the formation of blood vessels to and within the tumor, and to enhance the immune system. Studies are currently testing the effectiveness of shark cartilage in these two areas. The original theory was based on the observation that sharks do not appear to get cancer. Sharks do get cancer, however. Shark or bovine cartilage is used as an oral preparation. It is expensive and product purity is a concern. Potential side effects include mild gastrointestinal upset and flatulence.

MANUAL HEALING METHODS

Massage therapy is the specific manipulation of the body's soft tissues. Massage therapists use their hands, but sometimes forearms, elbows, and feet as well. The touch used in massage involves varying degrees of pressure. Massage therapy can be used in a variety of ways, but it has been controversial for cancer survivors. Fear of spreading cancer has kept many cancer patients and survivors from receiving

MOST COMMONLY USED HERBS IN THE UNITED STATES

HERB	INDICATIONS	SIDE EFFECTS AND CONTRAINDICATIONS
GINGKO BILOBA	Acts as an antioxidant. Has been used for vertigo and tinnitis. Believed to make platelets "slippery." Believed to improve memory.	Mild stomach upset and headache, allergic skin reactions, interferes with normal blood clotting. Has been linked to strokes caused by bleeding with higher doses. **Do not take with** anticoagulant drugs, NSAIDs, and aspirin.
ST. JOHN'S WORT	Has been useful in mild depression or Seasonal Affective Disorder (S.A.D.). Also known as "Nature's Prozac" because it has properties of Selective Serotonin Reuptake Inhibitors (SSRIs) or Monoamine Oxidase Inhibitors (MAOIs).	Photosensitivity, fatigue, itching, dizziness, and dry mouth. Avoid tyramine-containing foods. Avoid taking with prescription antidepressants and birth control pills. Can cause interactions with anesthesia. **Do not take with** Digoxin, cyclosporine, Indinavir, and other antidepressants. Should not be taken during cancer chemotherapy due to possible interaction with drugs used for treatment and symptom management.
GINSENG	Has been used to reduce fatigue and improve concentration. Has estrogenic properties.	Overstimulation, insomnia, and gastrointestinal upset may occur. Long-term use may cause Ginseng Abuse Syndrome, which is characterized by hypertension, nervousness, insomnia, and diarrhea. **Do not take** if you have high blood pressure or estrogen-influenced tumors.
GARLIC	Lowers cholesterol and triglycerides.	Heartburn and flatulence. Interferes with normal blood clotting. Check with health care professional if taking an anticoagulant (blood thinner). Some forms can cause symptoms of hypoglycemia and skin reactions.

{continued}

HERB	INDICATIONS	SIDE EFFECTS AND CONTRAINDICATIONS
ECHINACEA	Several kinds are believed to provide immune enhancement and to improve resistance to flu-like illnesses and colds.	**Do not take:** • if you have been diagnosed with an autoimmune illness, such as rheumatoid arthritis or lupus, or are taking medications that affect the immune system as part of your treatment; • if you are allergic to the daisy (compositae) family, due to cross hypersensitivity; • daily for indefinite periods of time because it can fatigue the immune system.
SAW PALMETTO	Helpful in reducing urinary symptoms, including nocturia in benign prostatic hyperplasia (BPH).	Generally well tolerated. Some reports of mild gastrointestinal upset. **Do not take** if you take any hormone therapy.
KAVA KAVA	Has been used for nervousness, anxiety, stress, and insomnia.	**Should not be used for depression.** Allergic reactions, gastrointestinal discomfort, decreased reflexes and motor judgment, changes in eye movement, liver toxicity, and rash. Drug interactions occur with alcohol (increased risk of toxicity), Xanax (risk of coma), and other prescription drugs.
VALERIAN	Used for restlessness, sleep disorders, mental strain, lack of concentration, and stress. Has a sedative effect.	Gastrointestinal distress, headache, and sleeplessness may occur. May cause heart dysfunction with long-term use. May interfere with ability to drive. **Do not take with** many prescription drugs.

{continued}

Most Commonly Used Herbs in the United States
(CONTINUED)

Herb	Indications	Side Effects and Contraindications
EVENING PRIMROSE OIL	Has been used for asthma, whooping cough, eczema, breast pain, premenstrual syndrome, multiple sclerosis, rheumatoid arthritis, high cholesterol. Also used for Raynaud's disease and Sjögren's Syndrome due to anti-inflammatory effect.	Gastrointestinal symptoms, nausea, vomiting, gas, diarrhea, bloating, and headaches. May lower the seizure threshold for patients on antiseizure medications.

Sources: Varro Tyler, 1999; Michael Blumenthal, 1998; PDR for Herbal Medicine, 1998

massage. Only certain types of massage are appropriate in certain situations. For example, massage directly over a tumor or surgical site is not appropriate. It is important to seek a massage therapist who is knowledgeable about cancer and its therapies. The key effects of massage include: 1) improved digestion, 2) increased range of motion, 3) improved lymphatic movement and circulation, 4) decreased muscle tension, and 5) decreased edema.

"Reiki" means *universal life energy.* It is an ancient healing art derived from the Japanese in which the healer is thought to manipulate energy. The energy, not the practitioner, effects healing. The practitioner will hold his or her hands in a series of positions on the patient but no pressure or massage is applied. The patient remains fully clothed at all times. The energy is believed to find its way wherever and however it is needed. The purpose of Reiki is to relieve the body of physical, emotional, and spiritual blockages. Healing also takes place on the emotional, mental, and spiritual levels, rather than only on the physical level. The environment is kept as quiet and soothing as possible. Reiki has been used for pain, nausea and other gastrointestinal disturbances, and in stress management.

Reflexology is the practice of applying specific pressure to specific points on the feet and/or hands. The pressure may vary from heavy to light depending on the practitioner. It is holistic because it looks at the needs of the whole body. Reflexology is more than a foot massage. The exact mechanism as to how reflexology works is not clear, but it is believed to restore balance to the body by restoring the flow of energy. Reflexology can be used for gastrointestinal problems, stress-related problems, chronic pain, and fatigue.

DIET, NUTRITION, AND LIFESTYLE CHANGES

Vegetarian diets include many health-promoting features because they are low in saturated fats and high in fiber, vitamins, and phytochemicals. Some vegetarian diets include no animal products, while others include dairy products, eggs, and fish.

PLANT-BASED DIET–This diet avoids all red meat but includes poultry and fish in a meal plan that contains most meals from plant sources. Additional protein can be obtained from milk and milk products, eggs, beans, lentils, nuts, and soy foods.

LACTO-OVO VEGETARIAN–This diet avoids meat, poultry, and fish, but will include dairy products and eggs.

FRUITARIANS–Representing one small group of vegetarians, fruitarians eat only raw fruits and vegetables because they believe that cooking fruit damages its nutritional properties.

PURE VEGETARIAN OR VEGAN–This diet avoids all meat and animal products.

Strict vegetarians may experience protein malnutrition, as well as Vitamin B_{12}, Vitamin D, calcium, zinc, and iron deficiencies. The amount of dietary fiber consumed can cause intestinal problems or discomfort unless introduced gradually. Some vegetarians may have difficulty maintaining a balanced diet, but with appropriate supplements they can achieve a state of balanced nutrition.

"Macrobiotic" means large life. Macrobiotic diets are based on the traditional Japanese diet consisting of approximately 50 percent whole-grain cereals, 20–30 percent vegetables, and small amounts of soup, beans, and sea vegetables. However, certain vegetables, such as all types of potatoes, tomatoes, eggplant, avocado, zucchini, asparagus, spinach, and peppers, are forbidden. White meat, fish, and fruits are limited. Coffee and tea are forbidden. All grains must be organically grown, and specific rules for preparation and cooking are also integral to this program.

Macrobiotics does not promote a single diet for everyone; it takes into account variations in age, geography, sex, levels of activity, and other factors to customize the diet. Because the macrobiotic regimens are so structured, it is very important that they be put into practice with the help of a specially trained professional. Cancer survivors are at risk for malnutrition, nutritional deficiencies, and electrolyte imbalances; therefore special attention to caloric and protein intake are especially important for survivors following this dietary regimen. Survivors following macrobiotic diets also may require specific nutritional supplements.

The *Gonzalez-Kelley (or Kelley-Gonzalez)* regimen is being studied at one of the NIH-designated research centers. It is based on the work of Donald Kelley, who believed that alterations in the body's proteins can result in cancer. Nicolas Gonzalez has evaluated Kelley's work and found that by applying Kelley's theory, many of his patients with pancreatic cancer had improved survival rates.

This regimen is composed of 10 basic diets. As with other nutritional programs, this regimen should be medically supervised to avoid complications such as protein malnutrition and other nutritional deficiencies.

Nutritional supplements have become popular because of the appeal of "natural" in treating or preventing disease. Megavitamin therapies appeal to many patients, although they have not yet proved to be effective. Much has been written about diet and its effect on health and disease. Recently, more Americans are taking nutritional supplements. Many medical experts are reluctant to recommend nutritional supplements, and the recommended dosages will vary from practitioner to practitioner. The Food and Nutrition Board of the National Research Council has been establishing Recommended Daily Allowances (RDAs) since the 1940s.

HOW TO KNOW IF CAM THERAPIES ARE RIGHT FOR YOU

Choosing to use a CAM therapy is a very personal decision. It must feel right to you. Research does not prove which therapies are right. Many well-meaning friends and acquaintances will offer advice about a therapy based on personal experience or the experience of a friend or relative. Each is physically and emotionally unique; you cannot assume that if a particular therapy was the right one for your neighbor, it will be the right one for you, too. For example, one person can take a certain antibiotic and another person cannot. Not all CAM therapies will complement your cancer therapies.

Read about any therapy before seeking a practitioner. Resources at the end of this chapter will help you gather information. It is very important that you not try a therapy just because someone recommends it. Many people will offer advice to you, but they may not know about you, your values and belief systems, or your diagnosis and treatment. They may mean well, but you must become personally informed. Before you choose any CAM, carefully weigh the benefits and drawbacks of the therapy. Tell your doctor about any therapy you consider.

CHOOSING A CAM PRACTITIONER

Carefully investigate the reputation of any practitioner you consider. When choosing a CAM practitioner, first check with your state's Education Department and/or Department of Health to learn if the state requires a license to perform the particular therapy. Also, the components of that practice must be defined. For example, in some states nutritional counseling can be provided by a chiropractor, and in others it is not considered to be within the scope of practice without additional training. When any CAM practitioner promises cure or speaks of a

MEASURING NUTRITIONAL SUPPLEMENTS

Recommended Daily Allowances (RDAs) were designed to provide a basis for evaluating the diet of groups, not individuals. The RDAs do not allow for those factors that may alter vitamins and minerals in foods, and the optimal level for many nutrients is controversial.

Reference Daily Intakes (RDI) are based on the RDA and represent intakes to achieve. Most labels use the RDI developed for adults and children four years and older.

Upper Tolerable Limits (UTL) are upper safe daily limits. They are listed for adults only. The UTL can be thought of as the highest daily intake over a prolonged time known to pose no risks to most members of the healthy population.

Vitamin C (ascorbic acid) is the most popular vitamin supplement in the United States and in many ways the most controversial. The best food sources include citrus fruits, broccoli, peppers, potatoes, and brussels sprouts. Taking antacids and smoking deplete vitamin C in the body. Much has been written regarding the benefits of vitamin C in fighting heart disease, high blood pressure, colds, and other diseases including cancer. The primary functions of vitamin C include the manufacture of collagen as an important element in immune function, absorption and utilization of other nutrients, and as an antioxidant. Vitamin C increases the absorption of iron, decreases the absorption of copper, and interferes with the blood test for B_{12} and the fecal occult blood test (the test to determine the presence of blood in the stool). Vitamin C also regenerates stored vitamin E (see vitamin E). The current dosage recommendation is 500 mg. of vitamin C daily. The side effect most commonly seen with higher doses is gastrointestinal distress and/or diarrhea.

Vitamin A was the first recognized fat-soluble vitamin. It was once known as the "anti-infective" vitamin and has recently been recognized as being important in immune function. Some carotenes can be converted into vitamin A (provitamin A carotenes). Conversion depends upon several things, including the presence of protein, zinc, and vitamin C. Food sources for vitamin A include liver, kidney, butter, whole milk, and fortified skim milk, while the best food sources for provitamin A carotenes include dark green leafy vegetables and yellow orange vegetables. Carotenes are also found in salmon and other fish, egg yolks, poultry, and milk. Carotenes are potent antioxidants. Vitamin E and zinc are needed for vitamin A function. *Beta carotene supplementation has been associated with an increased risk for lung cancer in those who smoke. Vitamin A supplementation has also been associated*

{continued}

MEASURING NUTRITIONAL SUPPLEMENTS (CONTINUED)

with an increased risk of birth defects. Vitamin A is best consumed as provitamin A carotenes in food, not as vitamin A supplementation. The current dosage recommendations vary and should be discussed with your health care professional. Toxicity is possible with higher doses. Symptoms of toxicity include: carotenodermia (yellow discoloration of skin), irritability, headache, fatigue, vomiting, and elevated liver enzymes.

Vitamin E is needed for a number of body processes. Best food sources include polyunsaturated vegetable oils, seeds, nuts, asparagus, green leafy vegetables, whole grains, and berries. The primary action of vitamin E is as an antioxidant; it protects the cell membrane from toxic compounds. It is also important in immune function. Vitamin E interacts with other antioxidants and improves the use of vitamin A. Vitamin E may increase the effects of anticoagulants (blood thinners) including aspirin and interfere with vitamin K's blood clotting effects. Do not take more than 400 IU/day if taking supplemental vitamin C (vitamin C regenerates stored vitamin E) unless medically supervised. Higher doses of vitamin E should be taken only with medical supervision. Vitamin E should be stopped one month prior to surgical procedures.

Folic acid has played a major role in the treatment of certain anemias and is necessary for cellular division. Folic acid deficiencies have been associated with birth defects, depression, atherosclerosis, and cervical dysplasia. Food sources include green leafy vegetables, whole grains, and legumes. Folic acid supplementation has the potential to mask an underlying B_{12} deficiency. Side effects at doses higher than 400 micrograms (mcg) per day may include nausea, flatulence, and anorexia. Higher doses have the potential to increase seizure activity in persons with seizure disorders. Estrogens, alcohol, methotrexate, barbiturates, and anticonvulsants interfere with the absorption of folic acid, and patients taking these medications are at risk for folic acid deficiency. The current dosage recommendation is 400 mcg of folic acid per day.

Selenium is a trace mineral that works with vitamin E to protect cell membranes. The primary action of selenium is that of an antioxidant. A daily dose of 200 mcg per day has been identified as appropriate to reduce the risk of colon and other cancers. Doses of greater than 1,000 mcg per day can be toxic. A symptom of toxicity is garlic odor especially noticeable on the breath. Heavy metals and high doses of vitamin C and zinc can decrease selenium absorption.

Coenzyme Q 10 (CoQ10) is also known by the name *ubiquinone* and occurs in every plant and animal cell. It is a fundamental component of a

{continued}

cell. CoQ10 is involved in the production of energy for all body processes. The heart is the most metabolically active organ of the body and therefore most vulnerable to CoQ10 deficiencies. CoQ10 levels naturally decline with age. The beneficial aspects of CoQ10 include energy production and antioxidant activity. Some evidence suggests that CoQ10 may be helpful when a patient is being treated with cancer chemotherapy that affects the heart. The recommended dosage is 100 mg/day.

Soy isoflavones and *soy protein* are plant sources of estrogen. These substances have estrogen-like effects and antioxidant effects. Genistein is the most researched of the isoflavones. Some may be helpful for reducing menopausal symptoms. Individuals who are hypersensitive to any component of soy should not take any soy product. Women with estrogen-influenced tumors should not use these as supplements unless they are closely monitored by a physician and should not eat foods containing soy.

"secret" curative formula, question this therapy. *There are no secrets.* Practitioners who are committed to improving health do not keep information secret.

Having a certificate does not make a practitioner certified. A certificate of attendance from a program or a series of programs is not the same as being certified. It takes time to learn and master these therapies and, in most cases, can take a minimum of a year and not weeks or months (in many cases it takes years). In addition to appropriate preparation in a particular CAM therapy, the practitioner also must have an understanding of cancer and its therapies. For example, an herbalist may be very knowledgeable about herbs, but have no understanding of cancer therapies and how the herbs might interfere with the therapy.

CAM Practitioners and Oncologists Working Together

You cannot ensure that your CAM practitioner and oncologist will work together. Survivors and health care providers are learning more about these therapies every day, but still have much to learn. In many cases, cancer survivors, oncologists, oncology nurses, and other members of the health care team are learning at the same time. Ask your CAM practitioners for written information about their particular therapy and a copy of any treatment plan they made for you. Give both to your oncologist to put in your medical record. Should any members of your health care team need additional information, they can, with your permission, contact the CAM practitioner. This creates an opportunity for communication, which can lead to collaboration.

Do not keep your CAM therapy a secret from your oncologist. A particular therapy may not be known to be safe during cancer treatment, but may pose no risk after the cancer treatment has been completed. Similarly, a particular therapy may be considered safe during treatment for one cancer diagnosis, but not known to be safe or unsafe for another diagnosis. *Safety trumps efficacy* is the advice offered by Dr. David Eisenberg of Harvard. That is, a particular therapy may be effective for a particular symptom, but it may not be safe for this particular person, at this particular time, under these particular circumstances.

STATES REQUIRING A LICENSE TO PRACTICE

This chart lists licensing requirements as of May 2002. Because licensing requirements change, you should check with your state licensing board to determine current licensing status for these disciplines and others.

STATE	CHIROPRACTOR	HOMEOPATHY	ACUPUNCTURE	MASSAGE	HYPNOSIS	NATUROPATHY
Alabama	X			X		X
Alaska	X		X			
Arizona	X	X	X			X
Arkansas	X		X	X		
California	X		X			
Colorado	X		X			
Connecticut	X	X	X	X		X
Delaware	X			X		
District of Columbia	X		X	X		
Florida	X		X	X		
Georgia	X					
Hawaii	X		X	X		X
Idaho	X		X			
Illinois	X		X			
Indiana	X		X		X	
Iowa	X		X	X		
Kansas	X					
Kentucky	X					
Louisiana	X		X	X		
Maine	X		X	X		X
Maryland	X		X	X		
Massachusetts	X		X			
Michigan	X					
Minnesota	X		X			
Mississippi	X			X		
Missouri	X		X	X		
Montana	X		X			X
Nebraska	X			X		
Nevada	X	X	X			
New Hampshire	X		X	X		X
New Jersey	X		X	X		

{continued}

STATE	CHIROPRACTOR	HOMEOPATHY	ACUPUNCTURE	MASSAGE	HYPNOSIS	NATUROPATHY
New Mexico	X		X	X	X	
New York	X		X	X	X	
North Carolina	X		X	X		
North Dakota	X			X	X	
Ohio	X			X	X	
Oklahoma	X					
Oregon	X		X	X	X	X
Pennsylvania	X		X			
Rhode Island	X		X	X	X	
South Carolina	X		X	X		
Tennessee	X			X		
Texas	X		X	X		
Utah	X		X	X		X
Vermont	X		X			X
Virginia	X		X	X		
Washington	X		X	X	X	X
West Virginia	X		X	X		
Wisconsin	X		X	X		
Wyoming	X					

Part Two

Taking Care of Your Emotional, Spiritual, and Social Needs

Chapter Six:

Mind and Body

Harnessing Your
Inner Resources

by Neil Fiore, Ph.D.

[S]eeing illness as an occasion to make positive changes in your life beyond the disease itself is a creative adaptation to a major life threat. . . . Your illness is an occasion to reevaluate life—a wake-up call, not a death knell. When your life is threatened, take hold and make the most of it; don't give up on it.

—David Spiegel, M.D., *Living Beyond Limits:*
New Hope and Help for Facing Life-Threatening Illness

A PERSONAL BATTLE AGAINST CANCER is, in many ways, like any other fight for survival. It requires a toughness of mind, an intense focus on the task, and a refusal to be deterred by the enemy, self-doubts, or seemingly rational fears. But more than toughness, it requires resilience, patience, humility, and flexibility. Surviving cancer and surviving with cancer is not a street fight that is over in a few seconds. Surviving is more like a spiritual journey that teaches how to change your life and your relationships.

Survivors often focus completely on their cancer and forget that they are more than a host to a serious illness. Even with advanced cancer, the healthy portion of the body continues to fight. Your inner mental and emotional resources, your immune system, and your very life force are poised to cooperate with your medical treatment to combat cancer.

In the course of coping with cancer, survivors can learn to respect their own emotions and to distinguish them from irrational and unhelpful worries. Survivors can learn different ways to express emotions—sometimes verbally, sometimes in writing, and sometimes with those fellow survivors who will understand.

Many survivors find it helpful to remind themselves: "I am more than my cancer. A healthy part of me is fighting for my life, wants to live my life—not someone else's image of who I should be and how I should feel. I intend to be fully alive in my life, moment to moment, until the last moment."

In charting the journey of survivorship, survivors can learn to protect their precious, limited energy to make it available for healing. As one colon cancer survivor said: "If I want to go to a party the day after my chemotherapy treatment, I make sure not to squander my energy on getting myself upset the way I used to. It is as if the elastic band of my emotions has been stretched. I can handle a lot more without snapping."

3

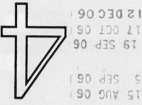

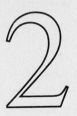

Keep this card in the book pocket
Book is due on the latest date stamped

Keep this card in the book pocket
Book is due on the latest date stamped

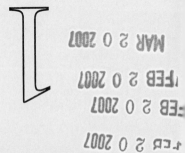

FEB 2 0 2007

FEB 2 0 2007

FEB 2 0 2007

MAR 2 0 2007

THE PERSONAL IMPACT OF CANCER

DISCOVERING STRATEGIES FOR HEALING

Learning to manage energy, time, and relationships is part of the empowerment that can come from surviving a crisis. Studies of survivors show that several activities appear to contribute to a healing of the spirit and often to a healing of the body:

- participating actively in your health care decisions and therapy—asking the doctor questions, learning about what you can do to lessen side effects and what additional help is available
- learning whether diet and exercise could enhance the effects of medical treatment
- expressing honest emotions—especially the more difficult emotions of anger and sadness, rather than stoic denial or false cheerfulness
- accepting the reality about your medical condition without minimizing it or assuming the worst
- mourning losses and moving on to adapting to the present condition, rather than struggling to hold onto the past
- practicing relaxation techniques, such as meditation, prayer, or yoga, to reduce stress and pain
- maintaining a sense of wonder about how your body will cooperate with medical treatment and how your emotional strength will see you through difficult times, rather than trying to predict the future. For example: "I wonder how I'll get through this one? This is going to be interesting. I wonder what unknown resources my body and mind will muster to cope with this?"

If, like most survivors, you do not know what caused your cancer, you may wonder whether your health habits and mental activity (thoughts, beliefs, and images) are related to your diagnosis and prognosis. However, Dr. Sandra Levy, former chief of behavioral medicine at the National Cancer Institute, states that "the most important determinant of cancer outcome is the biology of the tumor and the medical treatment."

Your thoughts, beliefs, and images do not *cause* cancer. You can do things, however—mostly behavioral (such as stopping smoking, eating more fruit and vegetables, and reducing fat in your diet) and some psychological—that *can improve your chances of surviving cancer.*

Research conducted at the University of California, San Francisco, found improved survival rates among patients who expressed their emotions, were realistic about their disease, and actively participated in their health care. These patients had significantly more healthy white cells at the site of their tumors, slower growing tumors, and a better prognosis than those patients who did not exhibit emotional expression, realism, and active participation.

While researchers in medicine and psychology continue to debate the physical and emotional factors that contribute to illness and health, most professionals agree:

- You can't wish away cancer, nor can you get cancer by having negative thoughts or painful emotions;
- Many factors and events beyond your control determine if and when you will get cancer;
- Supportive therapies—such as support groups, counseling, and meditation or prayer—can contribute to your peace of mind, emotional well-being, immune system strength, and improved survival time; and
- Unproven treatments often put patients through unnecessary expense and discomfort, and can be dangerous if they keep you from receiving prompt medical care.

In 1989, a study led by Dr. David Spiegel of Stanford University demonstrated that women with advanced breast cancer who participated in a support group survived eighteen months longer than those who did not. This research offers solid evidence that psychosocial treatments not only can make you feel better, they also can affect the length of survival with cancer. In his book, *Living Beyond Limits: New Hope and Help for Facing Life-Threatening Illness,* Dr. Spiegel summarizes much of the psychosocial research: "All of the studies . . . point in the same direction: You do better when you learn to take charge of the course of your illness realistically. You cannot control everything, you cannot undo what has been done (like getting the disease), but you will benefit by taking hold of your current situation in whatever way is possible. . . . When your life is threatened, take hold and make the most of it; don't give up on it." These findings encourage survivors to focus on what they can do after a cancer diagnosis to cope realistically with the situation and actively participate in their health care.

DIAGNOSING THE DIAGNOSIS—AND DISCOVERING YOUR BELIEFS

Many diseases are more severe, traumatic, and fatal than cancer. Yet the stigma attached to this disease makes the diagnosis of cancer disproportionately terrifying. The meaning of the word "cancer" is very different for the doctor who deals with it every day, for the person who has survived "terminal cancer" for eleven years, and for the patient hearing the diagnosis for the first time.

When the diagnosis is first presented, the emotional shock can be so great that survivors tend to look for an understandable cause to make some sense of what is unimaginable. Some people might even prefer self-blame and guilt to the greater discomfort of loss of control, unknown causes, and the feeling of being a random victim.

Everyone has remnants of a child's pattern of taking on inappropriate levels of responsibility for things beyond their control. For young children, the thought that their parents might be imperfect, unstable, or mortal is unthinkable. Because they must depend on adults for shelter, protection, and food, children frequently blame themselves for problems that occur in their families rather than imagining that parents and God may not be powerful enough to always keep them from harm.

In a time of crisis, adults may revert to this childlike illusion of control to explain how bad things can happen to good people. This protective device temporarily keeps adults from facing a chaotic world in which cancer and accidents randomly can touch anyone's life, regardless of how well we live, how we handle our emotions, or how positive or negative our outlook. Similar to children, adults feel safer blaming themselves rather than accepting vulnerability to a world that is not under their control.

Unfortunately, denying human limits leaves survivors feeling guilty about lack of control over uncontrollable events. Certain phrases in your internal dialogue may reflect a "refusal to mourn" the loss of the illusion of control. It is not unusual for survivors to say to themselves: "You should have known better. If only you had done things differently this wouldn't have happened. I don't believe it. I can't stand it." Statements such as these are symptoms of being stuck in a fantasy about how life should be and of finding it difficult to accept life on its terms.

Although you understandably may wonder what caused your cancer, self-blame as a means to explain uncontrollable events hurts your ability to cope with your illness. It can result in feelings of depression that contribute to a delay in seeking medical treatment, a reluctance to discuss worries and fear, and a diminished ability to form helpful relationships with doctors, social workers, and family members. Realistic information about cancer and its causes, however, can help you adjust to the unpleasant realities of a tough situation and can help you find support in doing something about it.

The strength and compassion of religious and spiritual beliefs are tested by the psychological and emotional stresses of cancer. Some survivors may find it helpful to reexamine the sources of their beliefs if they contribute to feelings of guilt rather than serve to comfort. In *When Bad Things Happen to Good People*, Rabbi Harold Kushner writes of his message to a young man in his community who was dying of a degenerative disease:

> I don't know why my friend and neighbor is sick and dying and in constant pain. From my religious perspective, I cannot tell him that God has His reasons for sending him this terrible fate, or that God must specially love him or admire his bravery to test him in this way. I can only tell him that the God I believe in did not send the disease and does not have a miraculous cure that He is withholding.

In his attempt to understand how bad things can happen to good people, Rabbi

Kushner concludes that the laws of nature impact on all alike and that not even God interferes with these laws.

You should carefully examine with clergy or counselors any beliefs that lead you to think of cancer as punishment from God. Personal and spiritual beliefs that accept human suffering as a natural part of life may help you adjust to and cope with your illness. Others, however, find similar comfort and guidance from spiritual or philosophical beliefs that are not religious.

The following exercise can help you identify troublesome beliefs that persist from your initial diagnosis, unnecessarily taxing your energy and clouding your thoughts. Developed at the University of California Medical Center, San Francisco, the following exercise may help you understand your initial reactions to cancer. To prepare for this exercise, read through it, and set aside 15 to 30 minutes to experience the exercise and talk about it with your family. You may want to tape record the instructions and play them back so you can be completely relaxed. Consider doing these exercises with someone with whom you can share your emotional reactions.

AN EXERCISE TO HELP IDENTIFY UNDERLYING BELIEFS

Begin by settling into a comfortable position, perhaps sitting in a chair with your feet flat on the floor. Take three slow, deep breaths, holding your breath briefly, and then exhaling slowly and completely.

With each exhalation, float down into the chair. Let the chair support you. Let go of holding with your muscles. Allow the relaxation to flow down over your body. Allow the chair to support your body and the floor to support your feet and legs. By breathing in this special way, you are letting your body know that it has no place to go for the next few minutes; that the strong part of you is choosing to face, resolve, and remove any blocks to living fully.

Now, simply drift back to that time and place when you first were told of the diagnosis. Imagine being in that place: Re-create for yourself that room, the furniture, the colors and lighting, and the sounds and the voices. Just be there and allow your mind to present what it will. Just let it happen.

Once you are there, in that place, at that time, focus your attention on three areas within yourself. Notice:
• What you are feeling physically—your muscles, your breathing, your heartbeat, and anything that makes itself physically evident.
• What thoughts and images are going through your mind. What you are saying to yourself—what your attitude is and how you are coaching yourself.
• What you are feeling emotionally. Just notice whatever emotions appear. Notice, too, that you can shift your focus from your emotions to your physical and cognitive reactions—showing that you can take control over your attention and feelings.

AN EXERCISE TO HELP IDENTIFY UNDERLYING BELIEFS
(CONTINUED)

All your reactions are legitimate and, whatever your reactions are, *simply note* them without judging them. You coped as well as you could under the circumstances given the information you had at the time.

Your job now is to reexamine those beliefs and attitudes to see which ones best serve you today. Identify and replace any beliefs that cause you only stress. Acknowledge that these old beliefs once helped you to adapt to your former situation. Now, equipped with "new ways of thinking," you are choosing to adjust to your illness, and focusing on those beliefs that make a positive contribution to your life.

REPLACING NEGATIVE REACTIONS

Examining your initial reactions to a cancer diagnosis and the beliefs that underlie them is the first crucial step toward developing other, more helpful attitudes toward cancer and discovering better ways of coping. Here are some common negative reactions to cancer and some suggestions for useful responses to them.

Negative reaction: Why me? Why now? Life is unfair. I feel pitiful.

Response: Now that it has happened and it is me, what can I do about it? As awful as this situation is, what can I do to improve my chances of beating cancer?

Negative reaction: Cancer is powerful and my body is weak. Cancer means death.

Response: Cancer cells are, in fact, abnormal cells that are weak. These confused cells cannot reproduce when exposed to chemotherapy or radiation. My immune system routinely identifies and destroys malformed cells and removes them from my body. My body can cooperate with medical treatment in destroying cancer.

Negative reaction: If I had lived life differently I wouldn't have cancer. If only I knew then what I know now. I wish I could do it over again.

Response: The past is over and I cannot control it or change it. It did happen. It does hurt. But brooding about what is beyond my current control only weakens my ability to deal with what I can do now. I do have control over how I make myself feel in this present moment and over my attitude in the future. I will focus on what I can do now.

COPING WITH STRONG EMOTIONS

If you have ever felt the ground shake beneath your feet from an earthquake or lived through a war or a near-fatal accident, you know how quickly feelings of tranquility can change to overwhelming anxiety. The emotional response of cancer survivors to their diagnosis is just as legitimate as the shock, anger, and depression expected in those who survive accidents and wars, and recovery involves similar steps of emotional and physical rehabilitation.

Worry about recurrence and wonder about changes in the rules of life make the task of "getting back to normal" a complex one for any cancer survivor. One survivor said, "Sometimes it feels like I'm living under a centipede, waiting for the other 99 shoes to drop." It takes the experience of many calm days that remain peaceful before we begin to relax our bracing for another catastrophe.

Over time, it is not so much the strong emotions themselves that cause difficulties as it is the fear of expressing them. With understanding and patience, physicians, family members, and survivors themselves can find helpful ways to express their feelings.

Anxiety. Feelings of anxiety are to be expected during any part of the cancer experience, but the time of diagnosis is often the most upsetting. During this time, thoughts about life and death predominate and survivors are most vulnerable to psychosocial problems. This is a period of monumental adjustment to

- the shocking news that your life is in danger
- the consideration of treatments that may be more severe than any of your cancer symptoms
- the loss of your physical integrity
- rapid changes in your work and relationships
- the possibility of a long period of rehabilitation

During this initial period, especially, the expression of anxiety, sadness, and anger are quite natural and potentially healing. Some studies suggest that survivors who were more expressive of their anger and sadness fared better than those who were less so, which does not mean that survivors should force themselves to be emotional, but that it may be better if they do not repress their natural feelings. After all, attempting to remain stoic during times of great trauma takes energy—energy that might better be used by the body to heal.

Other studies indicate that survivors who maintain a support network of friends and family are more likely to weather this difficult time without major psychological problems. The first months of cancer therapy are intense, but some comfort can be gathered from knowing that the second 100 days probably will be less stressful, as you adjust to your medical treatment and the process of healing.

Once the initial shock of the diagnosis is past, the next task will be to become familiar with the treatment steps and options—what you and your doctors can do. At that time, the disbelief and anxiety about having cancer generally will give way to the tasks of living and adapting to life with and after cancer. You may find that your actual cancer experience may differ considerably from your initial fears and beliefs.

Depression. Depression, a common reaction among cancer survivors and their supporters, is often regarded as a negative emotion, when in fact it may be a natural way to cope with shock by conserving energy and providing a time to think about ways of adjusting to change. Cancer survivors, says Dr. Jimmie Holland, chief of New York's Memorial Sloan-Kettering's Psychiatry Service, are no more depressed than people with other severe medical conditions. The type of depression experienced by cancer survivors, reactive depression, differs from that of patients suffering from chronic mental depression. The Psychiatry Service of Memorial Sloan-Kettering reports that half of the cancer patients they see have suffered from acute stress and "reactive" (as opposed to "chronic") depression.

The relatively short-term, reactive depression that often accompanies the stress of a cancer diagnosis and treatment can be handled more easily if it is accepted as natural and if a "mourning" process is allowed. Recovery from the depression of cancer is helped by acknowledging the loss—loss of control, loss of a physical function, and loss of self-image.

Another contributor to depression is the passivity that is required of patients as they follow orders and fall into the "sick role." Hospital regimes encourage dependence, adding to the sense of helplessness and reinforcing the negative image of "cancer victim."

When hospitals demand extreme compliance by patients and offer little opportunity for patient participation in their own health care, they can contribute to patient depression and rebellion. Studies have shown that some patients stop taking their chemotherapy, not simply because of side effects, but because they never had a chance to consider all their treatment options. A National Cancer Institute study demonstrated that the majority of those patients who turned to unconventional therapies had been told by their physicians that they had a "terminal disease" and that nothing else could be done (see Chapter 5 for a discussion of complementary and alternative medicine). These patients—who felt abandoned and unable to participate in conventional medicine—turned to treatments that required them to take an active role in getting involved and changing their lifestyles.

To lessen depression and hopelessness, you can accept some level of depression as normal, let go of trying to control everything, mourn your losses, and avoid assuming a passive role in your treatment. You can also talk to your doctor and health care team about ways to treat your depression and its possible causes. Counselors and support groups also can help you with the emotional components of surviving cancer. See Chapter 2 on how to communicate with your doctor and hospital staff. See Chapter 8 for information about support groups.

Once you have acknowledged that you are in a distressing situation and must face many hard choices, you can direct your thoughts toward the future by asking yourself, "Where do I go from here?" You do not have to be thrilled with where you are today, but to improve your situation, you do need to recognize the realistic paths that are available to you. By coping realistically with the emotional impact of cancer, you have prepared yourself to move beyond the initial reactions of "if only?" "what if?" and "why me?" to a more productive question: "What small steps can I take today to improve the quality and quantity of my life? What small pleasures can I find in this moment and this day?"

By understanding how cancer affects your emotions and relationships, you prepare yourself to master the skills of coping with trauma, transition, and survival. Concerns about life-and-death issues, while never totally dismissed from the thoughts of any cancer survivor, can give way to the challenges and joys of daily life.

THE SOCIAL IMPACT OF CANCER

Even though the shock of a cancer diagnosis primarily is physical, a major portion of the impact is emotional and social. It affects how you perceive yourself and how others react to you.

CHANGES IN SELF-PERCEPTION

If a cancer diagnosis is your first experience of being vulnerable to serious illness, its influence on your self-image can be especially traumatic. You may feel betrayed by your body, as if your cells have turned against you. In a very concrete way you realize that you are human and mortal, that life does end, and that your time is limited.

A dramatic change in self-image is most evident in teenagers with cancer. It makes them different from their carefree peers, who seldom believe that the threat of death or even serious illness applies to them. They have not had to face the body's gradual decline that many adults begin to experience in their forties. Usually they have not seen illness and death strike their peers, so they are unprepared for a life-threatening illness. It shocks them and makes them doubt their underlying assumptions about how the world is supposed to work. But this rapid change in perception can take place in people in their sixties who are accustomed to good health and energy. Some people maintain a teenager's sense of invulnerability and immortality well beyond the age of 60. For these older people whose self-image has remained stable for decades, a diagnosis of cancer can be dramatically inconsistent with their view of life.

The experience of facing a life-threatening event unites survivors around a new view of the world and the courage it takes to live every day. It also separates survivors from those who cannot appreciate the cancer experience. Cancer changes not only the self-perception of survivors, but how others perceive survivors.

Physicians will treat your physical losses, but you, your family and friends, and your psychosocial counselors must deal with the emotional and psychological changes. You can improve your self-image by accepting mortality and vulnerability to disease as facts for all human beings rather than as signs of personal weakness or failure. A more hardy and realistic self-image will enhance your ability to fight for your life. It will equip you with a better understanding of the social impact of cancer and will prepare you to cope in ways that contribute to your mental and physical well-being.

AFFIRMATIONS FOR A POSITIVE SELF-IMAGE

Cancer survivors often find personal affirmations helpful in making the transition to a new, robust self-image and greater strength to cope with changing relationships. These affirmations are a way of being there for yourself despite the events in your life. Affirmations can be like Ivan's credo in Dostoyevsky's The Brothers Karamazov: ". . . [i]f I lost faith in the order of things, if I were convinced that everything is a disorderly, damnable, devil-ridden chaos, if I were struck by every horror of man's disillusion—still I should want to live . . ." The part of us that still wants to live, even after so many losses, is the part that speaks the affirmations to the part of us that is understandably afraid and discouraged. The following are examples of affirmations you can write for yourself and say to yourself with compassion, to create a safe and comforting inner place.
- Regardless of what happens in life, you have worth with me.
- Regardless of who stays or who goes, I am on your side, always in your corner. I will never abandon you.
- Regardless of how intense your emotions become, I acknowledge their validity for you. All your emotions and thoughts are understandable and acceptable.
- Regardless of what happens out there, you always have a home in here. You are safe with me. I accept you, my body, and my life completely.

As a cancer survivor you may feel quite isolated at times, as if no one could possibly understand your shock and agony. In *Live with Pain, Learn the Hope*, William Keeling expressed his reactions to his cancer diagnosis as follows: "Self-doubts begin to play tricks with your head, like, 'Does anybody give a damn whether I live or die?' You begin to see and hear evidence that nobody does. No one else seems panicky, just you. The doctor seems cool, scientific. Your spouse and parents are cool, sad-looking. Your boss is cool and has a few sad, sympathetic words that sound like 'have a nice trip' (to wherever)." This young man felt that everyone was indifferent toward him, but some survivors feel they must be strong and repress their own needs because no one else seems capable of coping. They may even think that their doctor or spouse is too emotional about the diagnosis to consider the feelings and needs of the patient. Sometimes survivors find themselves comforting distraught family members, while wondering: "Who's going to listen to my feelings? I'm the one with cancer!"

Others in the survivor's community may attempt to help by offering a new "miracle cure" they have read about, or by giving unsolicited religious advice. Some may avoid the cancer survivor, because cancer for them is an uncomfortable reminder of their own mortality. Even doctors and nurses, at times, may have difficulty visiting patients whom they cannot help without showing their emotions.

Although a social stigma still is attached to having cancer, cancer is discussed more openly now than ever before. Some people may shy away during times of crisis, but you also may be pleasantly surprised by offers of help from unexpected sources. Survivors can lessen their own hurt and disappointment by appreciating the good intentions of others and by letting them help in whatever way they can. During the course of your cancer treatment you may need someone to give you rides, buy groceries, clean the house, and listen to your concerns. Accepting this type of help from people can ease your own burdens and reduce the feelings of inadequacy others may have concerning their inability to help.

Some people, even those with good intentions, may make you feel worse or you may feel more comfortable solving problems by yourself. Feel free to choose to be with people who make you feel better rather than with those who do not. Prepare yourself for a variety of social reactions to cancer, and try to accept the humanity and good intentions behind most people's actions.

A job or some form of work, paid or volunteer, can be a stabilizing influence for cancer survivors. It gives you the opportunity to focus your attention on something other than cancer and to experience yourself as more than someone with a dreaded disease. When work expands the roles you play in life, it can have a healthy effect on your self-image.

With some cancer treatments the disruption of the work schedule and the impact on coworkers are minimal. Many cancer treatments, however, do require lengthy periods of recuperation and rehabilitation. Survivors sometimes encounter prejudice on returning to work, with reactions ranging from avoidance to curiosity. Being prepared for a variety of reactions arms you with understanding so that you can be less shocked and hurt. The fear of cancer among colleagues and coworkers can result in additional feelings of isolation for the cancer survivor. When coworkers deny their vulnerability to the caprice of fate—and the same laws of nature that affect us all—they often attempt to support their erroneous view with attitudes such as: "He's different from us. He's no longer healthy; he's going to die. We who have lived life correctly don't have to worry about death."

Conventional misconceptions about the severity of the various types of cancer and their cure rates lead some people to wonder if and when you are going to die, or to be shocked that you look so well. Insensitive statements such as "You don't look like you're dying" and "Just my luck, I finally get some help in this department and he gets cancer" are not uncommon. Most people will not be that blunt or insensitive, but colleagues and employers may—even with good intentions—treat you as if you are preparing to die rather than fighting to stay alive.

Others may simply wonder about your ability to pull your share of the load, whether they will need to hire someone new, and if you will be a financial burden on the company. Such concerns can lead to overt and covert job discrimination and isolation from fellow workers who fear cancer. Prepare yourself to cope with the emotional, as well as the financial and legal consequences, of being a cancer survivor at work. See Chapter 13 for information about your employment rights and how to communicate with your employer and coworkers about your cancer.

CHANGES IN RELATIONSHIPS

Throughout the course of your treatment you probably will experience changes in your relationships. Some may become deeper, some more superficial, and some may end, while new ones may begin. When your treatment causes you to appear weak or sick, even some old friends may avoid you, resuming their friendship when you appear healthier. Whatever relationships remain will be intensified and strengthened during this challenging period of your life.

A healthy relationship should be a major source of support, not something that drains you emotionally. During the early stages of combating cancer, you will need to reduce the stress caused by your attitude, your diet, your job, and your relationships, making more energy available for coping with cancer and healing. This is a time when your first priority must be yourself and your health.

Loving friends and family will do what they can to be supportive of the way you want to fight cancer and of how you want to maintain the quality of your life. You may need to change those relationships that are not supportive of your commitment to survival. Changes in relationships need not be painful or negative. In fact, honest confrontation about your changing roles can heighten the quality of healthy relationships. A supportive family and understanding friends can lessen the devastation of cancer and clarify the importance of relationships in your life. See Chapter 7 for a discussion of the family's role in cancer survivorship.

One aspect of changes in relationships that people often avoid talking about is the place that sexual intimacy plays in the self-esteem and body image of a cancer survivor. While sex generally becomes a low priority during times of stress and preoccupation with survival, as physical energy and feelings of vitality return, so usually will the sense of attractiveness and interest in sex. See Chapter 4 for a more in-depth discussion of sexuality and cancer.

AUTOGENIC EXERCISE

"Autogenics" means "self-control of your body." This exercise is directed toward warming your hands and relaxing your entire body. It allows you to perform the amazing feat of dilating the blood vessels and capillaries in your hands and fingers. You cannot achieve this by commanding it to happen, the way you might command your hand to open or close. It is only possible when you speak in a language that your unconscious mind understands and allow the wisdom of your mind to bring you deep relaxation.

Start by sitting erect with your feet flat on the floor, with your hands on your thighs. Breathe deeply, hold your breath for a moment, and then exhale slowly and completely—floating down into the chair. Do this three times, counting each time you exhale. Let each exhalation be a signal that you are letting go of any remaining tension. Now allow your eyelids to close softly. You can try to keep them open, but may find that it is much more comfortable to allow them to float closed over your eyes. Now, allow that relaxation to flow down over your entire body.

Now you can focus your attention on the chair. Let yourself float down into the chair and let the chair support you. Let go of any unnecessary holding in those muscles. Shift your attention to the floor and let it support your feet. Continue to exhale away any remaining tension in those muscles. During these next few minutes, allow your conscious mind to be curious as your body and unconscious mind cooperate with the process of providing you deeper and deeper relaxation with each phrase.

As you repeat each phrase, just imagine, visualize, and feel the change happening. By imagining, visualizing, and feeling the direction given in each phrase, you are stating your will in a language your body can understand and cooperate with. You are letting the will give direction in a passive way, without using force and without trying to make anything happen.

Quietly let the change happen, using your body's natural tendency to cooperate. Now, you can be comfortable. Continue to breathe deeply and slowly and repeat quietly to yourself the following:

- "I feel quiet. I am beginning to feel quite relaxed—my feet feel quiet and relaxed. My ankles, my knees, and my hips feel light, calm, and comfortable. My stomach and the entire center of my body feel light, calm, and comfortable."
- "My entire body feels quiet, calm, and comfortable. My arms and my hands feel quiet and warm. My entire body feels quiet and warm. I feel calm and relaxed. My hands feel calm, relaxed, and warm. My hands are relaxed. My hands are warm. My hands are slowly becoming warmer and warmer as I continue to breathe deeply and slowly."

AUTOGENIC EXERCISE
(CONTINUED)

- "My entire body is quiet, calm, and comfortable. My mind is quiet. I draw myself from my surroundings and feel serene and still. My thoughts are turning inward. I feel at ease. Within myself I can visualize and experience myself as quiet, calm, and comfortable. In an easy, quiet, inward-turned way, I am quietly alert. My mind is calm and quiet. I feel an inward quietness."
- "I will continue with these thoughts for two minutes and then softly open my eyes feeling fine, relaxed, quietly alert, and better than before. It will be interesting to discover how deeply relaxed I can become in a time that normally would seem so short. But even a few minutes of clock time can be all the time in the world for the unconscious mind to dream, to problem-solve, and to achieve deep relaxation and recuperation." [Allow yourself two to five minutes of silence and sitting still.]

You can now open your eyes and feel alert, relaxed, comfortable, and better than before.

GAINING CONTROL OVER STRESS

The stress caused by cancer and cancer treatment is psychological and emotional as well as physical. Your usual strategies for coping with non-life-threatening events may prove inadequate for coping with the stress of cancer. (See Chapter 7 for a discussion of how families cope with stress.) The ability to manage stress, however, can be learned.

Stress management techniques can be used for (1) physical control over a body whose very cells seem to have gone awry, (2) cognitive control over the flood of distressing and counterproductive thoughts and images, and (3) assertiveness to maintain personal control and worth in an environment of strong social pressures.

Because we often experience illness as a loss of control over our bodies, learning how to calm anxiety and manage pain can restore a sense of connection with them that is revitalizing. The ability to relax deeply, to experience the release of tension, and to feel that your body can still provide pleasure is a powerful sign of hope when facing a life-threatening illness. Learning that you can achieve a state of relaxation at will brings a feeling of confidence that you are once again in touch with your body. In addition, relaxation itself is recuperative and can lead to less need for some types of medication.

Different methods for relaxing provide varying degrees of comfort: listening to music, warm baths, massage, exercise, yoga, meditation, autogenic training, self-hypnosis, and biofeedback. Your personal comfort with and preference for an activity that involves physical movement and contact or mental stillness will determine which method is best for you.

Thoughts, beliefs, and attitudes can lead to either calm or panicky feelings. Just as you can scare yourself by viewing horror films, you can soothe yourself by watching scenes of nature. You can, therefore, gain some control over your feelings by choosing the movies you permit to run in the theater of your mind. With some practice, you can learn to focus your attention on those thoughts, feelings, and behaviors that are the most beneficial, pushing aside—or considering later, when you have more information—those thoughts and beliefs that are disturbing.

You can learn mastery over your internal physical, mental, and emotional states. But to be effective in controlling external pressures, you will need to communicate your wishes in a forthright, assertive manner. Being assertive does not guarantee that you always will get what you want, but you will at least receive the satisfaction that comes from standing up for yourself. Moreover, communicating to your doctor and family your fears and preferences regarding your medical care may well lead to changes that reduce stress and worry.

COPING THROUGH IMAGERY

Most cancer survivors are exposed to negative images of their bodies as helpless victims of a virulent disease. Negative images arise from statements such as "the cancer has spread to your lymph nodes" or "chemotherapy is highly toxic and will cause your hair to fall out."

Healthy imagery combats these negative images and provides a way of reducing stress, enhancing well-being, and promoting cooperation with medical therapies that may save your life. Many survivors find comfort in actively replacing negative images with ones that promote realistic hope rather than distress. For example: "My body knows how to trap cancer cells in my lymph nodes or lungs. My immune system knows how to cooperate with medical treatment to destroy and remove the confused cancer cells, while my healthy hair and skin cells can recover and return to normal."

Healthy imagery encourages survivors to allow their bodies to work naturally without conscious direction. Instead of worrying about doing the "right kind" of imaging, you can delegate responsibility for maintaining the proper functioning of your immune system to the "wise, inner healer" (or "inner physician") of your body. You reduce stress and make more energy available to your body to continue its fight against cancer. For example, during stressful medical treatment, a survivor might say to himself or herself:

> I can relax my efforts and allow the superior wisdom of my body to do what it knows best. There's nothing much for the conscious me to do, except to allow the flow of relaxation, recuperation, and remission. I am letting go of tension as I exhale, and I'm turning that energy over to a part of me that knows more than

my conscious mind about washing away the cancer cells while protecting my healthy cells.

By delegating the task of fighting cancer to the "superior wisdom" of the body and its immune system, you can avoid concern about the correctness of the image, of sufficient "will to live" and "right thinking."

Three types of imagery are particularly useful for cancer survivors—autogenics, centering, and healthy imaging.

AUTOGENICS influences bodily functions, such as blood flow to warm your hands, by using a language with which your body and mind can cooperate. Through autogenics you learn to use "passive volition" to communicate in words and images that produce relaxation, recovery from fatigue, and improved circulation. In this first stage of gaining physical control through relaxation, you can achieve satisfactory levels of relaxation with increasingly improved results within a week or two of daily practice of 10 to 15 minutes. Resist the urge to test out your new skills against the most stressful events in your life until you have practiced and achieved a satisfactory level of relaxation.

CENTERING is a rapid, two-minute procedure that brings your mind back from fretting about the past and future into the present. This can help you clear your mind of past or future problems that cannot be addressed now. As you withdraw your thoughts from these problems, you can release their accompanying guilt and stress, and experience a stress-free moment in the present. You already are practicing centering your attention in the present whenever you experience moments of joyful abandonment or intense concentration. With the centering exercise, you can learn to bring about at will these relaxing and recuperative moments.

CENTERING EXERCISE

Begin by taking three slow breaths and just float down into your chair or bed. Let go of any unnecessary muscle tension. With your next three breaths, exhale away all thoughts and images from the past. Clear your mind and your body of all concerns about what "should have" or "shouldn't have" happened in the past. Just let them go.

With your next three breaths, let go of all images and thoughts about what you think may happen in the future—all the "what ifs." Clear your mind and body of all concerns about what you expect to happen.

And with your next three breaths, choose to be in the present where there is little for you to do now. Just allow the natural processes of your body to provide you with deep relaxation and recuperation. Let go of trying to be in any particular time or striving to be any particular way—just be here in this

> ### CENTERING EXERCISE　　*(CONTINUED)*
> moment, where it doesn't take much effort to breathe comfortably and to make more energy available for healing and recuperation.

Healthy imaging centers around the concept of the "inner healer." The inner healer is that wise part of you that knows more than all of modern science about cellular biology and the strength of your immune system. Use healthy imaging when you are ready to replace negative images about cancer and treatment with more relaxing, robust images. If you are new to imagery, you might first start with the autogenic exercise, the centering exercise, or your own form of meditation or prayer. Use any of these methods to become relaxed and to experience the way your body responds to your words and images.

As you practice these relaxation and imagery exercises, your ability to control stressful images will improve. You will find that you have more effective communications between your mind and body. With mind and body working together, your imagery exercises can become a mental shield, giving you time to push aside negative images, to let go of tension, and to make decisions about medical treatment.

> ### HEALTHY IMAGING EXERCISE
> Focus your attention on any part of your body about which you are concerned. Take a deep breath and exhale through that area, releasing any tension you may be holding there. As you let go, allow your muscles to relax, permitting your blood vessels to dilate, and your circulation to improve the flow of oxygen and potentially healing elements to that area. By exhaling and relaxing your conscious efforts and concerns, you are assisting your body in healing itself. Continue to breathe slowly and deeply and—changing these words to fit your own style—say to yourself:
>
> "Most of me is healthy and working for the removal of the weak, confused cancer cells. Even now, as I am sitting here, breathing easily, I am making millions and millions of healthy, new blood cells every minute . . . and I don't even know how I do it; but my mind and body do know how, and they do it for my protection and for my healing and recuperation, even while I sleep."
>
> "I imagine my body bathed in sunlight and clear water, washing and dissolving cancer cells out of my body while coating and protecting the healthy cells. I see and feel my chemotherapy as a powerful cleanser, and radiation as bullets of light removing cancer cells from my body, while doing little harm to my healthy cells. My body is strong and can rapidly heal and recover from surgery, chemotherapy, or radiation. My body welcomes the help of my medical treatment and works with it to free me of cancer."

TRANSFORMATION—NEW POTENTIAL FOR THE CANCER SURVIVOR

During the process of coping with the cancer diagnosis, treatment decisions, and adjustments to side effects, it is difficult to imagine any benefit coming from the experience of cancer. Yet those who have written and spoken of their survival experience often tell of the positive changes that have taken place in their outlook and character as a result of facing the challenges of cancer.

For many survivors, cancer calls forth a transformation in attitude, health habits, and self-image. They learn to replace ineffective and limited ways of coping with healthier methods of dealing with work and social challenges. In this sense, any crisis offers an opportunity for positive change. Facing a life-threatening experience stretches your abilities beyond previous limits and gives you a chance to achieve your greatest potential.

Most cancer survivors are forced to develop their latent skills, to refine their strengths, and to drop negative habits. Some survivors stop worrying about money and begin traveling around the world. Others leave destructive relationships and unsatisfying jobs. Some just take life a little less seriously.

The experience of cancer will not make you more powerful over nature, the economy, world events, or other people. But it can show you the power you have over your thoughts and attitudes, and that—regardless of the events in your life—you can affect how you feel.

Life-threatening experiences remind us that life is a precious, limited resource to be experienced fully each moment. For many survivors, discovering the ability to live fully in the present can bring about unexpected feelings of calm and power. For some, the possibility of death can bring freedom from worry about the future and about defending a former identity. Others may find that the power to change their lives comes more from a new appreciation of life once health and energy return after prolonged illness.

Some survivors have noted that they never had such an opportunity to change their roles with their families as when they had cancer. Even those who are shy find it easier to express their wishes, feeling, "Since I have nothing to lose, I have nothing to fear." The impact of cancer can shatter old roles and one's sense of identity and leave survivors without a set of rules on which to fall back. Many survivors must mourn the loss of the old securities and fashion new rules of life based on personal values and priorities. This focus turns survivors inward toward previously untapped reserves and resources. It gives survivors a second chance to discover and shape their "true self," apart from the family's and society's pressures.

In short, the cancer experience holds the possibility of making your life more meaningful. Learning to control your reaction to stress, worry, and social pressures can prepare you for the burdens imposed by cancer as well as energize you for a fuller life after cancer.

Chapter Seven

Family Challenges

Communication and Teamwork

by Elizabeth J. Clark, Ph.D., M.S.W., M.P.H.

After the usual biopsies and other tests, I was told that I had a potentially fatal disease. Now that gets your attention. The Big C. The word "cancer": it overwhelms the psyche—just the word. I couldn't believe it. I was unprepared for the enormous emotional jolt that I received from the diagnosis.

—Sandra Day O'Connor, Associate Justice,
U.S. Supreme Court

MOST CRISES ARE TIME LIMITED; the crisis period usually lasts from one to six weeks. By then, most people find a way to deal with the problem or become more used to it so that it no longer fits the definition of a crisis. One of the difficulties of living with cancer, however, is that the disease creates a series of crisis situations. The first crisis may result from the diagnosis and the initial treatment. A new crisis may be caused later by treatment failures, protocol changes, or recurrence of disease. The end of intensive treatment and the beginning of the waiting period to see if the treatment was successful may trigger yet another crisis.

Eventually, you become an expert about your own illness and treatment. You become familiar with your treatment and learn how to navigate the health care system. You develop the needed language and coping skills to manage the crisis periods. In short, you learn how to live with cancer. You may face recurrent crisis situations, both physical and psychosocial, but gradually the panic and lack of coping skills you first experienced after your diagnosis subside.

CANCER IS A FAMILY CRISIS

Because of your cancer, your family will have a similar crisis experience. A family is a social system. Change in one part of the system causes change in the other parts. Therefore, a cancer diagnosis for one family member significantly alters the pattern of the family system and affects all other family members. Many researchers have found that some of the most difficult problems faced by cancer survivors are the reactions of their family members, friends, and coworkers.

In times of individual crisis, families are often viewed as a refuge, a place of support when trouble occurs. Even the word "home" has special significance for most people in times of stress. Stress is an expected part of family life, but cancer is an extraordinary stressor. By virtue of its ability to threaten the continuity of family life, cancer results in a family crisis. The magnitude of the cancer crisis is such that the family system is thrown into distress, and family functioning and quality of family life can be compromised.

A diagnosis of cancer in one family member will impact each member of the family. The intensity of that impact will vary depending on individual factors such as closeness to the cancer survivor, developmental level, and personal strengths and coping abilities. Serious illness generally intensifies relationship patterns that already exist within the family, but excessive and prolonged stress can have a negative impact on even the strongest and closest family. Cancer can also offer the chance for personal growth and can strengthen a family.

During the initial cancer crisis, families face many tasks and challenges. Family members need adequate information to make treatment decisions. They must decide who to tell and what to tell them. They may need to reassign role responsibilities, at least on a temporary basis. They may have to make financial decisions. They have to find ways to support one another emotionally. As individuals and as a unit, they need to manage fear and uncertainty, and they need to maintain hope. Each of these tasks requires family communication.

FAMILY COMMUNICATION

The communication patterns of most families are well established; they may be functional or dysfunctional. If communication within the family is open and honest, it should serve a positive function in times of crisis. Some families, however, have less than optimal communication patterns, and serious illness may make communication even harder.

Your family may find it hard to talk about emotional subjects. For example, crying in front of others may not be acceptable in your family, yet a cancer diagnosis for yourself or for a loved one causes sadness. As a result, family members may be forced to cry alone in their cars, their offices, or in the shower. A lack of communication and the inability to express emotion in front of others can cause increased isolation and anxiety.

Open communication and the expression of feelings within the family are crucial to creating a healing environment and for helping one another gain the strength necessary to deal with the crises of cancer. Remember that while each cancer crisis is time limited, cancer is a chronic illness. You will need to maintain or develop good communication skills so your family can adapt over the long haul.

Good family communication skills can be learned, but you may need to seek specific training for dealing with cancer-related communication issues. This training often is available in your hospital or community through patient education programs or through mutual self-help and support groups. To improve family communication, you first need an understanding of what kinds of factors create communication barriers.

COMMUNICATING ABOUT HEALTH ISSUES

One difficult area for family communication often involves the health concerns of the person with cancer. Most people are not used to living with a chronic illness like cancer. First, the cancer survivor and family members must learn the "language of cancer." The vocabulary is not familiar; the terms, the tests, and treatment protocols can be difficult to understand, and it all seems overwhelming. Eventually, you will learn what you need to know and will become an expert in your own care and needs. In fact, you will have to become an expert so you can contribute vital information and monitor your treatment.

Asking questions is very important. Ask them again and again if you do not understand what your health care team is saying or suggesting. One excellent resource for helping you to determine the questions and how to ask them is *Teamwork: The Cancer Patient's Guide to Talking with Your Doctor.* This resource is available from the National Coalition for Cancer Survivorship. Another excellent resource is a free audio program called the Cancer Survivor Toolbox™. This self-advocacy training program teaches you the skills you need for living with cancer. It contains nine programs:

1. Communicating
2. Finding Information
3. Making Decisions
4. Solving Problems
5. Negotiating
6. Standing Up for Your Rights
7. Finding Ways to Pay for Care
8. Topics for Older Persons
9. Caring for the Caregivers

You can order a free copy by calling 1-877-TOOLS4U (1-877-866-5748) or listen to the Toolbox at **www.cancersurvivaltoolbox.org**. The communication section provides suggestions for better communication with your health care team and family.

Family members may have differing views about cancer and its treatment. They also are frightened and concerned for their loved ones. They may think that more aggressive treatment is desirable. Sometimes they may disagree with the physician's recommendations. Good communication and getting answers to their questions can help. The cancer survivor has the final word about health-related issues. Family disagreements and undue pressure only add to the stress level of the whole family.

Conflict about self-care also can be an issue. Only cancer survivors know how they feel, what their capacity for exercise is, or if they feel too nauseated to eat. Family members sometimes feel that the cancer survivor is not doing enough or trying hard enough to get better. This disagreement often centers around nutrition. Persons with cancer usually experience some weight loss. At the same time, chemotherapy can make food tasteless. The cancer survivor may not feel like eating, or simply cannot eat, leading to further weight loss. Nagging survivors to eat when they are having difficulty doing so is not useful. Instead, talk with your physician or oncology nurse or ask for a referral to a dietitian who specializes in oncology.

Pain control is another issue that requires good communication. That all cancer survivors experience severe pain is a myth. Almost all pain related to cancer can be controlled, but it may take a team effort to acquire the best pain control. The most important person on that team is the patient. Only the person experiencing the pain can know how severe it is.

Sometimes, cancer survivors hide their pain. Some may feel that acknowledging the pain may show weakness, or they fear that the cancer may be worsening. Living with pain is unnecessary and can cause other problems, including depression (see Chapter 6).

Another communication problem results when a family member mistakenly believes that the survivor will become addicted to the medication and suggests that their loved one use less pain medication than prescribed, or suggests waiting until the pain becomes severe before taking medication. This approach becomes self-defeating and leads to more difficulty in pain management.

Tell your doctor when you have pain and be honest about how severe and how frequent it is. Your health care team must have this essential information to plan your pain control. Also, ask your doctor or oncology nurse to reassure your family members about the proper use of pain medications and the low risk for addiction. Helpful suggestions about what you can do to control your pain can be found at the Web site for the American Pain Foundation at **www.painfoundation.org.**

One other problem area of communication for family members is talking about what happens if the disease is life-threatening and the loved one enters a terminal stage of illness. These conversations are very hard but important ones for families. Chapter 11 discusses maintaining hope and dealing with grief. Chapter 14 discusses health care directives and living wills.

These conversations are so difficult because family members are often not ready to acknowledge that their loved one might die. Sometimes, the cancer survivor wants to discuss issues surrounding end-of-life care and what he or she wants to happen when they die, but family members are emotionally unable to face these issues. Sometimes the family is ready for the discussion, but the cancer survivor is reluctant or emotionally unable to talk about it. It is probably one of the most important and meaningful discussions your family will ever have. It may take great courage and great caring to confront the issues directly, but doing so is like a gift for the family. Discussing end-of-life care and making plans frees family members to focus on their relationships, makes the remaining time special and meaningful, and maintains the cancer survivor's quality of life throughout the terminal period.

BARRIERS TO FAMILY COMMUNICATION

Many potential barriers can interfere with good family communication. These include fear, refusal to discuss sad topics, anger, guilt, gender difference, and a "conspiracy of silence."

FEAR–Fear is a major barrier to communication. When someone is first diagnosed with cancer, the major fear for the cancer survivor and the family is that cancer will lead to death. Even with unrealistic myths about cancer dispelled, and even when the prognosis and statistics are favorable, the fear of death requires some management. If not managed adequately, fear and sadness can drive a wedge into helpful family communications.

REFUSAL TO DISCUSS SAD TOPICS–Another burden is an almost instinctual need for family members to protect the cancer survivor from the realities of the cancer. This protection may extend to other family members who seem vulnerable and overburdened. The problem can be compounded by some therapies that encourage positive thinking as part of the cancer treatment. Because of these therapies, some family members do not want to hear sad or scared talk for fear of jeopardizing their loved one's recovery. The result is that the cancer survivor, as well as other family members, is cut off and isolated from talking about cancer-related fear and sadness. This isolation may increase the burden of the illness.

ANGER–Anger is inevitable during the cancer experience. Most cancer survivors and family members are angry at times. Try to look beyond the anger to its source. Anger usually is not a result of something someone has done; rather, it is a way of responding to the accumulated stress and helplessness that the cancer survivor or angry family member feels.

GUILT–Guilt, over real or imaginary events, can be another communication barrier. Family members may blame themselves for not insisting that the patient see a doctor sooner, or for various other illness-related concerns. Family members may feel guilty that they are well while another family member is ill, which especially may be the case among siblings when the cancer survivor is a child.

Guilt is often related to feelings of inadequacy. Perhaps a family member feels guilty because he or she is embarrassed by the way the cancer survivor looks during the treatment process. Hair loss, disfiguring surgery, or other changes in appearance take time to get used to. Questions and comments from friends or strangers may be difficult to handle.

GENDER DIFFERENCES–Family members often deal with problems differently. They usually rely on coping behaviors that they have found useful in the past. Men and women sometimes respond differently to fear and anxiety-producing situations. Men may present a brave front, denying the seriousness of the illness, especially when the female partner is the cancer survivor. This denial sometimes helps men cope with feelings of powerlessness and anxiety.

Some women also use a form of denial, but it generally relates to their own illness, not to that of their partner or child. They may find themselves trying so hard to calm the fears of their immediate family members and their relatives that they have little time to acknowledge the concerns and fears they have for themselves. They repress their own fears to help family members cope. Their responses to their own illness seem stoical, and others may comment about "how strong you seem," or that they "don't know how you do it." This "strong" behavior by female survivors eventually has a negative effect. Women who face a personal threat or poor physical health find it more difficult to provide the majority of the family support.

CONSPIRACY OF SILENCE–Both men and women with cancer may need help in voicing their fears and anger and in accepting emotional support and assistance. When communication is not possible among family members, confusion can result. The cancer survivor may resent that no one really understands the problems he or she faces. Family members feel they cannot let their guard down or discuss their real feelings. Sometimes this leads to a conspiracy of silence, a situation in which information is withheld from either the cancer survivor or family members for fear that they will not be able to deal with it.

FAMILY COPING STYLES

Family members respond to stress differently. One person may resort to anger as a response to feelings of helplessness. Another may withdraw emotionally or try to be out of the house as much as possible. Still another may appear not to care, or to act as if nothing has changed. These various coping styles may be misconstrued by other family members and may lead to conflict within the family.

Whatever their level of knowledge or understanding about cancer, children are aware that a tremendous change has occurred in the household. Changes in daily routine, long absences of one or both parents, preoccupation of parents or siblings, and feelings of tension are all obvious signals that something is wrong. Young children need to know that they will continue to be cared for and supported. In addition, they need to make sense out of the sadness, anxiety, and despair of the adults around them. If they are given inadequate information, they will make their own assumptions. They need to know what is happening or they will fill in the gaps with their own interpretations; what they imagine is often worse than the reality.

Teenagers in the family also need reassurances. Sometimes their needs are overlooked during family crises. Because they are approaching adulthood, their needs may be grouped with those of other adults. They may be expected to act like adults and take on adult responsibilities. This is not always possible for teenagers and may lead to increased stress and result in further family conflict.

A family crisis such as cancer disrupts normal adolescence. Just as adolescents begin a gradual emotional withdrawal from the family and start to establish individual identities, the illness of a parent forces them to have intensified family contact. They may be willing to accept increased household and babysitting responsibilities, but they also may act out their resentment in various ways. Teenagers need support and an opportunity to vent and talk about their mixed feelings. Perhaps a relative or close family friend could provide this support.

Sometimes adult children are initially left out of the family communication loop; this may be purposeful or accidental. While these children generally live outside the parents' home, they still remain a part of the extended family system and should know about a family problem as soon as it occurs. Not telling them about an illness isolates them and does not afford them the opportunity to receive or provide family support. You may think you have very good reasons for not informing your adult children about your diagnosis or for putting off telling them. Perhaps they are struggling with a crisis of their own, or are overwhelmed at work or school or with parenting issues. Regardless, they will be hurt if they find out about your diagnosis from a sibling or relative or an acquaintance. They may feel guilty that they were not able to support you sooner.

TIPS FOR CHILDREN TO COPE WITH CANCER IN THE FAMILY

- Don't be ashamed or afraid of the way you feel. Others in your situation have felt the same way.
- Sometimes things get better if you talk about them. Share your feelings with your parents or another adult or a friend you can trust.
- Learn about cancer and the way it is treated. What we first imagine about cancer is often far worse than what is really happening.
- Try to find other people your age who have a person in their family with cancer or another serious illness. You may be able to share your feelings with them.
- If you overhear someone talking and what you hear scares you, ask them to explain what they said. Don't assume that you heard everything and understood what it meant; ask about it.
- Don't forget the adults other than your parents who can help you.

Abstracted from the booklet *When Someone in Your Family Has Cancer.* Available from the National Cancer Institute (Publication No. 90-2685).

MULTIPLE FAMILY PROBLEMS

The crisis of serious illness seems to intensify the family relationship patterns that already are in place. Yet it also may intensify existing family problems. For example, if a child is not doing well in school, his or her grades will not likely improve when an additional family problem is introduced. Likewise, marital discord or financial problems may worsen when a serious illness is identified. Alcoholism, drug abuse, and eating disorders may also become more severe for a family member or the cancer survivor when new problems are introduced.

Sometimes, existing problems do seem to "self-correct" for a short time as everyone focuses on the immediate family crisis. Eventually, however, the increased stress will probably take its toll. If someone in your family has a personal problem or is engaging in destructive behavior, do all you can to get them to seek counseling or go together to see a family therapist so that your family energies are not fragmented and dispersed. If your loved one will not seek help, seek counseling without them so you can get help in managing your own responses to the ongoing family problem and to the new crisis.

ENHANCING FAMILY COMMUNICATION

The following are suggestions for avoiding some barriers to family communication:

TRY TO PUT CANCER IN PERSPECTIVE—Family members must recognize that cancer is a disease like any other disease. It can be cured, treated, controlled, and managed. Do not let the negative myths and fears about cancer impede communication. Both the cancer survivor and family members need accurate and honest information about the illness and the treatment plan.

Knowledge can increase personal control and can help minimize all family members' sense of helplessness. Family discussions about the type and extent of treatments and about expected side effects and changes in appearance are useful. Family members should discuss openly within the family worrisome statements that they hear from their friends or colleagues. Ask your health care team to explain troublesome comments and questions about suggested miracle therapies.

Educational materials to help your family understand cancer and its treatment are available from your hospital, your physician, your oncology nurse, or your social worker. Booklets related to specific types of cancer can be obtained free of charge from the local unit of your American Cancer Society at (800) 227-2345 and from the National Cancer Institute at (800)-4-CANCER. Excellent educational resources have been written for younger age groups. Two recommended resources for children include *It Helps to Have Friends When Mom or Dad Has Cancer* from the American Cancer Society, and *When Someone in Your Family Has Cancer,* available from the National Cancer Institute (NIH Publication No. 94-2685).

DISCUSS NEEDED CHANGES IN FAMILY ROLES AND ACTIVITIES–Will you need to delay or cancel a vacation or family event? Will the cancer survivor need to be absent from work for a period of time, and if so, will this affect family finances? What will remain the same—for example, your love for one another, honesty with each other, valuing family time, and continuing special activities? How will family chores and responsibilities be distributed during the treatment process? Who will be available to help with transportation, shopping, meal preparation, and homework?

The shifting of responsibilities for household tasks, managing family finances, and providing care for the cancer survivor or for children creates stress. Family members can feel overworked, unappreciated, or left out. Discussing these changes and related feelings openly and accepting anger, disappointment, and differences can help the family adapt to the crisis.

Even if a loved one is extremely ill, try not to exclude him or her from the family decision-making process. While illness may necessitate some role shifting, all family members, including the cancer survivor, need to feel that they are a respected and valued part of the family system.

DETERMINE WHAT IS ACCEPTABLE TO DISCUSS WITH FRIENDS AND EXTERNAL FAMILY MEMBERS ABOUT THE CANCER SURVIVOR AND THE ILLNESS–Many friends and neighbors will be curious about the illness and prognosis. Most will ask questions because they want to offer help and support. Some people, however, are simply interested in gossip. The cancer survivor has a right to privacy; you are not obligated to discuss the situation. With the survivor's input, practice answers to difficult questions that others may ask.

SEEK OUT ADDITIONAL RESOURCES FOR THE FAMILY–Classes like the American Cancer Society's "I Can Cope" and group meetings can provide education and support to meet the challenges of cancer. Mutual support and self-help groups and special programs designed to help individuals and families cope with family changes and problem solving are available in most communities (see Chapter 8). Let the cancer survivor and other family members know if you are planning to attend a support group or a cancer-related education program. Keeping attendance a secret will not foster family communication.

AVOIDING FAMILY BURNOUT

Most people think of burnout as an individual's problem, but families can suffer burnout too. Burnout is defined as a syndrome of emotional exhaustion that frequently occurs among individuals who do "people work," which means they spend considerable time in close encounters with others under conditions of chronic tension and stress. Two major clues to burnout are increased cynicism and feelings of being indispensable. This definition can easily fit family members during the initial cancer crisis and over the duration of a treatment regimen that may extend for many months or even years.

The signs and symptoms of burnout range from physical symptoms, such as fatigue and exhaustion, frequent headaches, or sleeplessness, to behavioral and psychological symptoms, such as being quick to anger, feelings of being unappreciated, and being unable to make decisions. Sometimes they result in escapist behavior; an individual may begin using alcohol or drugs to avoid the overwhelming feelings of stress. You may become cynical about the treatment plan or about the health care team or despair that the situation will ever get better. This cynicism may be linked to anger, and those angry feelings about the situation or your sense of hopelessness may be displaced onto others such as a physician, a family member, or even the cancer survivor.

Feeling indispensable can be equally dysfunctional. Family members who believe they have to be constantly present in a caregiving role will delay any personal gratification or plans so that they can be readily available to the cancer survivor and other family members. All family members must take care of their own health, which means eating right, exercising, and getting enough rest and relaxation. You do not need a family martyr—one person who sacrifices personal well-being for the family's sake.

A side effect of having one "indispensable" family member is that other family members may take advantage of the person, and after a while they stop asking to share the burden and are relieved that they do not have to be so constantly involved. Eventually, the constant caregiver will burn out, and the family will be unprepared for the consequences. Another outcome could be that the stress for the individual will be so great that he or she will become sick. A new illness will further compound the family crisis.

If you or a family member are feeling indispensable, have a family talk about the situation. To avoid burnout, you must know your own strengths and weaknesses, and freely admit these to others. When everyone is together, assess family skills and see how each person can contribute. Perhaps you will find that one person becomes panicky about being present at treatment procedures or simply cannot tolerate needles, yet that person's strength may be in planning family activities, managing finances, or preparing tax returns.

As time goes on, give individuals the opportunity to change assignments so that they do not become too burdened by any one task or responsibility. Avoid having all of the personal care tasks fall on only one person. Plan routine breaks for each family member. Let teenagers and close family friends share the burden. For example, a teenager who drives could take the cancer survivor for radiation treatments or to a doctor's appointment. This contribution will enable the teenager to learn something about the treatment process, will make him or her feel like a fully functioning member of the family, and will provide an opportunity for private and meaningful conversation between the teenager and the cancer survivor.

If you feel burned out, consider attending some educational programs or joining a support group (see Chapter 8). Maintain a personal support network that includes people outside of the family circle. Two people involved in the same crisis can seldom support one another equally because their emotional energy is going into managing the crisis. Look to friends and/or coworkers for emotional support. Take routine breaks from discussing and living the cancer crisis.

As much as possible, the family, including the cancer survivor, should try to maintain usual activities and routines. Continue outside interests, hobbies, sports, and exercise programs. If needed, recruit assistance from your extended family and friends for carpooling and other services. They will be glad they can be useful.

TAKE TIME OUT–Vacations, even if only for a day or two, are essential so that you can maintain perspective. Guilt because you take a day or two off from the family crisis suggests that you may feel indispensable and may be a strong warning sign for burnout. Encourage the cancer survivor to give up the patient role as soon as possible. Too often families become overly protective during the treatment phase. They continue to limit or discourage individual and family activities even when no physical limitations warrant doing so.

ASK FOR WHAT YOU NEED–Another task for family members is asking assertively for what they need. At times of serious illness and tension, many persons put their own needs on hold and feel that it would be selfish to ask for something they personally want or require. After a while, this denial of personal needs can become the family norm, and resentment builds up. Do not assume that other family members know what you think, feel, or need. They are as involved in the crisis as you are and probably have not taken your needs into account. Similarly, you may have overlooked their needs and concerns.

While acute crises are time-limited, the burden of caregiving for family members can extend over long periods. The family, as a whole, may become worn down, depressed, or less functional than it was at the beginning of the illness. If this is the case, you may need some professional advice or counseling to help you move beyond family burnout. You may also need additional tangible support from home health aides or community agencies.

LIFE AFTER THE CANCER CRISIS

Cancer permanently changes families. Although everyone longs to "get back to normal," a "new normal" must evolve to move forward. The new normal includes elements of the cancer crisis, such as increased medical checkups, living with uncertainty, and fear of a cancer recurrence or the end of a remission. Some experts liken the aftermath of an acute cancer experience to a post-traumatic stress reaction. It may take years for the cancer survivor and the family to feel safe again. Periodic episodes of flashbacks and heightened anxiety that are unrelated to cancer often arise around periodic checkups or minor illness episodes.

Uncertainty may result in a hesitation to give up your patient identity and dependency on the health care team. You may be frightened to start over and to trust the future again. Thinking about living after experiencing an acute fear of death is a difficult transition. The ability to make long-range plans can take months or even years. To move forward, you must take the experiences and the related skills and strengths you have acquired and integrate them into your "new norm" life.

Managing a crisis frequently leads both cancer survivors and family members to function at a higher level. Families may have drawn closer together and can now handle minor problems and stressors more easily. They may be able to communicate more directly. They may know one another better and be able to recognize and acknowledge one another's strengths and weaknesses and provide support as needed. In some cases, though, the stress of the illness is too great, and family members become alienated and more distanced than before the crisis. If the family infrastructure was weak before the illness, adversity may not strengthen it.

If your family has inadequate communication, seek assistance from your health care team, attend mutual support groups or community programs specific to cancer-related problem-solving, or seek individual or family counseling. As a family, you probably will retain an interest in cancer-related topics for a long time. You may follow developments in cancer research and may serve as a resource for other individuals and families who are in the midst of a cancer crisis. Frequently, cancer survivors and their family members want to give something back and turn to personal and community advocacy on behalf of other survivors. For a discussion on how to become an advocate, see Chapter 16.

In summary, persons diagnosed with cancer must become their own best advocates. With good communication, family members can join in these advocacy efforts, and the family can face cancer together—as a strong team. This approach can result in enhanced relationships, better care, and a higher quality of life for all members of the family.

CHECKLIST FOR THE FAMILY

Are you pressuring the person with cancer to—
- stop talking about his health because it is morbid?
- stop feeling sorry for himself?
- prove that he is feeling great even when he is not?

Instead, help by—
- letting him talk about his problems and finding positive topics to talk about
- keeping his interest up about home, work, and world affairs
- being sympathetic but emphasizing the good things about life
- not pressuring him to be a cheerleader for you to keep up your spirits
- letting him level with you about his feelings

Marion Morra and Eve Potts, *Triumph: Getting Back to Normal When You Have Cancer,* 1990: 211.

Chapter Eight

The Power of
Peer Support

How to Benefit from
the Wisdom of Other
Survivors

by Catherine Logan-Carrillo and Gena Love

*S*OMETHING VERY SPECIAL HAPPENS when people facing cancer turn to one another for help. The resulting peer support can have a profound impact on how they feel about themselves and on how well they manage their lives during and after cancer.

Peer support can take many forms: support groups, one-to-one consultations, telephone hotlines, newsletters, and connections through the Internet. It also can be found at week-long retreats with intimate groups and in larger groups, such as educational workshops and conferences.

Whatever its form and whether the participants are cancer survivors or their loved ones, peer support is empowering. Seeking help from your peers is an act of faith in people just like you and in your own ability to deal effectively with the crisis of cancer. Members of cancer support networks are eager to share their experiences with you and to learn what they can from you. This chapter will help you make the most of this valuable resource.

PEER SUPPORT IN THE CANCER SURVIVORSHIP MOVEMENT: A BRIEF HISTORY

Cancer is only one of many life situations that motivate people to create peer support networks and mutual aid groups. Historically, people who have shared political, social, medical, and other mutual concerns have worked together to create resources to meet their needs. Alcoholics Anonymous is one of the oldest and best known of these peer support networks.

The United Ostomy Association is another peer support organization with a long and effective history. In 1949, five people who had ostomies (surgery to construct an artificial opening in response to colon cancer and other illnesses) met in Philadelphia to share their experiences and knowledge. By 2001, the United Ostomy Association had 25,000 members and 400 chapters in the United States. Although many of the United Ostomy Association members have had cancer, the organization's primary focus is on the common experience of having an ostomy.

Other peer support organizations concentrating exclusively on cancer issues began to evolve in the early 1970s. The Candlelighters Childhood Cancer Foundation is one of the oldest of these organizations. In 1970, parents of children who had cancer founded the Candlelighters Childhood Cancer Foundation to address the needs of their families. By 2001, Candlelighters had become an international organization with more than 250 local chapters. On a local level, Candlelighters chapters provide opportunities for sharing experiences and information about the needs of children with cancer and their families. Some local chapters provide financial assistance, camps, and parties. On a national level, the organization serves as a clearinghouse for information on childhood cancer, develops resources to address members' concerns, and advocates for adequate funding for childhood cancers and for the legal rights of childhood cancer survivors.

Many organizations that offer education and support programs have both a professional and a peer support component. The largest and best known of these organizations is the American Cancer Society, founded in 1945. In addition to its other activities, such as funding cancer research and promoting cancer prevention and early detection, the American Cancer Society distributes information about cancer to the public and to cancer survivors and their families. One of its most popular educational programs is I Can Cope, an educational program for newly diagnosed survivors and family members. Over the years the American Cancer Society has developed a number of peer support programs, such as Reach to Recovery, which provides peer support to women who have been diagnosed with breast cancer and to their families. The American Cancer Society also provides many opportunities for cancer survivors and family members to become involved in cancer-related advocacy.

THE EMERGENCE OF THE CANCER SURVIVORSHIP MOVEMENT

Although cancer survivors have always exchanged mutual aid, the peer support movement began to gather momentum in the early 1980s. In 1986, the National Coalition for Cancer Survivorship (NCCS) was started to coordinate and encourage communication between newly emerging survivor-driven activities, including peer support programs. A grassroots social movement evolved as survivors and survivor organizations across the country began to communicate. NCCS was the first to identify this survivorship movement and to develop a national survivorship agenda.

Initially working out of the offices of People Living Through Cancer, an Albuquerque peer support organization, NCCS was the first successful attempt at providing a national organization to represent the concerns of all cancer survivors, their loved ones, and their organizations. In 1991, NCCS moved its office to Washington, D.C., where it became one of the primary organizations advocating on behalf of cancer survivorship.

In the early 1990s, cancer survivors in organizations like NCCS and the National Breast Cancer Coalition, founded in 1991, became the cutting edge of a new wave of cancer survivor organizations with a primary focus on advocacy.

These organizations raise the visibility of cancer issues and demand that more of the nation's resources be dedicated to eradicating the disease.

QT ALUMNI

In 1950, Mount Sinai Hospital in New York had two wards, Q and T, for patients recovering from life-saving ileostomy surgery. Although surgeons had learned how to perform ileostomies successfully, being a patient who was living with one was quite another matter. People living with ileostomies faced a lack of adequate appliances to collect bodily waste and to prevent its corrosive nature from injuring the skin around the ileostomy. Not content to live with appliances that leaked and fell off, patients on both wards began to share ideas about how to improve their quality.

Once they returned to their homes, QT Alumni and ostomy patients from other cities kept in touch. Driven by a need to create better appliances, some group members made models of improved appliances in their garages. They shared their discoveries with others as their ideas developed from drawing-board sketches to effective appliances.

The QT Alumni were pioneer survivors who had in common practical adversity and, sometimes, social isolation. The drive to find practical solutions to mutual problems led to the first peer support network for people with ostomies, and laid the foundation for the development of other health-related mutual aid organizations.

THE VALUE OF PEER SUPPORT

Dealing with cancer is one of the most difficult challenges a person can face; facing cancer alone is an even greater challenge. One of the most important things you can do for yourself when going through a cancer experience is to find people who can give you adequate emotional support. Support can come from many different places, but perhaps the most abundant and most natural source for it is the vast population of cancer survivors and their loved ones.

Approximately 9 million people in the United States have had cancer. Many of them have joined together in support networks to ensure that no one has to go through cancer alone. They have just the right experiences to understand and respect your needs.

Even survivors with supportive friends and families often feel they need more; they want to talk with someone who knows what they are experiencing. Relationships with family members and friends may become strained and uncomfortable after a cancer diagnosis. At the very time the need for support increases, familiar ways of support may not work anymore, and faithful friends may not know how best to help.

People facing cancer seek out peer support for different reasons. Most often, they simply want to feel better—to ease the emotional distress caused by the diagnosis. Support networks offer inspiration from the courage of others and the motivation to fight for your life. They provide role models who can help you accept a changed life, a new identity, and an uncertain future. Networks can provide a place to gain control of some aspects of your life again and to vent and validate feelings. They offer hope—sometimes hope for cure or improved health, sometimes hope for a good life, sometimes hope for a good death.

Cancer support groups cannot guarantee a cancer-free future. Members can inspire and motivate survivors, however, by facing difficult issues together and sharing experiences. Some people find support groups difficult because they closely identify with others whose disease is advancing or with someone who dies.

Survivors and their family members also reach out to peers for information or for help in making difficult decisions. Cancer veterans have a wealth of knowledge that can help others find their own path through the cancer experience.

WEAVING STORIES INTO THE FABRIC OF SURVIVORSHIP

In a support group, one story after another describes the very personal experiences of survivors and family members—feelings and problems, hopes and fears, victories and disappointments. Often these experiences are so all-consuming that they isolate survivors from the people around them.

Each person's unique cancer story tells of the profound, life-changing impact of cancer. At first each group member knows cancer only through his or her own experiences. As they share their stories, common themes and intimate bonds evolve and begin to weave the stories together. Like individual threads stretched side by side in a loom, the stories are woven into a strong fabric. The same powerful experiences that once isolated survivors now link them to those who share their experiences. They gain strength from one another as each story becomes part of the fabric of survivorship.

The story tellers also gain a much broader understanding of the cancer experience. This understanding not only allows group members to help one another, but it builds a foundation for advocacy.

SHARING THE JOURNEY

Interdependence
not independence
is the reality of this world.
I have a shared destiny
touching the lives of countless others
as ripples in a pond
fan out in ever widening circles.
We live in

one another's company.
Together we can diffuse the pain
and multiply the
joy
of being.

Brenda Neal
© 1985
People Living Through Cancer Journal

THE VALUE OF SHARING YOUR STORY—Telling your story and listening to others' stories can be the foundation both for personal healing and for building a sense of community. Sharing your story is healing because it breaks through isolation and allows you to express your feelings to others. Hearing others' stories connects your life to theirs. It also can help you sort out which of your responses are natural reactions to the stresses of dealing with cancer and which might be signs of special problems that deserve professional attention.

Sharing stories also builds a foundation for advocacy. It helps survivors in the following ways:
- understanding survivorship in the broader sense—beyond just their own unique experience
- identifying the kinds of problems that survivors and family members face
- preparing them to work with others for necessary changes

PEER SUPPORT ISSUES—Many issues surface after a cancer diagnosis. Peer support can help you address

Emotional, social, spiritual, and financial issues such as
- feelings of fear, depression, and anger
- isolation
- reclaiming a sense of control over your life
- strained relationships with family and friends
- loss, grief, and facing the possibility of death
- changing values and beliefs
- financial, insurance, and employment issues

Treatment issues such as
- side effects (immediate, long-term, and delayed)
- effective use of medical resources
- relationships with health care providers
- pain management
- complementary and integrative therapies

Wellness issues such as
- changes in physical appearance and body image

- sexuality
- diet and nutrition
- long-term health maintenance

HOW PEER SUPPORT DIFFERS FROM PROFESSIONAL COUNSELING

Peer support is a process of sharing feelings and practical information learned through personal experiences—sharing between people who have similar life experiences. Professional counseling promotes personal exploration and change and is guided by a trained counselor or therapist. The chart on page 154 summarizes these two approaches in a group setting.

Many cancer survivors and family members benefit from both kinds of help. They find that peer support and professional counseling complement each other. Support group members commonly encourage each other to get professional help; counselors and therapists often recommend peer support groups.

Peer support is not a substitute for professional counseling; it has a distinct value of its own. It builds a sense of community and empowers people through creating social structures that provide opportunities to improve their own survivorship and to help others.

THE ROLE OF HEALTH CARE PROVIDERS IN PEER SUPPORT ORGANIZATIONS

Health care providers are valuable contributors to, as well as advocates of, peer support groups. Some peer groups have a philosophy that endorses peer leadership only. Health care providers should be sensitive to these views; they might ask how a group views the role of professionals when they offer their assistance.

Maintaining the balance between peer ownership and taking advantage of valuable services offered by professionals can be difficult. "Professionalization" of peer networks deserves careful thought both by the peer network leaders and the health care providers, because the group's identity will change if peers lose ownership. Nevertheless, peer support networks look to professionals for help in a variety of ways including direct referrals, consultation, technical assistance, and help with educational programs. Professionals also can help peer groups by advocating on their behalf to other health care providers.

PEER-LED SUPPORT GROUPS COMPARED WITH PROFESSIONALLY LED GROUPS

"I want to be my own expert. Having a health care provider as the group leader implies that they are an expert and, somehow, that reduces my own expertise. For me, it changes the group process into fixing something that is wrong, instead of learning to live through this difficult life experience with others who share the experience."

Julie Reichert
breast cancer survivor
Albuquerque, NM

How Peer Support Groups Differ from Professional Counseling and Therapy Groups

This chart describes some of the basic attributes of peer support and therapy groups. Groups do not always fall precisely under either type.

Peer Support Groups

Leader
- contributes to the group from personal experience
- balances flow and content of exchanges
- keeps group safe
- comes from within the group, on the same path as other members but may be further along
- no profit orientation

Purpose
- helps members manage their lives, cope with emotional and other issues, and educate themselves
- social support is means and end; therapeutic results are by-product

Process
- self-governed: goals and format established by group
- members accept responsibility for selves; no expectation of others
- usually ongoing, open-ended
- new members may be added or drop out at any time

Professional Counseling Groups

Leader
- has special expertise founded on professional, theoretical education
- directs flow and content of exchanges
- keeps group safe
- trained to maintain professional distance and usually not from the group
- usually has fee-for-services agreement with group members or is paid through salary

Purpose
- helps members with personal exploration and change of basic perceptions and behaviors
- therapy is purpose; social support is by-product

Process
- group goals and format set by leader before group meets
- leader guides and encourages members to set personal goals and to move toward those goals
- usually time-limited
- restrictions on adding new members after group begins; members make a commitment to attend all sessions

Peer support groups have two models: (1) "pure" peer support, where everyone in the group, including the leader, shares the cancer experience, and (2) peer support groups led by health care providers—social workers, nurses, counselors, psychologists, and psychiatrists. Professionally led peer support groups are not therapy groups and more closely resemble the description of peer groups on the left side of the chart on page 154. In these groups, the leader facilitates the peer support process between group members.

Some survivors prefer "pure" peer support groups, which are led by others who share the cancer experience. They believe that peer-led groups function differently from those led by health care providers who have not had a personal or family cancer experience. One reason may be because the level of intimacy in a group deepens when everyone in the group, including the leaders, shares personal feelings and experiences.

Professional therapists and counselors often have valuable theoretical understandings of healing during and after a cancer experience. Peer leaders may or may not have the technical knowledge, but can be living examples—proof that one can heal and feel whole again. They can be valuable models of how to address the difficult issues that follow a cancer diagnosis.

Sometimes people dealing with cancer prefer to join support groups with peer facilitators as evidence of their confidence that they can handle their own lives. Some feel that it is more comfortable and more empowering to belong to a group without the guidance and oversight of an outside expert. After medical experiences where they have felt a significant loss of control of their lives, with little choice but dependence on outside experts, they want to reclaim control of their lives. Peer support can be a tool for doing just that.

At times, survivors and family members need to express anger and frustration with health care providers and the health care system. The expression of these feelings may be inhibited in the presence of a health care provider, although a skilled and sensitive professional will be sympathetic to this kind of anger and frustration.

On balance, both peer-led and professionally led groups have their merits. One way to benefit from the best of both peer support and professional expertise is to have the group led by a health care professional who also has a personal cancer history and is willing to share those experiences with the group.

Choosing the Right Peer Support Service for You

You are the only one who knows what is best for you. Different kinds of peer support are appropriate for different people, or even for the same person at different times in his or her survivorship. Your decisions should be based on your own values and beliefs, as well as on your physical and financial situation. Think about your experience with giving and receiving support in previous difficult situations. Trust what your experience tells you about your own style of seeking help; at the same time, do not be afraid to try something new.

If available, you may want to look for a group that focuses on your particular kind of cancer, especially if you have a more common diagnosis like breast cancer or prostate cancer. You may decide to attend a group that includes people with all kinds of cancer, one that includes survivors and family members, or, if available in your community, a specialty group like one for long-term survivors or young adults. Are you looking for emotional support, information about medical care, or advice in handling financial issues? Whatever your reasons for seeking support, remember that your needs may change, and allow yourself to respond to that change.

Because no single source will have information about all the peer support resources available to you, ask about support resources from more than one of the following places:

- social service departments or discharge planners at local hospitals or treatment centers
- state self-help clearinghouses
- yellow pages of the telephone directory under "social service organizations" or "support groups," or the white pages under "cancer"
- psychologists, counselors, social workers, clergy
- newspaper listings of support groups and help lines
- reference libraries
- public health offices and mental health associations
- national organizations that have direct relationships with local peer support programs (see Chapter 17 for contact information), such as:
    Alliance for Lung Cancer, Advocacy, Support, & Education
    American Cancer Society
    CancerCare
    Candlelighters Childhood Cancer Foundation
    Colon Cancer Alliance
    The Colorectal Cancer Network
    Leukemia & Lymphoma Society
    National Alliance of Breast Cancer Organizations
    National Brain Tumor Foundation
    NCCS
    Ovarian Cancer National Alliance
    United Ostomy Association
    US TOO! International (prostate cancer groups)

If you decide to try a peer support group, call ahead, if possible, to talk with the group's contact person. You also can ask to speak to group members and ask for print material with a description or history of the group. Some groups list only a time and location for meetings, so you will have to save questions until you meet someone from the group.

You may want to ask the group's contact person the following questions:

- How many people attend and what is the makeup of the group (survivors, family members, age range, kind and stage of cancer diagnoses, etc.)?
- Who leads the group sessions and what is his or her experience or training? Do group leaders have a personal experience with cancer?
- What is the format of the group meetings? Does the group have guidelines or ground rules?
- What kinds of subjects are discussed?
- Are group members expected to share a particular philosophy or approach to cancer?

These questions have no right or wrong answers, but the responses should give you a feeling for whether the group is for you and whether its leaders are thoughtful about providing a quality group that is sensitive to group members' needs.

Have You Found the Right Group?

When you first try a cancer support group, look for the following:

- The atmosphere is welcoming to newcomers.
- The group's process encourages constructive solutions and does not dwell only on problems.
- Group members participate actively in supporting each other and do not look to the group leader as the expert.
- The group has a sense of shared ownership; one or two members do not dominate the group process.

Groups have different personalities. Not everyone is a good match for every group, no matter how well a group functions. Does the group feel comfortable to you? Trust your own instincts, but give a group a second and third try, unless you are absolutely sure it is not for you. One or two meetings may not be enough to get the feel of a group. If you decided this group is not for you, check out another group, if possible. It may be a better fit.

Guiding Principles of Effective Peer Support Groups

No universally accepted standards guide the quality of mutual aid or peer support groups, and the quality varies. Many cancer veterans, however, look for several simple guiding principles in peer support groups as well as other peer support programs. These two ground rules should be discussed as part of orienting new members to groups; they should be repeated to all group members on a regular basis.

- *All participants are asked to give nonjudgmental support and to respect others' rights to make their own decisions based on their own values and lifestyles.* This

STANDARDS OF EXCELLENCE FOR CANCER PEER SUPPORT PROGRAMS*

To ensure consistent, high-quality services and long-term viability, cancer peer support programs should have the following:

I.   Sound Structure
   • leaders who support the program's purpose, philosophy, mission, and scope of work
   • formal ground rules for support, including confidentiality and non-judgmental interaction among participants
   • annual program evaluation
   • strategies for ensuring cultural diversity and competence at all levels of the program

II. Collaboration
   • maintaining relationships with other cancer survivorship organizations locally, regionally, and nationally
   • fostering relationships with other health care consumer groups and providers, and government agencies offering survivorship resources

III. Appropriate and Skilled Leadership
   • majority of leaders are cancer survivors or family members of cancer survivors
   • shared leadership and a system in place to cultivate, recruit, and train leaders
   • training for all staff, support volunteers, and group facilitators, including:
       • the program's philosophy, mission, and scope of work
       • emotional preparation for functioning within the program
       • commitment to nonjudgmental support
       • information on cancer and cancer treatment
       • national, regional, and local resources
       • information about a wide range of psychosocial and survivorship issues, such as:
           • psychological and emotional issues
           • family issues
           • spiritual issues
           • financial, employment, and insurance issues
           • pain management
           • death and dying, grief and loss
           • cultural differences that affect survivorship

* These standards were authored by Catherine Logan-Carrillo, People Living Through Cancer, Inc. © People Living Through Cancer, 1995. For the complete document, contact People Living Through Cancer, Inc., 3939 San Pedro, NE, Building C, Suite 8, Albuquerque, NM 87110, (888) 441-4439; Web site: **www.pltc.org**; e-mail: **pltc@pltc.org**.

principle is reflected in acceptance of different approaches to dealing with cancer and an expectation and appreciation of diversity among those in the support group or network.

• *All information shared is kept confidential.* Confidentiality enhances honesty and openness, the most basic requirements for adequate support.

REWARDS OF GIVING BACK TO YOUR SUPPORT GROUP

Most survivors attend support groups for only as long as they need support. Some survivors, however, stay with a group for months or years to help sustain and improve the group so it will remain available for others. A group that has developed a mature core of cancer veterans is in a unique position to help group members, even those in great distress. Few things are as healing as helping others who share your experience.

CREATING YOUR OWN PEER SUPPORT

In your search for peer support, you may find that none exists in your community, or that existing groups do not meet your needs. As a result, you may consider creating your own.

LOOK BEFORE YOU LEAP

Before creating a new group, your first task is to look at what already exists. Creating a support program can be both energizing and exhausting. To begin and sustain a group demands personal energy as well as financial resources, which are limited commodities in the cancer community that should be conserved. Because a new group may even undermine existing groups by competing for group members and resources, consider working within an existing network rather than creating a new one. Start a new group only if you are sure your new program does not duplicate existing services or if more people are in need of services than existing programs can accommodate.

To decide whether a new resource is truly needed, thoroughly search the cancer support resources in your community. Then determine what needs, if any, they do not address, and what services, if any, they do not provide. Does your community need a telephone hotline, a support group, a newsletter, a hospital visitation program, or some other service? Are only certain populations within the cancer community served by existing programs? If you are a 65-year-old man with prostate cancer, support groups that cater to young adults or women with breast cancer may be of little value to you.

Other programs can serve as models, but as the creator, you decide what will work for you and your particular community. The requirements for a program in a large city where people live closely together, have access to transportation, and may have defensive mistrust of strangers will be different from the requirements for a new organization in a rural area, with a strong sense of community trust but a lack of transportation.

Before you begin the difficult task of founding a new group, clearly define the concerns your group will address and be sure that others share those concerns. In addition, your group must be accessible to prospective members. Find the best way to link people to your resource. Many cancer survivors who want to participate in your group may be too busy or too ill to do so. Traditional programs like group meetings can be adapted and expanded to accommodate survivors who are homebound, have physical limitations, are isolated in rural communities, or have limited financial means. If you do not have the resources to start a group on your own, then look to other survivors, supportive professionals, and hospitals or other organizations to work with you.

DEVELOPING A PEER SUPPORT GROUP

The following are suggestions that have worked for a variety of peer support groups. They offer general guidelines that can be adapted to fit the circumstances in your community.

Getting Started. Before you consider starting a cancer support group, examine the history of peer support groups. Even more important than library research, however, is field research. If possible, visit other programs, especially those that serve cancer survivors and their families. Note what you like and dislike, how the group members interact, and how the structure of the group addresses—or fails to address—its goals.

If you are interested in becoming a chapter or an affiliate of an existing organization, first make sure that a similar group does not already have a chapter serving your community. Contact the organization to learn whether it has specific guidelines you must follow. If you want to form an independent group, you may still wish to model your organization on a successful peer support program.

Identify a core working group of people who are interested in working with you. To help ensure the success of your group and to prevent burnout, develop a core working group that includes several people with commitment to the program. Working group members can be survivors, family members, oncology professionals, and experienced community organizers. Look for individuals who have strengths that complement yours and who can assist in everything from designing the organizational structure to addressing envelopes.

The first meeting. Before you determine the structure of the first meeting, the core members must decide what services you want your group to provide. A group whose purpose is to offer emotional and social support to a limited group of participants may start with an informal gathering in a member's home. If your goal is to provide education about surviving cancer, you may wish to begin with a meeting to plan a community-wide program, such as a conference on a current survivorship topic.

Tasks in planning the first meeting should be shared by working group members. They may include arranging the meeting space, preparing a presentation, and advertising the meeting to your target audience. You can attract participants by advertising in local newspapers; placing flyers in community, health, and religious institutions; speaking with survivors in other cancer programs; and encouraging local health care providers to tell their patients about your plans.

Planning for the future of your group. At the close of the first meeting, the group should reach a consensus on whether and how to continue. Future meetings must strike a balance between focusing on the purpose of the group and tending to the business of developing a structure that will sustain the program. Participants should be invited to contribute time or resources to the group.

In planning the future of your group, you should resolve a number of questions to ensure that the purpose is defined clearly and the means exist to work toward that purpose.

- What are the specific goals?
- Who may be a member of your group? Anyone? Only cancer survivors and their families? Only survivors of a specific type of cancer?
- When, where, and how often will you meet?
- How will you publicize the group?
- Will group discussions be facilitated by cancer survivors, health care providers, or both?
- What will be the focus of your first activities? Support group meetings? Newsletter? Public education program? An editorial in the local newspaper?
- How will you handle the business aspects of your group? Will you charge a membership fee? Will you elect officers? Will you adopt bylaws? Will you seek federal tax-exempt status so that donors can deduct their financial contributions from their income taxes and group purchases will not be subject to sales tax? How will you finance the group's activities?

Maintaining the Group. Expect the group to experience a natural flux in attendance and enthusiasm. New problems and issues will arise. What do you do if members of the group disagree on its purpose? How do you handle a member who dominates the discussion? Where do you go if you lose your meeting space? What do you do if a fund-raiser is a flop? Be prepared to respond to these and other problems in a way that supports the goals and unity of the group.

On a regular schedule, evaluate the effectiveness of your group. Have you accomplished your initial goals? Have your goals changed? Are your services still needed? Does the group need mid-course redirection? Are the members of the core group working together, or is all the work falling on the shoulders of one or two people?

It may take longer than you plan for the program to attract members on a consistent basis. Give your new group sufficient time to develop, grow, and become known in your community. Three things will help you maintain enough members for your group:
- consistent, long-term, and widespread promotions of the group to sustain enough new members
- thoughtful cultivation and support of group members to encourage attendance
- skillfully led group meetings

An open-ended, long-term group will need the following:
- a core of members, including group leaders, who attend regularly and have been in the group long enough to form close and caring relationships
- new group members who are in more immediate need of the support that the group is formed to provide

Groups with these two kinds of members can create a dynamic group process that keeps participants interested and feeling fulfilled.

Peer support programs are rather complex. They take skill, experience, and savvy to sustain and to develop consistent quality. But they are worth everything it takes, and they can make a tremendous difference in the lives of those who lead and those who participate.

RESOURCES TO HELP YOU BUILD AND SUSTAIN YOUR GROUP

You are not alone in your effort to create a survivorship organization. The first place to turn for help is in your own backyard. Medical centers, churches, synagogues, community centers, and private businesses may provide space and advisors. Ask your oncologist, social worker, or nurse to help. In addition to providing meeting space, your community may be a source of enough donated materials and personal assistance to get you started. A printing company may donate flyers that advertise your meetings, or a business supply company may give you office equipment. A social worker or an accountant may offer advice for free or at a discount.

In addition to local resources, several regional and national sources offer assistance. The National Coalition for Cancer Survivorship offers technical assistance to individuals and communities organizing around cancer survivorship. NCCS draws from its experience as a bridge between peer leaders and health care providers to provide a balanced list of suggestions to new organizations.

NCCS helps new groups in three ways. First, it helps leaders of new groups explore successful models represented by other cancer organizations. Second, it links new and established groups with other local, regional, or national groups that have similar survivorship programs. Third, NCCS sponsors events that unite survivors with one another and introduces survivors, their families, and caregivers to community organizations, resources, and advocacy. These events have fostered the development of dynamic organizations that continue to partner with NCCS to help shape local and national cancer policy.

Other important resources include self-help clearinghouses—nonprofit organizations that help callers locate mutual aid organizations and provide assistance to peer support networks. They sponsor training, conferences, newsletters, speakers, and consultation on developing and maintaining groups, developing resource materials, assisting with coalition building, and conducting outreach efforts with professionals and the media. Make sure your group is listed with any local self-help clearinghouse so it can refer survivors to your programs.

The American Self-Help Group Clearinghouse has some of the best available resources for support groups, including:
- a Web site that includes lists of self-help group clearinghouses in the United States, Canada, and other countries; general information on self-help groups; and information on starting new groups
- *The Self-Help Sourcebook,* which lists national peer support groups and detailed "how-to" materials with practical help for developing and managing support groups
- free online consultation on starting a national self-help group for any condition that has no established national self-help group

American Self-Help Group Clearinghouse
100 Hanover Avenue, Suite 202
Cedar Knolls, NJ 07927
(973) 326-6789
www.selfhelpgroups.org

One of the most difficult tasks of creating a new organization is managing the business aspects. Should you obtain tax-exempt status? How should you raise funds? Should you rent an office or work out of your home? Should you have a volunteer or paid staff?

Several resources in your community or region may help you answer these questions and can give guidance if you decide to create a nonprofit organization. Contact your closest United Way organization, community foundation, or self-help clearinghouse to ask what local services will help you get started. For more information, contact www.library.wisc.edu/libraries/Memorial/grants/npsrce1.htm, which has an alphabetical listing of resources.

ROLE MODELS—EXAMPLES OF PEER SUPPORT ORGANIZATIONS

The cancer survivorship movement represents the diverse experiences of hundreds of peer support organizations. Older, more established groups serve as models for newer ones. The following are examples of community-based peer support, national peer support, and other support groups that address the needs of special populations.

COMMUNITY-BASED PEER SUPPORT

CanCare of Houston, Inc.

9575 Katy Freeway, Suite 428
Houston, TX 77024
(713) 461-0028
www.cancare.org

CanCare of Houston, Inc., is an interfaith cancer support network. CanCare trains cancer survivors as volunteers to provide one-on-one, long-term emotional support to cancer patients and their families at any stage in the cancer experience for as long as needed. CanCare volunteers are matched with individuals according to type of cancer, treatment method, age, gender, and family situation.

CanCare's services include
- matched referrals, one-on-one support by a trained volunteer
- volunteer training
- an annual retreat and continuing education
- educational events and information services
- a Library of Hope
- a newsletter titled *About Life*
- a speaker's bureau
- a hospital visitation program

People Living Through Cancer, Inc.

3939 San Pedro, NE
Building C, Suite C8
Albuquerque, NM 87110
(888) 441-4439
(505) 242-3263
Web site: www.pltc.org
E-mail: pltc@pltc.org

People Living Through Cancer is a peer support organization that offers comprehensive support and education services to New Mexican families facing cancer. It does not endorse any single approach to managing life after cancer, but supports its members in making informed choices based on their own beliefs, values, and experiences. People Living Through Cancer's peer-led peer support programs serve about 2,000 families each year through:
- ongoing cancer support groups in New Mexico

- one-to-one support
- a statewide outreach program to develop peer support activities serving New Mexico's culturally diverse and rural communities
- a Telephone LifeLine, providing immediate support, information, and referrals
- the *Living Through Cancer Journal,* a quarterly publication
- New Mexico's largest library of cancer-related materials for health care consumers
- an annual statewide survivorship conference
- training sessions on support group facilitation and organizational development, including a national training program for American Indians

Operation Uplift

P.O. Box 547
Port Angeles, WA 98362
(360) 457-5141
Web site: http://operationuplift.org
E-mail: info@operationuplift.org

Operation Uplift is a nonprofit, grassroots, community-based organization that encourages people to make informed decisions and to participate in their own health care. The all-volunteer staff does not promote any particular kind of cancer treatment. It encourages a positive approach to cancer survivorship by providing support, education, and information through

- monthly peer-facilitated support meetings
- one-to-one support in person and through a 24-hour message line, with calls returned by volunteers
- volunteer training
- lending library of books and tapes
- bimonthly newsletter
- community cancer education programs
- semiannual free breast health clinics
- workshops on cancer-related subjects
- annual Celebrations of Life Picnic/Walk

NATIONAL PEER SUPPORT ORGANIZATIONS

Some national peer support organizations encourage the development of local affiliates. Two of the most established of these organizations are Y-ME and US TOO. Both are based in the Chicago area where Y-ME's successful peer support programs influenced both the US TOO name and the peer support model they developed.

Y-ME

National Breast Cancer Organization
212 West Van Buren, Suite 500
Chicago, IL 60607
800-221-2141 (English)
800-986-9505 (Spanish)
Web site: www.y-me.org
E-mail: help@y-me.org

In 2001, Y-ME had affiliate partners in 27 states, although it probably is best known for its national peer support hot line. In 1978, twelve women met at the YWCA in Park Forest, Illinois, for Y-ME's first support group. The following year, the organization established a 24-hour hotline, at first offering local help and then expanding to a national service in 1987. The national hotline now has a Spanish/English bilingual line and a men's line for partners of women diagnosed with breast cancer. All of the more than 100 trained volunteer telephone counselors are breast cancer survivors or, in the case of the men's line, partners of breast cancer survivors. Y-ME also has educational brochures and some local support groups.

US-TOO International, Inc.

Prostate Cancer Support Groups
5003 Fairview Avenue
Downers Grove, IL 60515
800-808-7866
Web site: www.ustoo.com
E-mail: ustoo@ustoo.com

In 1990, responding to patients' requests, a Chicago urologist brought together a group of prostate cancer survivors. As a result of this meeting and inspired by the Y-ME model, US TOO was founded by five prostate cancer survivors. US TOO is a grassroots, self-help organization of prostate cancer survivors. By 2001, the organization had grown to hundreds of independent chapters, mostly in the United States, but also in many other countries. US-TOO offers prostate cancer survivors and their families education and support programs, as well as help with establishing local chapters.

PEER SUPPORT IN SPECIAL POPULATIONS

In the early 1990s, an increasing number of peer support programs and national networks serving specific racial/ethnic communities began to emerge. Although many established peer support organizations have outreach programs tailored for diverse populations, they have not always been successful. Sometimes new programs serving special populations have emerged after someone goes to existing peer support groups and finds that no one there looks like them.

Although many of the issues addressed by peer support programs are basic human needs, different populations have different approaches to support. For example, some African Americans may look for stronger spiritual components than they find in most standard support groups. Some Hispanics may want a support group that invites the whole family.

Low-income and medically underserved populations, no matter what the racial or ethnic makeup, are often more concerned with access to health care and navigating the health care system. By necessity, emotional support is not always a primary concern. Some programs started by survivors from these populations combine peer support services with a strong emphasis on education about cancer, resources, and the health care system.

Two examples of peer support programs serving special populations include Sisters Network and the Native American Breast Cancer Survivors' Network.

Sisters Network

National Headquarters
8787 Woodway Drive, Suite 4206
Houston, TX 77063
(713) 781-0255
Web site: www.sistersnetworkinc.org
E-mail: sisnet4@aol.com

Founded in 1994 as a national network for African American breast cancer survivors, Sisters Network identifies strongly with individual and group peer support and also conducts community education, advocacy, and research. In 2001, the organization had 35 affiliate chapters and over 2,000 members who are breast cancer survivors.

Native American Cancer Survivor Support Circles

Native American Cancer Research
3022 South Nova Road
Pine, CO 80470-7830
(303) 838-9359
Web site: http://members.aol.com/natamcan
E-mail: natamacan2@aol.com

This network addresses various support issues for those dealing with cancer in Native American communities. It has a prepaid, long-distance telephone peer support system and also focuses on improving the understanding of how cancer affects Native communities.

See Chapter 9 for a discussion of cancer survivorship issues in special populations.

PEER SUPPORT ON THE INTERNET AND RADIO

Internet. As the Internet grows in scope and accessibility, more survivors are finding peer support online. Chat rooms, listservs, and message boards are common avenues for cancer survivors to get information and support.

A listserv is an e-mail group that you must join to participate. Some are private (invitation only) and some are open to anyone who enrolls. The Association of Cancer On-line Resources (ACOR) is a reputable and well-known organization that hosts more than 100 cancer-related listservs. Its Web site, **www.ACOR.org**, offers a variety of listservs open to anyone. Some private listservs are hosted by ACOR, but they are not listed for public enrollment.

To join a particular listserv you will be asked to complete a registration form. ACOR will send a confirmation to your e-mail address, to which you must reply within 48 hours. Then you can visit your chosen listserv at any time. All messages sent to the listserv from other members will arrive in your e-mail.

ACOR listservs are hosted, which means someone will read postings from every member before they are distributed to the listserv. This provides some measure of quality control and privacy for the list members, so the information you receive may be more factual and reliable than from other similar sources.

Message boards, usually hosted by large national cancer organizations from their own Web site (for example, **www.candlelighters.org**) provide another avenue for survivors to connect with each other. Survivors can post requests for information or support to the message board. Other visitors to the Web site may read the request and add their own postings to the board. Most message boards are open to anyone (no enrollment required) and are not monitored. Message boards allow survivors to give and receive information without receiving all the postings through their e-mail accounts.

Another option for peer support through the Internet is a chat room focusing on cancer and survivorship issues. A chat room is a forum where participants can converse in real time by typing back and forth to others. Some national survivorship organizations host chat rooms as part of their Web site services. Internet providers, such as America Online, also offer chat room participation to their members.

Chat rooms can be a quick way to get information and support from others currently visiting the site, but most are not monitored in any way. While this provides freedom and complete anonymity for all participants, it also allows anyone to post anything with no accountability. In general, visitors to chat rooms, message boards, and listservs should be skeptical of any claims for cure or requests for personal information (except when registering for a listserv).

While the Internet provides great opportunities for increasing physical access to information and peer support, it cannot replace the quality of support you receive from meeting with and talking to other survivors face-to-face. The

Internet offers information and support in the privacy of your home, at any time of day or night, whenever you most need it. But seeing the faces, looking in the eyes, and holding the hands of others who are speaking the words you hear echoing in your own head are powerful gifts no computer can offer.

Radio. One national radio show, "The Group Room," serves as a talk-radio support group. The show is hosted by Selma Schimmel, a cancer survivor and advocate who founded Vital Options, a not-for-profit organization that provides cancer information and support. "The Group Room" offers guidance and advice from physicians, therapists, other health care professionals, and survivors. The program features interviews with guest experts and Group Room staff who respond to callers' questions. For more information, contact:

Vital Options International
800-477-7666
www.vitaloptions.org

CONCLUSION

Cancer survivors and their family members choose peer support for many different reasons, from relieving feelings of isolation and dealing with the emotional impact of cancer to learning more about the cancer experience and discussing options for difficult decisions. Peer support can take many different forms: support groups, sharing one-on-one in person or by phone, retreats, conferences, and Internet communications. Peer support also can help address a myriad of difficult issues related to life beyond a cancer diagnosis.

Peer support can be a valuable part of a comprehensive approach to cancer survivorship. Choose peer support, like any resource, after you carefully evaluate available services, as well as your own needs and values. Peer support may not be for everyone, but most cancer survivors who participate in peer support find it an empowering and rewarding experience.

Chapter Nine

How Culture Affects Cancer Survivorship

by Jody Pelusi, Ph.D., F.N.P., A.O.C.N.

*C*ULTURE IS SAID TO BE the lens through which we view the world, other people, and ourselves. Our culture influences how we assign meaning and value to each person and experience, as well as guides our behavior and responses to life situations. Therefore, culture is individual, personal, and unique to each of us, as well as collective in nature as we share many of the same values, rules to live by, and life experiences.

Our culture is shaped by our life experiences, upbringing, family, friends, community, and society as a whole. It not only guides the way we act, but it also influences the way we set priorities, develop trust, and make decisions. In essence, culture is who we are, how we identify ourselves, and how we choose to live. Thus, your culture should provide the basic framework for your cancer care and be respected in every setting. The purpose of this chapter is to help you understand how your culture may be assessed and used to provide you with the best cancer care possible.

Many people think of culture in terms of one's ethnicity. Most people, however, identify with several cultural groups, such as those related to ethnicity, gender, age, religion/faith/spirituality, sexual orientation, socioeconomic status, occupation, cancer survivor status, and many others. Regardless of which cultures you identify with, sharing how your cultural identities affect your response to cancer and how you make decisions helps your health care team develop a treatment and follow-up plan based on your individual and community identity.

Your culture and geographical location may affect your access to preventive cancer care and treatment, and ultimately affect the outcome of your treatment. For example, some survivors have poor access to quality cancer care because they are physically isolated from medical care or have little or no health insurance. This may cause individuals to have higher mortality rates for all types of cancer because they have less access than others to preventive medical care and quality cancer care. Some individuals are at higher risks for certain cancers because of socioeconomic status and lifestyle factors, such as diet, exercise, and smoking.

Cultural bias or misunderstanding by health care providers may also affect the quality of cancer care. For example, some individuals may receive less pain medication than others as they may not express or describe pain in the same way. Thus their providers may not realize they are in pain and therefore do not provide sufficient pain treatment. Similarly, members of the health care team may have problems explaining treatment options effectively, because every survivor and family member has their own style of communicating, making decisions, and sharing information within the family. Your health care team must know who you are and what your needs are so they can address your needs and give you the best care possible.

During the last several years most hospitals, oncology facilities, providers, and oncology-related organizations have attempted to incorporate culturally competent cancer care into their practices. But what does that mean to you as a cancer survivor, and how should you expect your culture to be woven into your overall care plan? If your care is not provided in a way that accommodates and respects your culture, then you are not likely to participate in your care, obtain the best results possible, or trust in the health care system that provides it. Cancer treatment and long-term follow-up is a partnership between cancer survivors, their family and friends, and the health care team. The Oncology Nursing Society (ONS) was the first professional organization to develop a set of guidelines for culturally competent cancer care. These guidelines are considered the standard of care you should expect regardless of where you receive your cancer treatment and follow-up.

Josepha Campinha-Bacote developed a Cultural Competency Model of Care, which consists of four steps that health care providers, such as your physicians, nurses, social workers, and others, should take to provide culturally competent care.

1. *Cultural self awareness.* Health care providers must assess their own personal beliefs and values. They must also ask themselves how their own values and beliefs could influence the care they provide. Your health care providers should not impose their own values and beliefs on you or your family, but rather ensure that they can separate their culture from yours.

2. *Cultural knowledge.* Your providers must take the time to learn about how different cultures view health and illness, promote prevention, and use health care systems (traditional, Western, etc.).

3. *Developing cultural skills.* Your health care team must be able to do a cultural assessment to obtain the best information about you and your culture. Larry Purnell and Betty Paulanka identified 11 areas that providers should assess for every individual to ensure they know each individual's cultural beliefs and practices. Your health care team can then provide cancer care that is relevant to you. (See *Questions Your Health Care Provider Can Ask about Your Culture,* developed by the Oncology Nursing Society, on pages 174–177, which reflects the 11 area/domains of culture and what types of questions you might be asked for each area.) You should feel free

to share any other information about yourself and your beliefs to ensure that you receive care based on your individual needs.

4. *Cultural encounters.* This step is the time in which you and your health care team interact. Tell them what you liked about your cancer care and whether anything else could be improved. Your ability to articulate your needs and desires is crucial to receiving culturally competent quality cancer care. You should understand the culture of the health care system and what it can and cannot do. Listening is a key skill both for you and the health care team members because it facilitates true partnership and understanding.

QUESTIONS YOUR HEALTH CARE PROVIDERS CAN ASK ABOUT YOUR CULTURE

TOPIC	POTENTIAL QUESTIONS
ETHNIC IDENTITY	• What ethnic group do you identify with? • What is your country of origin? • How long have you been in the United States? • What was your motivation to come to the United States? • Do you currently spend time, communicate, and participate in activities with other individuals from your ethnic group? • Do you feel you follow the majority of your country's traditions and practices more than you follow American traditions and practices?
COMMUNICATION	• What languages do you speak (specific dialects)? • What language do you usually speak at home and with your family and friends? • What languages do you read and write? • Who is the main communicator in your family? • How are decisions made in your family? • Who makes the majority of the decisions in your family? • Who would you prefer to provide you information and physical care (male or female, physician or nurse, older or younger person, etc.)? • If a translator is needed, who would be the most appropriate?

{continued}

TOPIC	POTENTIAL QUESTIONS
COMMUNICATION (CONTINUED)	• What is the most effective way to communicate with you? • What do you consider rude (eye contact, tone of voice, touch, etc.)?
TIME AND SPACE	• When you are talking with someone (a member of your health care team, family, friends, strangers, etc.), at what distance should they be from you? • Are you more focused on what has happened in the past, what is currently happening, or what will happen in the future?
SOCIAL ORGANIZATION	• Who is in your family? • Who do you live with? • Are there specifically identified roles within your family (who is the head of the house, who makes the decisions, how are decisions made, who works, who manages the family's health, etc.)? • What is the structure of your community? • How involved are you within your community? • What types of activities do you participate in? • Are you expected to participate in certain activities? • Do you like to participate in certain activities? • Does the cancer diagnosis change how you are viewed in your community or what you are allowed to do? • Have you told others about your cancer diagnosis?
FINANCIAL ISSUES	• Who is the primary wage earner in your family? • Has your cancer affected your ability to work? • Has your cancer affected others' work abilities? • How has the cancer impacted your finances? • Will your diagnosis impact the finances of family members in the long term? • Will your diagnosis affect your ability to work in the future? • Due to family work schedules, do you anticipate any problems getting to treatments? • Do you understand your legal rights to medical leave, insurance, and freedom from cancer-based discrimination?

{continued}

QUESTIONS YOUR HEALTH CARE PROVIDERS CAN ASK ABOUT YOUR CULTURE *(CONTINUED)*

TOPIC	POTENTIAL QUESTIONS
FINANCIAL ISSUES *(CONTINUED)*	• Are any physical or psychosocial issues related to your cancer causing you problems at work or at home?
HEALTH BELIEFS, PRACTICES, AND PRACTITIONERS	• What do you think caused your cancer? • What do you need to do to fight your cancer? • Do you see yourself as healthy or as ill? • Who do you usually see when you are not feeling well? • Are you currently using any herbs, vitamins, or other treatments to help fight cancer? • Do you see a healer in your community? • How do other cancer survivors act in your community? • Should any special rituals, healing ceremonies, or food and drink be considered in your treatment? • What has been your experience with others who have had cancer? • What are your thoughts and beliefs about transfusions, genetic testing, transplantation, surgery, and clinical research trials?
NUTRITION	• Do you consider any foods or drinks to be helpful or harmful to your health? • Are you currently on a special diet, supplements, or nutrition regime? • Who prepares your food? • Should it be prepared in a special way? • Do you ever fast, and if so, when and for how long? • How does cancer affect your nutrition? • Do you view foods in terms of hot or cold, and how they interact with different types of illnesses? • What weight and body size do you consider good for you?
PERSONAL HEALTH	• How do you currently care for your mouth, teeth, skin, hair, and private areas? • Have you ever been told that your ethnicity may increase your risk for certain illnesses?

{continued}

TOPIC	POTENTIAL QUESTIONS
SEXUALITY AND REPRODUCTION	• Has your cancer or treatment changed the way you see yourself or how you respond to loved ones, family, friends, or your community? • Has your cancer, cancer treatments, or any other illness or medication affected your ability to have sexual relations? • Do you want to have children now or in the future? • How do you get information about your sexuality and sexual function?
RELIGION, FAITH, AND SPIRITUALITY	• How do you identify your religion, faith, or spirituality? • If you are involved in a religious group, do you want to contact any members about your illness? • How would you describe what gives you meaning in life? • Who or what is your source of strength? • Are any symbols, items, foods, activities, prayers, or meditation important to you? • Do you need time to be alone or participate in a ceremony or prayer at a particular time?
DEATH AND DYING	• How do you view death and dying in terms of meaning, significance, and afterlife? • What are your thoughts on resuscitation? • Are certain preparations or care needs, either prior to or after death, important to you and your family? • Whom do you consider the most appropriate person to care for a body after death? • How is one talked about in relationship to dying or once they are dead? • How do family and friends from your culture usually react to someone dying or when they have died? • Who needs to be notified when one dies? • What type of funeral, wake, or other ceremony should take place once death has occurred? What is the time frame for such activities?

Based on information from Larry Purnell and Betty Pavlanka, *Transcultural Health Care: A Culturally Competent Approach* (FA Davis, Philadelphia: 1998); J. Brandt, et al., *Oncology Nursing Society Multicultural Outcomes: Guidelines for Cultural Competence* (Oncology Nursing Society, Pittsburgh: 2001); and K. Jennings-Dozier, et al., *Multicultural Tool Kit: Moving Toward Cultural Competence* (Oncology Nursing Society, Pittsburgh).

A person's culture is a dynamic process, as it changes daily in some way based on personal experiences and interactions. Many cancer survivors share common traits, experiences, and concerns over time, despite their individual cultural differences. They share a unique culture: the culture of survivorship. Common traits of cancer survivorship have been identified, such as

- uncertainty about the future
- loss of the "pre-cancer" life
- sense of abandonment by health care professionals at the end of treatment
- sanctuaries during the cancer journey (people, rest, resources that provide comfort and guidance during cancer treatment)
- survivors' lifelines (resources, activities, and individuals who assist in helping after treatment is completed)
- self-transcendence (personal growth from the experience)
- facing the financial cost of cancer
- circle of influence (how cancer survivors help others manage their cancer care)

Many survivors want to share their experience and knowledge with others like them. They want to give back to their communities, help community members with their cancer experiences, and dispel myths that cancer is not a death sentence. Learning from their own experiences, cancer survivors can give back by teaching health care teams how to provide culturally sensitive care, participating in peer support, and advocating on behalf of survivors with whom they share a common culture. Many cancer-related service groups and organizations strive to include a diversity of individuals to ensure that everyone has access to someone with whom they share a common culture and can comfortably discuss their cancer experience. Health care providers and other cancer survivors can benefit from learning about your cultural experiences. Do not hesitate to share your knowledge and skills with others. See Chapter 8 for suggestions on how to participate in peer support.

Many cancer resources are designed to address your specific cultural needs. These resources include educational material printed or spoken in many different languages, support groups, survivors' conferences, and services based on cultural groups (type of cancer diagnosis, ethnic group, age, gender, etc.). See Chapter 17 for a list of cancer resources. In addition, clinical trials and research activities are exploring the role of culture on cancer incidence, health practices, and treatment response. Your input and participation in these studies would help improve culturally competent cancer care.

Most survivors see their cancer experience as a journey that constantly changes and continues throughout life. One cancer survivor described how his newly acquired survivorship culture affected him as an individual:

I am a cancer survivor, but I am more than a s
part of who I am now, but not all of me. It ha
define what is important to me. It has shaped
things, and how I choose to live my life. I am
am. I have shared this journey with many othe
me, those I travel with now, and those who wil
We share many common paths, emotions, and
journey. . . . I am better for this as I have had t
and grow in ways I might never have imagined
am sure there will be more challenges in the fu
ney and who I am now.

In summary, when you are challenged with
ture of cancer survivorship, keep in mind that
and gives you strength to travel on the cancer j
meaning within the experience and shapes your
fore, your culture must be identified, assessed,
the framework for your cancer care.

I am a cancer survivor, but I am more than a survivor as cancer is not me. It is part of who I am now, but not all of me. It has made me look at myself and define what is important to me. It has shaped how I look at things, respond to things, and how I choose to live my life. I am more than the cancer; I am who I am. I have shared this journey with many others, those who have come before me, those I travel with now, and those who will travel the journey in the future. We share many common paths, emotions, and concerns, but we continue the journey. . . . I am better for this as I have had the chance to see my life and learn and grow in ways I might never have imagined. It hasn't always been easy, and I am sure there will be more challenges in the future, but I am proud of the journey and who I am now.

In summary, when you are challenged with a cancer diagnosis and the new culture of cancer survivorship, keep in mind that your culture keeps you grounded and gives you strength to travel on the cancer journey. Your culture helps you find meaning within the experience and shapes your responses to life situations. Therefore, your culture must be identified, assessed, respected, and ultimately become the framework for your cancer care.

Chapter Ten

Special Issues for the Older Survivor

by Elizabeth J. Clark, Ph.D., M.S.W., M.P.H.

$\mathcal{S}$OME READERS MIGHT WONDER why we need a separate chapter about the needs of older cancer survivors. Isn't cancer the same for everyone? First of all, cancer primarily is a disease of aging. According to the American Cancer Society, each year more than 60 percent of all newly diagnosed cancers occur in people over 65 years of age. In fact, the President's Cancer Panel in 1997 discussed the significance of the connection between cancer and the aging population and concluded that age is the single greatest risk factor for cancer. Every year almost three-quarters of a million people over 65—two of every 100 Americans—get cancer. If you are in this age group, many of your friends or relatives your age probably have had a cancer.

Managing cancer for older survivors can be more complicated than for younger survivors because many older persons already have at least one chronic health problem. Other issues for older cancer survivors include finding quality cancer care despite your age or other health problems, getting help paying for needed outpatient medications that are not covered under your insurance, and standing up for your rights in a health care system that sometimes discriminates against the elderly.

AGE DISCRIMINATION

Our society is reluctant to admit that our elderly are treated differently. But in American society we value youth more than the wisdom and contributions of older citizens. Discrimination against someone on the basis of age, called *ageism* or *age discrimination,* can be found in some of our health care institutions and care settings. Like racism or sexism, ageism is a negative view that some people attach to all persons of a certain age. Ageism assumes that the desires, fears, or concerns of older people are different from those of younger persons, and that they may not deserve the same credence or attention. Thus, you may have to work harder to get access to care, to get your concerns listened to, or to get excellent treatment.

For example, many people over 65 have had the experience of being called "grannie" or "gramps" instead of their own names. Frequently, the person using these greetings feels that they are being friendly or familiar. What they do not realize is that they are denying you your own identity. They are seeing you as just another older person with no uniqueness or diversity. Similarly, when care providers speak loudly when they talk to you, they assume that at your age you must have hearing problems.

More seriously, when you have a younger family member with you, your health care professional may speak directly to them, as though you were not in the room or were unable to understand the conversation. Worse yet, your health care team may decide, based solely on your age, that you cannot tolerate aggressive life-saving cancer therapies. Some health care institutions limit procedures such as bone marrow transplants to patients under 65 years of age, and some clinical trials exclude older patients.

The Alliance for Aging Research completed a study in 1999 asking women with early-stage breast cancer if they would prefer a mastectomy or a lumpectomy with radiation therapy. A majority of older women, as well as younger women, said they would prefer the lumpectomy. Yet data from the National Cancer Institute found that older women were more likely than younger women to get mastectomies for early-stage breast cancer. Some surgeons do not offer breast-sparing surgical options to older women, performing mastectomies rather than the less deforming lumpectomies. Some older women complain that they are not routinely offered breast reconstruction options, yet a majority of younger women are told of these options. These decisions may be the result of age discrimination, a belief that older women do not care as much about their body image as younger women, or the mistaken belief that older women are no longer sexually active, and so care less about sparing their breasts.

BEING AN ACTIVE OR PASSIVE PATIENT

Years ago, if you were sick, the doctor made all of the decisions about your care, often without consulting you. As recently as 25 years ago, some doctors would not tell patients that they had cancer. They would tell a family member, but not the patient, in an attempt to "spare them the bad news" or to protect them from the reality of the disease.

Fortunately, very few doctors act this way now. The patients' rights movement fostered change by demanding that patients be fully informed about their illnesses and that they have some input into decisions about their treatment and care. Additionally, stronger informed-consent laws required that patients must be fully informed not only about their illness and treatment, but also about any possible side effects that might result from the surgery or the medicines.

The other movement that has improved cancer care is the cancer survivorship movement. Numerous advocacy groups work to ensure that persons diagnosed with cancer receive quality care regardless of the type or stage of disease, their age, their ethnic background, or their insurance coverage.

These changes seem to be accepted more readily by younger cancer survivors. Many older persons still feel that the doctor is in charge. They are reluctant to question anything the doctor says or does. Older people are not as likely to question people in authority; some would see this as rude or disrespectful behavior.

Some older persons delegate their health care decisions to a child because they know their children have their best interests at heart. It is very important to identify a health care proxy for making decisions *if you are unable to do so,* to get the care and the treatments that are best for you (see chapter 14), but sometimes having a child make these decisions can lead to conflict. You may feel that you are unable to take a certain treatment, or do not want additional surgery, or do not want to change treatment to start a clinical trial. Your child may be willing to try anything to help you survive or live longer, but you may be ready to stop such aggressive measures and enjoy what remaining time you have left. Chapter 7 discusses managing family communication issues such as these.

Research confirms that informed patients usually do better in treatment. They know what they can tolerate, what to expect, what side effects to look for, and when to call their doctor or nurse with a question or problem. To live with a disease as serious as cancer, you must be willing to be an active participant in your care. Because of ageism, you may have to work harder than a younger survivor to advocate for quality medical care. You must voice your opinions, your concerns, and your wishes. You will find that most doctors and other care providers will be receptive to your concerns.

You may have other barriers to being an active participant, which can range from hearing or vision problems to not being able to read.

What If You Cannot Read, See, or Hear Well?

Most cancer survivors value information about their disease and treatment. Much of this information is provided in written format that has an average reading level of the tenth grade. Yet, 20 percent of the U.S. population read no higher than at a fifth-grade reading level. In fact, the average reading skill of adult Americans is the eighth-grade level. People who do not read well often are older, are members of an ethnic minority group, or speak a language other than English as their first language.

If you are older and do not read well, you may have found various ways to compensate. Limitations in literacy skills are rarely obvious. Persons with low literacy skills usually have normal intelligence. Reading problems, though, can affect good communication with your health care team, and thus the quality of your care. Health reading tasks include reading and signing informed-consent forms; understanding preoperative and postoperative instructions; and reading health education materials, discharge instructions, appointment slips, prescription labels, and insurance forms.

If you cannot read, see, or hear well, you must tell your health care team. While you may be embarrassed to tell people that you read poorly or not at all, that you do not speak or understand English well, or that you do not see or hear well, they must know this so they can better explain, and you can better understand, instructions and health materials. Sometimes it is easiest to have this conversation in private with your nurse. Oncology nurses have had experience with other cancer survivors with similar problems. They can make the health care team aware of your concerns and create an education program tailored to your needs.

KEEPING YOUR SPIRITS UP

If you are older, you likely have memories of relatives and friends who died from cancer many years ago. Some died without the benefit of good pain or symptom control. Others did not live very long after diagnosis. So, if you are diagnosed with cancer, you may be very fearful and still believe that cancer is an automatic death sentence. You may believe that nothing can be done for you or that the treatments are too horrendous to take. In fact, you may think, "What's the use? Why bother with treatment at all? Years ago I watched my aunt (or grandmother or sister) go through treatment, and she suffered greatly, and it didn't do her any good."

This type of thinking is dangerous and self-defeating. Cancer is now diagnosed at very early stages. More than one-half of those diagnosed are cured. Many others live with their cancer as a chronic illness for many years. Tremendous advances in cancer therapies and cancer management have been made in the past few years. Many drugs alleviate nausea and vomiting, reduce cancer-related fatigue, and control pain. Cancer-related depression is now successfully treated.

If you believe that your cancer is untreatable or that nothing can be done for you, you may doubt what your health care team or family members tell you. This can lead to family conflict and further sadness. Maintaining hope and a positive future outlook is essential to managing your cancer. Chapter 11 discusses hope in detail and gives you tips for remaining positive.

You also may have trouble deciding who to tell about your cancer diagnosis and when. You may be able to talk to your doctor and health care team, but find it hard to tell loved ones or friends. You may need to decide in advance what you want to say. Sometimes writing it down helps. It is okay to say, "I'm scared, but hopeful," or, "I'm relieved to finally know what is wrong." Consider setting ground rules for your family's involvement. You may need to ask them not to call your doctor or nurse without your permission, or to respect your privacy by not discussing your condition with friends or coworkers.

Dealing with acquaintances may be harder. Too often, especially in small towns, news of someone's illness becomes public. Also, some effects of cancer treatment, like hair loss, may be hard to hide. Many of your friends will be well meaning and will want to help in any way they can. Others, though, will be nosy and negative.

You may find that many people tell you a cancer story—about someone they knew with cancer who either died from it or had a terrible time with treatment. When you hear negative stories, advocate for yourself, even if you must be abrupt, perhaps even rude. Tell them that their comments are not helpful or that you do not want to hear about others whose situation may be very different from yours.

DEALING WITH DEPRESSION

Depression is not a normal consequence of aging. Most older people experience different losses as they age, but these do not routinely result in depression. For example, when a couple retires, they often have a reduced income. But this reduced income may have been planned for, and may be offset by their ability to travel or do things they love.

Similarly, health conditions such as arthritis or diabetes may have some limiting factors, but generally, individuals learn to live with and compensate for these limitations. Likewise older age brings changes in hearing and vision, but these, too, can be compensated for with the help of hearing aids and glasses.

Other losses might be more difficult to overcome. For example, older people who can no longer drive may lose independence. They may need to rely more on their network of friends and relatives for transportation and assistance, or make a major change such as moving into a child's home, an assisted living facility, or a nursing home. Giving up one's own home is a further loss.

As individuals age, they also lose loved ones and friends, sometimes several in a fairly short time period. They may lose a child, spouse, longtime partner, or best friend. These losses are especially hard to deal with, and being depressed about them is quite natural. It is called "reactive depression"—reacting normally to a loss in your environment. Chapter 11 discusses ways to manage loss and grief.

Despite losses, most older people are resilient. They find new interests and even new relationships. They have much experience in dealing with life crises and have strong coping mechanisms. They grieve and move on.

If, however, you have been living with chronic stress or constant worry, have pain or physical symptoms that are not well controlled, or have suffered several major losses in a fairly short period, you may develop a serious depression. Clinical depression is different from reactive depression or sadness. It is so major or so sustained that you cannot overcome it yourself. You will need professional help and perhaps antidepressant medicines. Research estimates that 5 to 10 percent of the elderly who visit primary care physicians have major depression, but only about one out of six who need help get it.

If, in addition to any of the problems discussed above, you now are diagnosed with cancer, you may feel that life is hopeless and that cancer is simply too much to deal with at this point in your life. You may be frightened and not think clearly.

When a person becomes hopeless, he or she also becomes powerless and helpless. People with clinical depression slow down, do less, and can be less hopeful.

Many good medications help manage depression. In addition to treating depression, these medications can help treat pain and control side effects from other medicines you may take for cancer.

If you have signs of depression, please find help. Talk to your doctor or nurse. Ask them how you can get your depression under control. Your doctor may give you a prescription for a special medication, or your nurse may refer you to a social worker or a psychologist specially trained to deal with cancer-related depression. When depression is treated, you will feel more hopeful. Also, depression can actually interfere with the healing process, which is the last thing you need when you are trying to recover from cancer.

Managing and Paying for Your Medications

As noted earlier, many people over age 65 have several chronic or acute medical conditions. When you are a cancer survivor, these other illnesses are referred to as comorbidities. Having several illnesses often means that you are taking many daily medications, which puts you at greater risk for adverse drug reactions.

The 1998 report "When Medicine Hurts Instead of Helps: Preventing Medication Problems in Older Persons," published by the Alliance for Aging Research, found that medication-related problems are particularly acute for the elderly. These problems include drowsiness, loss of coordination, and confusion—conditions that can result in serious accidents and hospitalizations.

The average older person uses four to five prescription medications and two over-the-counter drugs at the same time. As the number of prescription and nonprescription medications increases, so does the risk for problems. Drug-drug, drug-food, and drug-botanical interactions create serious concerns. Older Americans use 25 percent of all over-the-counter drugs purchased in this country. They also use many herbal and botanical products.

Keep good records of what medications, including the dosage, have been prescribed for you. Chapter 3 emphasizes the importance of using one pharmacy so that a professional monitors potential drug interactions for you. You must also tell your doctor and health care team what medications you are, and are not, taking, including all vitamins, herbal and botanical products, and old medications. People often keep unused portions of old prescriptions and then self-medicate when they think their symptoms are similar to past illnesses or problems. This can cause serious problems, especially if you are taking powerful chemotherapy drugs.

Cancer drugs are very expensive. Their high cost may cause you to take less medication than your doctor prescribes or to not fill a prescription. You may be embarrassed to tell your doctors or nurses you cannot afford the drugs they prescribe. Do not tell your doctor you are taking your drugs if you are not, and do not take less medication than prescribed.

Several options are available to help you pay for medication. First, your state may have a pharmaceutical assistance program that helps older persons pay for prescription drugs. Some of these programs are funded by state lottery programs and have been in existence for many years. Ask your local pharmacist if this is available in your state, or call your local or state Department on Aging to apply for these programs.

Also, most large drug companies have an indigent drug program that helps provide medications to people who cannot afford them. Do not be put off by the word "indigent." Cancer is an expensive disease. Many older persons live on restricted incomes. Cancer survivors cannot apply directly for these drug programs themselves, but your doctor, nurse, or social worker can help you get your drug costs covered. See Chapter 17 for a list of organizations that provide financial support to cancer survivors.

Finally, suggest to your children and others with whom you exchange gifts that you would enjoy gift certificates from your pharmacy or drugstore. You may resist asking for assistance, but your health is too important to let pride stand in the way of treatment.

TAKING CONTROL OF YOUR PAIN

Chronic pain is common in older persons. It frequently goes undetected or untreated. Many family members, cancer survivors, and even health care professionals believe that pain is an unavoidable consequence of aging. Many older people believe that you have to put up with pain and that it is a sign of weakness to talk about it or complain about it. Furthermore, many people believe that pain medication should be used very sparingly, if at all, because it can be addictive.

Uncontrolled pain creates numerous serious problems. It limits your social interactions, causing isolation. It compounds or causes depression. It may cause sleeplessness, increase your fatigue, and decrease your overall quality of life.

Pain can be safely controlled, but it requires a partnership between you and your health care team. Only you know how much pain you experience. Everyone has different tolerance levels for pain. Your level of tolerance cannot be compared to a friend's or relative's pain. Think carefully about how to describe your pain to your doctor or nurse. Is it continuous or intermittent (comes and goes)? Is it dull or does it throb? Is it related to movement or is it worse at night when you are lying down? These clues are important for your health care team. Consider keeping a record of your pain—how frequently you have it and its duration. By treating pain as any other symptom, such as a fever, you can more readily control it.

If your spouse, partner, or children are concerned about your taking pain medication, or are fearful of your becoming addicted, have them accompany you to an appointment and ask your doctor or nurse to reassure them about how unlikely addiction is. Chapter 7 discusses the challenges of good family communication.

TRANSPORTATION ISSUES

Transportation issues can be a concern for cancer survivors of any age, but they may be a special problem for the older survivor. Older persons may already have some problems driving, such as limited night vision or slower reflexes. When cancer treatment is added to the equation, at times the survivor may feel too shaky or weak to drive. Transportation often can be provided by family and friends.

Some older cancer survivors do not have others who can help, which may be especially true if the survivor has daily radiation treatments for several weeks or lengthy chemotherapy treatments. Also, your cancer treatment may be offered only at a cancer center that is far from your home.

First, ask your doctor's office or oncology nurse about transportation. Some agencies may have resources to assist you with your transportation needs. Call your local American Cancer Society, local unit of the Leukemia and Lymphoma Society, or the United Ostomy Association. If you have breast cancer, a community breast cancer group may help. If you have prostate cancer, a branch of US TOO, International may provide transportation.

You can also call your local area Agency on Aging or your state Department on Aging for assistance. Finally call the Eldercare Locator at 1-800-677-1116 or www.eldercare.gov. It is a nationwide directory assistance service designed to help older persons and caregivers locate local support resources. It links you with state and local agencies on aging that offer information about services such as transportation, home care, meals, housing alternatives, legal issues, and social activities.

SELF-ADVOCACY

All cancer survivors, regardless of age, can improve their quality of life during treatment by becoming informed self-advocates. One resource to help you learn how to collect information and advocate for yourself is the *Cancer Survival Toolbox: Building Skills That Work for You,* a training program written by cancer survivors, oncology social workers, and oncology nurses. It is available both by Internet and by ordering a set of audiotapes or CDs. You can read the content at www.cancersurvivaltoolbox.org. To order a free set of audiotapes or CDs, call 1-877-TOOLS-4-U (1-877-866-5748).

One of the nine programs of the *Cancer Survival Toolbox* is "Skills for the Older

Person with Cancer." It covers many of the same topics covered in this chapter, but in much more detail. The *Toolbox* gives case examples and exercises that you can practice so you can stand up for your rights and receive the best possible care. The *Toolbox* also comes with a comprehensive resource booklet to help you find assistance for a variety of problems.

Older cancer survivors have faced many life challenges, are resilient, have excellent coping strategies, and are often quite able to deal effectively with cancer. Today many millions of people of all ages are living full, productive lives after a cancer diagnosis. Age should not be a limiting factor in cancer survivorship.

Chapter Eleven

Confronting the
End of Life

by Elizabeth J. Clark, Ph.D., A.C.S.W., M.P.H.

S OME CANCER SURVIVORS and their families live with a chronic state of illness for many years; other cancer survivors never achieve remission of their cancer. Still others, despite excellent care and good initial responses to treatment, experience one or more recurrences or even develop a second, unrelated cancer. These situations sometimes become life-threatening; approximately one-half of all persons diagnosed with cancer eventually die from their disease.

Loss is a recurrent theme in cancer. While undergoing cancer treatment, you may experience physical and psychological losses, such as hair loss and loss of autonomy. Families also experience losses, such as loss of security, income, and dreams. Nothing, though, ever prepares us for the most severe loss, such as our own death or the death of a loved one.

Most people find it hard to think about death. Death usually is something that happens far in the future, when we are very old. In fact, in our society, advances in medicine and technology make it quite possible to reach middle adulthood without witnessing death or experiencing the loss of a loved one.

As a result, Americans are unfamiliar with dying and death. Frequently, patients ask health care professionals what it is like to die and what they can expect. Television provides the most frequent framework for death. As a result, death is often portrayed in unrealistic ways.

TASKS FOR THE PERSON WHO IS DYING

Elisabeth Kübler-Ross's groundbreaking study in the late 1960s set some guidelines about dying. Kübler-Ross identified five stages that most persons pass through when they reach a terminal stage of illness: denial, anger, bargaining, depression, and acceptance. Her work was not meant to be a directive for dying. Not everyone goes through all of the stages, nor in the order listed. Some people skip or repeat a stage. For example, not everyone reaches a stage of acceptance. However, the stages can help demystify dying.

Initially after learning of a terminal illness, people commonly deny bad news, believing that the test results or the doctor are wrong. Being told that an illness can no longer be cured or controlled creates great anxiety for most people. It takes time to absorb that information, to recognize the consequences, and to realize that your life will be shortened. Even though most people realize that they will eventually die, they still experience shock when the time draws near.

Anger is a common response to learning that your cancer cannot be successfully treated. Frequently, by the time people enter the terminal phase of an illness, they have gone through much treatment, followed medical instructions, and tried everything to survive. It seems unfair and unjust to have tried so hard, yet not be able to overcome the disease. This anger may be directed at the health care team, at God, at family or friends, or it may be internalized. Some people are angry because they feel they were misled or because they were naïve. They may even feel foolish because they undertook that last round of treatment when they themselves believed it would not help.

Anger frequently gives way to bargaining. Most people bargain in private, thinking, "If I can just live another year, or five years, or ten years I will..." or "I will not complain anymore if I can only do...." Learning that you are in a terminal stage of illness almost always causes some depression. You may feel great sadness and feel overwhelmed and immobilized. See pages 120–122 for more guidance on how to cope with cancer-related depression.

Depression can result because you are mourning your own losses; mourning is a normal, healthy response to loss. When you know your life is going to end in the next few months or weeks, you realize all that you will lose and miss. You had hoped to achieve or experience things that will not be possible now. You find it difficult to watch your loved ones mourn the impending loss of you in their everyday lives. When you are mourning your own losses, you may not be able to support others. Sometimes family members are so caught up in their own grief that they are unaware that the person who is dying is also mourning.

Some family members and friends become uncomfortable around a person who is dying. They may stop visiting or calling. They too are inexperienced with dying and death, and do not know what to do or what to say. So they stay away. Their inaccessibility can add to your own loss and can increase depression and feelings of isolation.

Often, the person who is dying must find a way to make others comfortable. This seems like an added and unfair burden. Sometimes you can help put the person at ease and improve your relationship by saying something like, "I may look different, but I am still the same person, and I want our relationship to remain the same as it was for whatever time I have left."

At the same time, as your illness progresses, you may find that you do not want many visitors, or that you want to be with only close family members or a special friend or two. Withdrawing from the outside world is a normal part of terminal illness.

Be honest with your own feelings and assess what you want to accomplish within the time you have left. If you know you have a life-ending illness, you usually have the benefit of some time to say good-byes, to make amends, to put your affairs in order, and even to plan your own funeral if you so desire.

You may have specific questions about dying. Doctors cannot pinpoint when people will die, so asking how much time you have left is not always the best question. It might be better to ask for a range of time: what is the shortest to the longest time expected? Other common questions for people in a terminal stage of illness include:

- Where will I die?
- What will dying be like?
- How will I know when the end is near?
- Will I suffer or be in pain?
- Will I be alert until the end?
- Who will care for me at the end?
- Should I be hospitalized or can I die at home?
- Do I want someone to be with me at the time of death?
- If so, who do I want this to be?
- What will happen to my body when I die?

Your doctor and health care team can answer some of these questions. You should also discuss these issues with your loved ones. These conversations are often difficult. It saddens your loved ones to talk about losing you, so you may find it is easier to avoid such conversations. However, making your wishes known and having plans in place regarding caregiving, pain control, and whether you will be hospitalized or will remain at home usually relieves anxiety for you and your family. See Chapter 7 for guidance on communicating with your family.

Family Tasks during Terminal Illness

Survivors must make most cancer-related decisions themselves. Some decisions and tasks, however, especially those concerning terminal illness, fall to family members. During the terminal phase, family members have many tasks to prepare for their loved one's death. Family members should address the following questions:

- What kind of medical care does our loved one want?
- Is the family in agreement about the death taking place at home?
- Can family members handle the caregiving and be available around the clock?
- Should we ask for a referral to a freestanding hospice or to a home-care hospice program?
- Even with home-care hospice services, if our loved one dies at home, how will death be pronounced and by whom?

Legal considerations need attention. Has your loved one signed an advance directive, durable power of attorney, or updated will? Does your loved one want to donate any organs? Chapter 14 discusses many of the legal decisions that should be made in advance to avoid legal and financial problems after death.

Perhaps the most difficult tasks facing the family are making preparations for the final weeks of life and planning the funeral. If your loved one is staying at home, will you need to make changes in sleeping arrangements or other home accommodations? How will caregiving duties be shared? How will you know when death is near? How and when will you notify family and close friends about impending death? Who will notify the funeral home?

Your local hospice or health care team can help you with many of these questions. They can also tell you what to expect during the final hours and how to deal with the physical changes as death occurs. An excellent resource that helps families prepare for a loved one's death at home is called "Dying at Home." You can get a copy of the booklet, which was written by professionals at the Massey Cancer Center in Virginia, by calling (804) 828-0450.

Your loved one may have expressed desired funeral arrangements. Decisions must be made about burial or cremation. If burial is chosen, a cemetery must be selected and a plot must be purchased.

- Will you have a tombstone or a grave marker, and how should it be engraved?
- Do you want a wake or viewing?
- Will you have a religious ceremony or a memorial service?
- Will the burial be private or open to the public?
- Does your loved one want flowers or prefer that memorial contributions be made to a favorite charity or community agency?
- Will the death be announced in the newspaper, and what information will be included in the obituary?

Reading the above paragraphs may make you think that you cannot handle the death-related tasks. You may even think that you cannot broach the subject of death with your loved one, but you can. Almost all persons in the terminal phase of life realize that they are going to die. They can feel themselves getting weaker. They may have asked a member of their health care team if they are dying. You do not want to waste the time you have left together trying to keep the truth from one another. Instead, use this time to say all of the important things you want to say: how much you have loved the person and how wonderful it has been to have him or her in your life. Express how much you will miss them. If possible, resolve past issues and make peace with the conditions that were not always right with your relationship.

Most people do not make significant changes during their final weeks or days of life. A person who has a lot of anger will probably die angry. Persons who have had a difficult time expressing personal feelings may still be unable to say all of the things they would like to say. The best you can do is approach the final hours with as much openness as is possible for you and your loved one. Sometimes touching, a very important form of communication, takes the place of talking.

HOSPICE CARE

Hospice care, sometimes called *palliative* care, is available to people with terminal illness who want to focus on comfort and control of symptoms. Your doctor, nurse, and social worker should work with you to make a decision about hospice care and to coordinate hospice services for you. Most people choose hospice care when they decide that they do not want treatment, such as chemotherapy or radiation therapy, but do want pain control and support. At this time, your doctor will refer you to a hospice in your area. The hospice will evaluate your medical and emotional needs and will work with you and your family to develop a plan of care.

Hospice care usually is provided in your home with backup care in the hospital or in a special unit of a hospital *(hospice care unit* or *palliative care unit)*. Some hospices that are separate from hospitals and have their own buildings are called *freestanding hospices.*

The purpose of hospice care is to provide physical comfort, especially pain control and emotional support, for you and your family. A nurse is usually your primary contact with a hospice program, but hospice staff includes physicians, social workers, clergy, and volunteers. All of these people may visit you at home. Someone is always on call to assist you and your caregivers. A hospice also provides bereavement counseling to family and friends after a person dies.

Many families who have participated in hospice care find that it offers tremendous comfort and relief to them as they deal with terminal illness. Families report that hospice care helps them provide comfort and a sense of peacefulness in addition to preparing them for the death of a loved one. However, home hospice care is not for everyone, particularly when the family feels it would be too difficult for them to provide care at home to someone who is very sick, when the caregivers are faced with too many other demands, or when it would be too upsetting to have someone die at home.

Sometimes, people want to keep treating the cancer and view hospice as a form of giving up. The decision to stop active treatment and focus on comfort is a complicated, emotional one for many families. You should gather information about local hospice services, discuss the options with everyone involved, and come to a decision that is shared by the patient and loved ones.

One other consideration is the timing of selecting hospice care. Hospice is designed to provide services for people with six months or less to live. All too often, hospice services do not begin until weeks or days before the death occurs, which does not give you enough time to plan the best death possible and help family members who need more assistance as the death of their loved one approaches. The members of your health care team should be involved in this process and should be able to offer you information and support as you deal with this difficult decision.

MAINTAINING HOPE

Most people forget that while a person may be dying, they are also living. They should live life as fully as possible in whatever time they have left. To do that, they must avoid despair and hopelessness. Despite the stage of illness or the direness of the situation, you always have something to hope for.

Hope is a way of thinking, feeling, and acting. It functions as a protective mechanism and is essential for managing and adapting to an illness as serious as cancer. Maintaining hope is not always easy. At times of crisis you may need additional support and assistance from your family, your health care team, and other cancer survivors.

Many people have never thought much about what role hope plays in their lives, about how they hope, or even how they learned to hope. Yet research shows that people hope very differently and that our personal hope is affected by various social factors. One of these factors is the way your family hopes.

Families have well-established ways of hoping. These patterns are called *family hope constellations.* They contain your family's values and norms regarding hope, and the strategies used to maintain hope. For example, some families use a religious or spiritual basis for their hope. As a result, statistics and medical facts may not be as important to this family because they believe God or a higher power will determine the outcome. These family members may draw great strength from prayer, clergy, and attending religious services.

Another family may use an educational or information basis for their hope. Their hoping strategies center on fact gathering. They read about cancer and its treatment. They seek second, third, and fourth opinions. For them, information provides control and hope.

No one family hope constellation is the best or most functional. You should consider how your own family thinks about hope and what strategies they use to maintain it. You should recognize, though, that individuals within your family may hope differently, particularly if they are part of your family through marriage and were raised differently.

Hope is broader than just the therapeutic aspect of treatment and control of disease. Hope has many dimensions. It changes over time as situations and reality change. Even when hope for survival dims, individuals and families can find something else to maintain hope. Perhaps you are hoping to have a family reunion, to see a child graduate from college, to welcome the birth of a new grandchild, or for a peaceful death. Always choose hope, because hopelessness leads to despair and helplessness. For more guidance on how to maintain hope during a cancer experience, see *You Have the Right to Be Hopeful* by Elizabeth J.

Clark, available from the National Coalition for Cancer Survivorship at (877) 622-7937.

MANAGING GRIEF

If you are the loved one of someone who dies, you need to grieve. Perhaps you began to grieve while you were preparing for the death and the funeral. Even if you did, the reality of the actual death is still overwhelming. For the first two weeks or so, you may feel numb. You may not accept the reality of the loss and may move through the days following the death and funeral as if you are in a fog.

After the numbness wears off, you may begin to acknowledge the finality of the loss and enter a period of despair. While people vary in how they deal with grief, the syndrome of acute grief is remarkably uniform. Most people have periods of crying and sadness, problems eating and sleeping, and restless pacing and sighing. You probably will engage in *searching behavior,* where you search for your loved one's face on passing buses and cars. You also may have auditory and visual hallucinations; you may think you briefly see your loved one, hear his or her voice, or hear the car pull into the garage at the usual time. These thoughts are caused by psychological cues and will decrease in time. They do not mean that you are going crazy; they are a normal part of the grieving process.

You also may find comfort in an object that links you to your loved one. You may wear a piece of his or her clothing or sleep in your loved one's bathrobe. This, too, is normal grieving behavior. Your need for the linking object will lessen over time.

RECOMMENDED GRIEVING BEHAVIORS

Four major tasks of mourning were identified over 50 years ago. They are to (1) accept the reality of the loss, (2) experience the pain of grief, (3) adjust to a changed environment in which your loved one is missing, and (4) emotionally relocate the loss in your life and move forward.

Grief counselors recommend certain behaviors for the period immediately following the death of a loved one:

- *Be gentle with yourself*—The experience of caring for a loved one over an extended period of time and witnessing his or her suffering and death is extremely difficult and draining. You will need time to recover physically and even more time to recover emotionally.
- *Do not expect too much of yourself* or of other family members who are grieving. Defer making important family and personal decisions, such as moving to a different location or making major purchases, for several months or even a year or more.
- *Recognize that grief cannot be postponed*—Grief has to reach expression in some way. If you cannot express your grief openly, your grief will come out in other emotions, such as displaced anger, guilt, anxiety, or physical symptoms.

- *Allow variation in grieving patterns* among family members. Grief, like hope, is individualistic; each person has to grieve in his or her own way.

HIDING GRIEF

American society is uncomfortable with grief. Individuals hide their feelings and emotions. Many persons reach adulthood without having experienced a loss by death. As a result, most people do not know what to say when someone dies and are unfamiliar with the normal grieving process. Additionally, many employers give their employees less than a week to bury a loved one and mourn the loss.

Denial of the significance of the loss makes grief harder. Bereaved persons are forced to hide their grief in public and act as though they have completed their grieving process and are "back to normal." This inability to be open about grief may extend the grief process.

Many people ask how long grief lasts. Others ask if it ever ends. The answer is different for everybody. Death ends a life; it changes, but does not end, a relationship. Researchers estimate that many people need at least one year to work through the grief process. Because grieving is an ongoing experience, researchers do not use terms like "finish grieving," "resolve the grief," or "get over the loss." Many people work through grief for many years. Most need at least one year because it takes a year to experience all of the anniversary dates for the first time with the loved one missing. These dates include holidays, birthdays, wedding and other anniversaries, and finally, the anniversary of the date of the death. You probably will have more difficulty during these periods, which is a normal reaction.

You can tell that your acute grieving is coming to an end when you can think about your loved one without feelings of intense pain. One woman was able to describe eloquently the pain she felt when her daughter died. She said that at first it felt like total body pain. Everything about her hurt. Eventually, it did not hurt quite so much, and after a longer time, she could think about her daughter without being consumed by painful feelings. She said that several years after her loss, she kept her pain in a special place in her heart. It was always with her; it just did not hurt as much anymore.

Some people who lose loved ones will benefit from grief counseling. Ask your doctor or other members of the health care team to recommend a counselor who specializes in helping people deal with grief. Ask your local hospice what services it provides. Most hospices provide mutual support groups for persons who have lost loved ones. You may find that a support group is right for you.

Perhaps the most important thing others can do to help friends or loved ones who are grieving is to recognize their need to grieve and to encourage them to express their feelings and sadness. Through expression comes healing.

Though cancer is no longer an automatic death sentence, and more than one-half of those diagnosed will be cured, more than 500,000 people die from cancer each year in the United States. Terminal illness is one of the most difficult crises faced by families. Yet, with open communication and through caring and support, family members can handle death in a positive way and gain a new perception and appreciation of each other. They can be enriched by the gifts of love they give and receive during their final days together.

RIGHTS OF THE BEREAVED

The bereaved have a right to expect optimal and considerate care for their dying loved one.

The bereaved have the right to a compassionate pronouncement of the death and to respectful and professional care of the body of their loved one.

The bereaved have the right to view the body, and to grieve at the bedside immediately following the death, if this is their wish.

The bereaved have the right to expect adequate and respectful professional care (both physical and emotional) for themselves at the time of their loved one's death.

The bereaved have a right not to consent to an autopsy and not to be coerced into consenting to an autopsy, regardless of how interesting or baffling the patient's disease, unless an autopsy is required by law.

The bereaved have the right to an adequate explanation of the cause of their loved one's death and to answers regarding the illness, treatment procedures, and treatment failures.

The bereaved have the right to choose the type of funeral service most consistent with their wishes and financial means and not to be coerced into something they do not want.

The bereaved have the right not to be exploited for financial gain or for education or research purposes.

The bereaved have a right to observe religious and social mourning rituals according to their wishes and customs.

The bereaved have a right to express openly their grief regardless of the cause of the loved one's death, even if by suicide or violence.

The bereaved have a right to expect health professionals to understand the process and characteristics of grief.

The bereaved have a right to education regarding coping with the process of grief.

The bereaved have a right to professional and lay bereavement support including assistance with insurance, medical bills, and legal concerns.

Elizabeth J. Clark, "Bereaved Persons Have Rights That Should Be Respected," in A. Kutscher et al., eds. (New York: Columbia University Press, 1987).

Part Three

Taking Care of Business: Insurance, Employment, Legal, and Financial Matters

Chapter Twelve

Straight Talk about Insurance and Health Plans

by Irene C. Card

*N*O LAW GUARANTEES that all cancer survivors can buy adequate, affordable health and life insurance. A number of laws, resources, and helpful suggestions, however, can make your search for insurance more productive. This chapter is intended to guide you through your right to health, disability, and life insurance. Terminology you may not be familiar with is defined in the glossary at the end of the chapter. In addition, Chapter 17 includes organizations and information, and a list of state insurance departments.

INTRODUCTION—HEALTH INSURANCE IN TRANSFORMATION

How we buy and use health insurance has changed dramatically during the past few decades. Your relationship with your insurance provider continues to be in a state of flux as states and the federal government pass new laws and as insurance companies respond to the market. This chapter provides a guide to help you understand your health insurance rights. Because laws often change, however, use the resources in this chapter and in Chapter 17 to ensure you have the most current information about your rights.

Insurance is sold to groups or individuals whom private companies consider a sufficient economic risk. Most companies consider cancer survivors to be a high risk. Cancer survivors often feel trapped and confused by the insurance system. They can resent a system that seems to prioritize cost controls over good medical care. Obstacles to obtaining, collecting on, and keeping insurance can hinder cancer survivors' efforts to receive needed medical care. Cancer survivors have to be very savvy consumers to make the system work for them. You must arm yourself with information about your rights and options for you and your dependents.

State and federal officials are increasingly aware of the need to reform the health insurance system so that cancer survivors and others can be assured it will include them and their health care needs. Carefully consider the impact of buying new insurance or changing your coverage in any way. You may find it useful to consult with an advocacy or patient service organization, an attorney or financial planner, your state insurance department, or other governmental agencies.

Types of Health Insurance

The market offers many different types of health insurance: fee-for-service or indemnity policies (what most people think of as traditional, private insurance); health maintenance organizations and their variations, known collectively as managed care plans; and public health insurance programs (Medicaid and Medicare).

Fee-for-Service (or Indemnity) Policies

It is exceedingly difficult to purchase what was known as traditional, fee-for-service health insurance. The doctor provided a service and was paid for it; insurance reimbursed the doctor or the patient according to "reasonable and customary fee schedules," and the patient was responsible for paying the doctor whatever amount was not covered by insurance. Those days are pretty much gone.

Today, even health insurance that individuals purchase themselves is connected to networks for reimbursement purposes. The plans may be known as *comprehensive major medical policies* or *comprehensive fee-for-service health insurance.* Reimbursement is based on contractual agreements between the provider and the insurer.

When a provider (hospital, doctor, therapist, etc.) is part of a network, it has signed a contract agreeing to accept a lesser fee for services that it provides to any member (patient) participating in the network plan. You may first have to meet a very high deductible. For example: You have a policy with a $1,500 deductible, and then it pays 70 percent. Your doctor, who is part of the network, charges you $125. Your doctor's office submits the claim to your insurance company. The "allowable" charge is only $75 (the amount the doctor agreed to when he or she signed the contract with the insurer). If you have not yet met your deductible, you must pay your doctor $75. If you have met your deductible, the insurance company will pay your doctor $75. Either way, your doctor cannot charge you the remaining $50 because he or she is in the network. If you went to a doctor out of the network, however, you would be responsible for the entire $125.

Managed Care Plans

The term "managed care" describes a mechanism designed to bring about cost-effective, quality health care. An HMO (health maintenance organization) is an example of a managed care plan.

Although the term "health maintenance organization" (HMO) was not coined until the 1970s, HMOs were first established in the United States before World War II to serve as both an insurer and a provider of medical care for their members. Today, many variations of the classic HMO model exist and new forms are emerging continually, although all HMOs can be characterized as various types of managed care. The most common managed care plans are HMOs, POSs, and PPOs.

HMO—Health Maintenance Organization

An HMO is a highly structured managed care plan. Members of an HMO receive health services only from the health professionals and hospitals that are under contract with the HMO. The HMO may employ the health care providers or they may be under contract with the plan as a member of the plan's network. With an HMO, you must choose a primary care physician (PCP) (either a family or general practitioner or an internist) from the directory of HMO providers. Many HMOs also will allow a female patient to choose a gynecologist as well. Your primary care physician will coordinate all of your medical care and can refer you only to specialists who are in the network of providers. Some states require HMOs to allow you to go out of network if the specialist you need is not part of the HMO network of providers.

With an HMO, you have very little, if any, freedom of choice. The advantage of an HMO is that you do not have to submit claim forms and wait for reimbursement. You usually are required to make a copayment at the time the service is rendered, ranging from $5 to $30 per visit. HMOs provide some routine services each year, such as a routine annual physical. In contrast, many other health insurance plans will pay only for a routine physical if you have a diagnosis. The major disadvantage of an HMO is that you have limited choices for receiving health care. You may wish to review the more comprehensive list of pros and cons of choosing an HMO on pages 218–219.

POS—Point-of-Service HMO

A POS plan is an HMO with the opportunity to go out of network. You still choose a primary care physician from the directory of physicians in the network, and this provider will coordinate all of your medical care. You simply make your copayment at the time of the visit. However, should you desire to see a provider who is not in the network, you may do so. The POS plan then works like a traditional indemnity plan. You reach a deductible first, and then the plan pays a certain percentage of the allowable charge (70 or 80 percent is the most common). You must submit a claim to the point-of-service plan to be reimbursed. The advantage of a point-of-service plan compared with an HMO is that you have more freedom of choice. It will cost you more money out of your pocket, but at least you can go where you desire to get another opinion. This flexibility is especially important for cancer patients.

PPO—Preferred Provider Organization

A PPO is a network of providers and facilities that have contracted with an insurance company to provide services to its members at discounted prices. You will be given a directory of providers and may choose anyone in the directory, including specialists. This is known as an "in-network" benefit. Most PPOs have a small copayment ranging from $5 to $25 per visit, depending on the plan. PPOs have no primary care physician; you choose anyone in the directory. Should you choose a provider who is not in the network, you must first meet a deductible before the plan will pay for the services. Although you may also have to pay a deductible if you choose a network provider, your total costs will be lower if you stay within the network. After the deductible, reimbursement will be at a fixed percentage, ranging from 60 to 80 percent, depending on the plan.

A PPO is often a bit more expensive than an HMO or POS, but the big advantage is freedom of choice and "no permission needed."

FINDING THE RIGHT MANAGED CARE PLAN—Shopping for the best managed care plan to care for you and your family can be difficult under the best of circumstances. Some managed care plans may restrict your access to the best oncology care tailored for your needs. These organizations also are notorious for their unwillingness to disclose information about their plans before a contract has been signed. Information about which health care providers and hospitals are in their networks, however, can be critically important to cancer survivors. Some states have passed laws requiring managed care organizations to make information available to the public to help prospective customers choose a plan. Before choosing a managed care plan, review the pros and cons of Medicare HMOs on page 218–219, and consider the following suggestions:

Look for a network where your physicians practice—If you have a choice between managed care plans, ask your doctor which managed care plans he or she has joined. Ideally, your entire health care team has joined a managed care plan at the same time. Thus, that plan may guarantee you coverage of services provided by any member of the team at less cost than you were paying under traditional fee-for-service insurance.

Learn whether the services and specialists you may need at some point during your treatment are included in the plan—These could include a comprehensive cancer center; a selection of board-certified oncologists, including at least one who is particularly experienced in treating your type of cancer; conveniently located radiation therapy services; pain specialists; and home care, mental health, and prescription drug coverage. If any of these features are not guaranteed by the plan, you may want to choose a point-of-service (POS) or a PPO plan that provides coverage for services outside the network of approved providers.

Determine what requirements the plan will impose on you—Will you have to select a primary care provider who must preapprove all of your care, even during chemotherapy or radiation therapy, or will the plan allow your oncologist to act as your care coordinator during a course of treatment? Who will monitor you after your treatment?

Determine if the plan guarantees coverage of a specialist or service outside of the network if no provider in the plan can provide that service.

What percentage of your premiums actually goes toward medical care versus administrative fees?—The term for this in the insurance industry is medical loss ratio. For example, if the loss ratio is 80 percent, 20 percent of the premiums are being used to conduct the business of administering the plan, and 80 percent goes toward medical care. Typical loss ratios in traditional insurance are in the 70 to 80 percent range, although some nonprofit insurers maintain ratios closer to 90 percent.

What specifically is excluded from the plan?—What are your rights and responsibilities if you wanted to appeal a decision by the plan that denied coverage of something your doctor recommended?

Is the plan accredited by the National Committee for Quality Assurance (NCQA)?—Arguably, NCQA accreditation does not guarantee that it is the best plan for you and your family, but it may indicate a better plan than a competing one that does not have NCQA accreditation. The most telling piece of information about NCQA accreditation may be if the plan has been turned down for it. See **www.NCQA.org** for more information.

What provisions or limitations would the plan impose if you needed medical care when traveling?

SELF-FUNDED (SELF-INSURED) INSURANCE PLANS

Large companies usually find it more cost effective to self-fund their health insurance benefits plan. The employer pays claims based on actual expenses rather than anticipated claims. Funds are set aside from which to pay claims to a certain dollar limit per person and for the entire group. This is the portion of the plan that is self-funded. A good self-funded plan will have a reinsurance policy to pick up after an individual's or the entire group's expenses reach a certain dollar limit.

The claims employees file to obtain their reimbursement through these plans are likely to be administered by commercial insurance companies. Most people covered through self-insured plans, therefore, do not realize their health insurance is somewhat different from insurance purchased by an insurance company. Generally, large employer groups and unions find it beneficial to self-insure, while smaller employer groups choose to finance employee health benefits through commercial insurers. Ask your employer whether your health insurance policy is self-insured, because self-insured plans are exempt from most state and some federal laws. See page 224 for more information on your legal rights if you have a self-insured plan.

HOSPITAL INDEMNITY POLICIES

A hospital indemnity policy pays a daily benefit for each 24-hour period that you are in a hospital. These policies are a source of extra cash during an illness because benefits are paid directly to you in cash for you to use as you see fit. Hospital indemnity policies are relatively inexpensive and simple; you only need to submit proof of how many days you were hospitalized to collect. A fixed amount is paid for each day you were in the hospital, regardless of the actual charges, although some policies may not pay for the first few days. Try to find a policy that pays benefits starting the first day of your hospitalization. An inpatient hospital policy is a "nice little extra" for high-risk individuals who are very likely to be hospitalized numerous times. Many of these policies have a two-year waiting period for persons with preexisting conditions. The American Association of Retired Persons (AARP) will sell hospital indemnity policies to anyone 50 years of age or older. Their policies have only a three-month waiting period for preexisting conditions. A hospital indemnity policy does not take the place of your comprehensive or managed care insurance plan; it is something extra.

CANCER INSURANCE

Some insurance companies market cancer policies, which pay benefits only for cancer treatment. Such policies generally are sold only to people who have no previous history of cancer. Because of the many disadvantages of cancer policies, many states have banned or restricted their sale. Most insurance experts recommend buying good basic and major medical plans instead of disease-specific policies for five reasons:

1. Major medical plans usually cover the costs of cancer treatment; additional cancer policies usually duplicate other policies and are an unnecessary expense.
2. Premiums are very high for limited benefits.
3. Cancer policies often exclude coverage of complications from cancer treatment.
4. Some policy salespersons try to mislead consumers and prey on their fears about cancer.
5. Sales and administrative expenses for cancer policies tend to be much higher than other policies.

DISABILITY INSURANCE

Disability insurance is a type of indemnity health insurance. You may receive disability insurance as an employee benefit or buy it yourself. It will pay you a cash amount representing a percentage of your regular income should you become unable to work due to illness. However, many provisions of these policies can differ quite dramatically; you will want to comparison shop. The chart below can help you compare different plans.

ANALYZING AND EVALUATING DISABILITY INSURANCE

FEATURE	VERY GOOD	FAIR	POOR
Elimination period	1–3 mos.	6 mos.	12 mos.
Benefit period	Lifetime, or to age 65	5–10 yrs.	1–2 yrs.
Noncancellable?	Yes		No
Guaranteed renewable?	Yes		No
Benefits for partial disability?	Yes	Yes, following total disability	No
Contract definition of disability	Inability to perform the major tasks of your occupation	Inability to engage in any occupation for which one is reasonably suited by education, training, and experience	Unable to engage in any occupation
Taxable income?	No	Partially	Yes
Pre-existing condition exclusion?	None	All preex. conditions excluded 6–12 months	Requires 12 months treatment-free period
A.M. Best Rating	A+, A	B+, B	C or lower

Excerpted and copied with permission of Affording Care.

LONG-TERM CARE INSURANCE

Long-term care insurance provides you with a daily benefit when you need substantial assistance with two out of six of the activities of daily living, such as eating, bathing, dressing, transferring, continence, or toileting. It also is available if you have a cognitive impairment. A good long-term care insurance policy will provide you with a daily benefit regardless of where you receive the care. It can be at your home, in an assisted living facility, an adult day care center, or in a nursing home receiving either skilled, intermediate, or custodial care.

The ideal time to purchase long-term care insurance is in your 50s or 60s as part of your retirement planning. You must be in fairly good health to purchase it. It is not for everyone. Cancer survivors can purchase long-term care insurance, depending on the type of cancer they have had and how long they have been in remission. As a general rule, insurance companies want you to be five years post-treatment, but this varies depending on the type of cancer you had. All of these policies are medically underwritten, which means that the insurance company will review your medical records, which they will request from your physician. The premium is determined by your age and your medical history. You can request a copy of "A Shopper's Guide to Long-Term Care Insurance" from:

The National Association of Insurance Commissioners
120 W. 12th Street, Suite 1100
Kansas City, MO 64105-1925
816-842-3600
www.naic.org

MEDICARE

Medicare and Medicaid are sometimes referred to as "public health insurance." Medicare is health insurance provided by the federal government and funded through the Social Security program. Any person who meets any of the following criteria qualifies for Medicare:

- Sixty-five years or older and entitled to either Social Security, Widow's, or Railroad Retirement benefits;
- Totally disabled and, regardless of age, collecting Social Security benefits for at least 24 months;
- Legally blind; or
- On renal dialysis regardless of age.

Medicare Part A covers the hospital bill and charges from other health care facilities if eligibility requirements are met. Part A, which has no premium, is provided free and paid through the Social Security program (as long as you are 65 or older and have contributed to at least 40 Social Security quarters). If you are 65 or older

MEDICARE PREVENTIVE SERVICES HELPFUL TO CANCER SURVIVORS

COVERED SERVICE	WHO IS COVERED	WHAT YOU PAY
BONE MASS MEASUREMENTS Varies with your health status.	Certain people with Medicare who are at risk for losing bone mass.	20 percent of the Medicare-approved amount or a set coinsurance amount after the yearly Part B deductible.
COLORECTAL CANCER SCREENINGS • Fecal Occult Blood Test—Once every 12 months. • Flexibility Sigmoidoscopy—Once every 48 months. • Colonoscopy—Once every 24 months if you are at high risk for colon cancer. • Barium Enema—Doctor can substitute for sigmoidoscopy or colonoscopy.	All people with Medicare age 50 and older. However, there is no age limit for having a colonoscopy.	Nothing for the fecal occult blood test. For all other tests, 20 percent of the Medicare-approved amount after the yearly Part B deductible. Your costs may be different if you get these services in a hospital.
MAMMOGRAM SCREENING Once every 12 months. You can get one baseline mammogram between ages 35 and 39.	All women with Medicare age 40 and older.	20 percent of the Medicare-approved amount with no Part B deductible.
PAP SMEAR AND PELVIC EXAMINATION (Includes a clinical breast exam) Once every 36 months.	All women with Medicare.	Nothing for the Pap smear lab test. For Pap smear collection, pelvic and breast exams, 20 percent of the Medicare-

{continued}

COVERED SERVICE	WHO IS COVERED	WHAT YOU PAY
Once every 12 months if you are at high risk for cervical or vaginal cancer, or are of child-bearing age and had an abnormal Pap smear in the past 36 months.		approved amount or a set coinsurance amount with no Part B deductible.
PROSTATE CANCER SCREENING • Digital Rectal Examination—Once every 12 months • Prostate Specific Antigen (PSA) Test—Once every 12 months	All men with Medicare age 50 and older.	20 percent of the Medicare-approved amount after the yearly Part B deductible. No coinsurance and no Part B deductible for the PSA Test.

but have made fewer than 40 quarters' worth of contributions to Social Security, you are eligible for Medicare Part A, but you will have to pay a premium.

A benefit period consists of 60 days. If you are out of the hospital for more than 60 days, a new period begins and you must meet the deductible all over again. If you reenter the hospital within 60 days of your last discharge date, you do not have to meet the deductible again. After the deductible-per-benefit period, Part A will pay the hospital bill in full for the first 60 days.

Medicare Part B covers your medical expenses, durable medical equipment, and certain other supplies. For example, Part B pays for incontinence products for ostomy patients. Part B has a small deductible. A monthly premium is deducted directly from your Social Security check.

Part B Medicare will pay for most medically necessary services rendered, but will not pay for

- Routine annual physicals unless you have a diagnosis.
- Experimental treatment.
- Any services rendered outside of the United States, unless the individual is close to a border (Canada or Mexico) and the nearest hospital is outside of the United States.
- Prescription drugs, with one exception: Chemotherapy drugs that are injected intravenously or by intravenous pump are covered by Medicare. If the doctor provides the drug, Part B will cover it. If the doctor gives the

patient a prescription to get filled and the patient takes the drug to the office for injection, a copy of the actual prescription must be sent to Medicare with the pharmacy receipt.
- Syringes or insulin for diabetic patients.

When Medicare first started in 1965, it was intended for acute care only, but over the years, many more benefits have been added. Medicare now covers certain routine services, although it does not pay for a routine annual physical unless you have a diagnosis. In late 2003, Congress amended Medicare to permit an optional, limited prescription benefit effective January 1, 2006.

MEDICARE COVERAGE FOR CLINICAL TRIALS

If you are in a clinical trial for cancer treatment, Medicare will pay anything normally covered by Medicare, including the following:
- Tests, procedures, and doctors' visits.
- Experimental treatment. For example, Medicare will pay for giving you a new drug intravenously, including therapy to prevent side effects from the new drug.
- A test or hospitalization resulting from a side effect of new treatment provided in the clinical trial.

Medicare will not cover:
- Investigational items or services being tested in a clinical trial. Sponsors of clinical trials often provide new drugs for free, but ask your doctor before you begin treatment.
- Items or services used solely for the data collection needs of the trial.
- Anything being provided free by the trial's sponsor.

Medicare will cover cancer treatment and diagnosis during clinical trials if:
- They are funded by the National Cancer Institute (NCI), NCI-Designated Cancer Centers, NCI-Sponsored Clinical Trials Cooperative Groups, or any other federal agency that funds cancer research. Other trials may be eligible for coverage, and doctors can ask Medicare to pay patients' costs.
- They are designed to treat or diagnose your cancer.
- The purpose or subject of the trial is within a Medicare benefit category. For example, cancer diagnoses and treatment are covered; cancer prevention is not covered.

Clinical laboratory procedures—such as blood tests, urinalyses, and cultures—are covered. If the doctor processes the blood and receives the results, he or she must accept assignment, and Medicare will pay the doctor 100 percent of whatever it approves. Doctors who draw blood at their offices can charge $3 for collection and interpretation. In most cases, the doctor draws the blood and sends it to an outside laboratory. The laboratory must then bill Medicare, and Medicare pays the laboratory 100 percent of the approved amount. Many times laboratories are not notified that the patient is on Medicare. If you receive a bill from a laboratory, you should simply write your Medicare number on the bill and send it back to the laboratory.

A participating physician accepts assignment on all Medicare patients. The physician can charge only what Medicare approves. Medicare pays 80 percent of the approved amount, and you are responsible for 20 percent of the approved amount. When the doctor accepts assignment, Medicare mails the check to the doctor.

A nonparticipating physician does not accept assignment. You are responsible for the entire charge. However, the doctor is not allowed to charge you more than 15 percent above that which Medicare approves for the service, although some states require you to pay a smaller percentage. Nonparticipating doctors can still choose to accept assignment on a case-by-case basis. On no-assignment claims, the Medicare payments are mailed directly to the patient, and the patient is responsible for paying the doctor.

TEFRA/DEFRA–If you continue to be actively employed when you become eligible for Medicare, TEFRA and DEFRA are two federal laws that govern which of your claims will be paid by your group health insurance and which will be paid by Medicare.

If you continue to be employed actively 30 hours per week or more for a company with 20 or more employees, your group insurance is primary and Medicare is secondary. If you are retired and your spouse is employed 30 hours or more per week by a company with 20 or more employees, and you are covered under your spouse's health insurance policy, the group insurance plan is primary and Medicare is secondary.

If you are TEFRA/DEFRA eligible, you probably do not require Part B Medicare. Once you or your spouse decides to retire, however, the employer must write a letter to the Social Security Administration giving your Social Security

---

MEDICARE RESOURCES

Medicare and You, published annually by the Centers for Medicaid and Medicare (formerly the Health Care Financing Administration), is an excellent guidebook to understanding Medicare. You can get a copy in any Social Security office or call 1-800-633-4227. The Web site address for Medicare is www.Medicare.gov.

The Centers for Medicaid and Medicare (formerly the Health Care Financing Administration) also publishes an annual *Guide to Health Insurance for People with Medicare.* Obtain a copy at any Social Security office or by calling the Medicare Hotline at 1-800-638-6833.

number and the effective date of your retirement, stating you will no longer be covered under the group insurance plan as primary insurer. Take this letter to your Social Security office. This is very important so that you may obtain Part B (medical) benefits effective the date of your retirement. If you neglect to do this, you can purchase Part B Medicare only during the open enrollment period in January, February, or March of each calendar year, and the benefits become effective July 1 of that year. In addition, you will have to pay a 10 percent increase in premium for each year you did not have Medicare. You can save this added expense and waiting period by having your employer notify the Social Security Administration in writing of your retirement or your spouse's retirement. Then your Medicare benefits are effective immediately, and you are not penalized by having to pay additional premiums.

MEDICARE SUPPLEMENTAL OR "MEDIGAP" PLANS—When you retire and are eligible for Medicare, you may or may not be able to continue your group health insurance plan as secondary to Medicare. If you are able to continue your group benefits once you are eligible for Medicare, it will be secondary to Medicare and it may or may not provide prescription benefits. If you cannot continue your group health insurance benefits (and most people cannot), then you should consider purchasing a Medigap policy to "fill in the gaps" and pick up where Medicare leaves off.

Congress has standardized the Medigap market. Since 1992, insurance companies that sell Medigap policies can sell only standard Medigap plans identified as Plans A through J. Every state insurance commissioner determines which of the 10 plans will be available for sale in their state. Plan A consists of the very basic benefits and Plan J the most deluxe, including up to $3,000 in prescription benefits. For complete details on the 10 standard plans and the benefits provided by each, request a copy of the *Guide to Health Insurance for People with Medicare* from the Centers for Medicaid and Medicare.

Congress mandated that the benefits be identical on all of these plans regardless of where you purchase the policy. The only differences will be the premium and the service you receive from the companies. Some companies waive any waiting period for preexisting conditions if you buy the supplement the month you turn 65, and some waive the waiting period for preexisting conditions if the policy is replacing another Medicare supplement or other medical coverage. Congress has further mandated a six-month open-enrollment period for buying Medicare supplemental health insurance. This law guarantees that for the six months immediately following enrollment in Part B, persons age 65 or older cannot be denied Medigap insurance because of their health status or history. Thus, you must be issued a Medigap policy regardless of your health, and the waiting period for preexisting conditions cannot be longer than six months.

Each of the ten plans has a letter designation ranging from "A" through "J."

MEDIGAP PLAN BENEFITS

					PLAN					
	A	B	C	D	E	F	G	H	I	J
CORE BENEFITS										
Part A hospital (days 61–90)	X	X	X	X	X	X	X	X	X	X
Lifetime reserve (days 91–150)	X	X	X	X	X	X	X	X	X	X
365 Life hosp. days—100%	X	X	X	X	X	X	X	X	X	X
Part B coinsurance	X	X	X	X	X	X	X	X	X	X
ADDITIONAL BENEFITS										
Skilled nursing facility coinsurance			X	X	X	X	X	X	X	X
Part A deductible		X	X	X	X	X	X	X	X	X
Part B deductible			X			X				X
Part B excess charges						100%	80%		100%	100%
Foreign travel emergency			X	X	X	X	X	X	X	X
Recovery at home				X			X		X	X
Prescription drugs*								1	1	2
Preventive medical care					X				X	X

*Two plans provide some prescription drug benefits: Plans H and I offer a basic benefit with a $250 deductible, 50 percent coinsurance, and a $1,250 maximum annual benefit.

Plan J has a $250 annual deductible, 50 percent coinsurance, and a $3,000 maximum annual benefit.

Core benefits pay the patient's share of Medicare's approved amount for physician services (20 percent) after 100 percent annual deductible, the patient's cost of a long hospital stays and charges for the first three pints of blood not covered by Medicare.

Insurance companies are not permitted to change these designations or to substitute other names or titles. They may, however, add names or titles to these letter designations. While companies are not required to offer all of the plans approved for sale by the individual states, they must make Plan A available if they sell any of the other nine plans in a state.

Medigap policies can be problematic for people who are on Medicare because of a disability and are under age 65. Most states require any company selling Medigap policies must sell Plan A or Plan C to anyone eligible for Medicare under the age of 65. Plan C is the better choice because it pays the Part A inpatient deductible. Plan A does not cover it.

MEDICARE HMOs–When you become eligible for Medicare, you have two choices. You can participate in the traditional or "original" Medicare program, as described on page 211. If so, consider buying a Medicare supplement policy or group health insurance from a former employer to supplement the traditional or "original" Medicare benefits. As another option, you may choose an HMO instead of the "original" Medicare program.

Medicare HMOs contract with Medicare to provide the full range of Medicare-covered services to Medicare beneficiaries. To be a member, you must continue to pay your Part B monthly premium to Medicare. Medicare, in turn, pays the HMO for providing you with health care. Certain HMOs also require you to pay some additional fees. Most Medicare HMOs are risk-based HMOs, meaning the HMO will receive a set fee from Medicare for each enrollee, regardless of the number of services received or the cost of delivering those services. The HMOs assume the "risk" that caring for you will not cost more than they receive from Medicare to do so.

As a Medicare risk member, you will pick a primary care physician who will coordinate your care, and in conjunction with plan administrators, decide when you may see a specialist or go to the hospital. Like traditional HMOs, in Medicare HMOs, you can use only the health professionals in the HMO network. HMOs offer some clear advantages and disadvantages to cancer survivors.

Medicare HMOs are not for everyone. In exchange for some additional benefits, you give up freedom to choose your health care provider.

DISADVANTAGES OF MEDICARE HMOs:
- You will lose some control over your health care decisions.
- You will be covered only for health care services received through the HMO, except in emergency and urgent care situations. Generally, if you take long trips or spend part of the year outside the HMO plan area, or expect to be away for more than 90 days, joining an HMO is not in your best interest.
- You will not be able to see a specialist or be admitted to the hospital (except in emergencies) without authorization from your HMO primary care physician.

- No system measures the quality of treatment options paid for by HMOs. An HMO will limit your freedom of choice and may compromise the level of care you receive.

ADVANTAGES OF MEDICARE HMOS:
- You may receive coverage for services that Medicare does not cover. HMOs generally offer free checkups and other preventive care services. They may also offer limited routine eye care, limited hearing care, free transportation to and from the HMO, and limited prescription drug coverage.
- You will not need Medigap insurance.
- You will not have to pay the Medicare deductibles or coinsurance.
- Your premium may be less than that of a Medicare supplement (Medigap).

Generally, HMOs work best for young, healthy people in their childbearing years because of all of the routine and wellness benefits they offer. People dealing with diagnoses and serious or life-threatening illnesses may prefer to have complete freedom of choice. For example, one cancer survivor was faced with the following situation:

> At age 65 Tom was healthy and could not see the need to spend $75 a month on a Medigap policy, so he chose an HMO instead of the traditional Medicare program. Three months later he was diagnosed with a rare cancer. A major cancer treatment center in New York City had a branch in one of the suburban hospitals near his home. The HMO covered his treatment at the local "branch" hospital, but when its doctors wanted him to go to the New York facility for a week to get started on a regimen, the HMO refused to pay for the New York hospital. He had to take out a home equity loan to cover the week in the New York hospital.

Many HMOs are withdrawing from the "senior" Medicare market. On January 1, 2000, nearly 1 million seniors were unilaterally dropped from their Medicare HMOs; 700,000 seniors were dropped from their HMOs between 1998 and 1999. If this happens to you, you will automatically be enrolled in the traditional Medicare program on the date that the HMO withdraws from your state. Any company selling Medigap policies must sell you a policy, regardless of your health, with no waiting period for preexisting conditions.

PRESCRIPTION BENEFITS FOR SENIORS

A significant problem for seniors is that Medicare does not cover oral medications. Medicare pays only for certain chemotherapy drugs (and a few others) that are injected intravenously or with a pump by a physician.

You may be able to continue your group health insurance benefits from your former employer as secondary to Medicare. Most people, however, lose their comprehensive major medical benefits when they retire and must purchase Medigap or supplemental insurance to pick up where Medicare leaves off. See page 216 for a discussion of Medigap.

Until Medicare provides prescription benefits, or if you choose not to participate in Medicare's optional prescription plans, here are some options if you are ineligible to stay on a group health insurance plan:

1. Three Medigap policies (*H, I,* and *J*) provide limited prescription benefits, but they are quite expensive. You cannot be refused these plans if you buy them within six months of becoming eligible for Part B Medicare once you are age 65. If you wait beyond that time, insurance companies selling these plans do not have to sell them to you if you are already taking prescription medications.

2. Comparison shopping is very important. You can save as much as 40 percent when comparing one pharmacy with another.

3. Purchase a discount prescription card, which will entitle you to a discount on the drug. Some of these cards work well in your local pharmacy but the discount will be much greater if you use mail order services. You should not pay more than $40 a year for such a card.

4. If you are a veteran (this does not mean you saw combat; it means you wore a uniform in the service of your country and received an honorable or general discharge), you can obtain your prescriptions through a Veterans Administration (VA) medical center for only $2. Look in the blue pages of your telephone directory for the number of the nearest VA facility to call for information.

MEDICAID

Medicaid is a jointly financed federal-state insurance program for low-income families. The federal government administers Medicaid through the Centers for Medicaid and Medicare of the Department of Health and Human Services. Each state has a single agency (usually the Department of Social Services or the Department of Public Welfare) that administers Medicaid in that state.

The federal government requires certain basic benefits; each state then determines what additional benefits it will provide and who is eligible. Because states have some role in determining who is eligible for Medicaid and what benefits are paid, Medicaid coverage varies widely from state to state. Every state, however, must give you a fair hearing before its state agency if your Medicaid claim is denied. The types of expenses covered by Medicaid may include hospitals, physicians, prescription drugs, and home aids. For more information about Medicaid, contact your state public welfare department.

MEDICARE/MEDICAID DUAL ELIGIBILITY—Through the Qualified Medicare Beneficiary (QMB) or "Medicare Buy-in" Program, Medicare beneficiaries can get Medicaid to pay their Medicare premiums, deductibles, and coinsurance.

However, not all physicians will agree to accept the Medicaid reimbursement rates. If a doctor does not accept Medicaid, Medicare will pay 80 percent and you will be responsible for any unmet deductible and the 20 percent coinsurance. Under the Specified Low-Income Medicare Beneficiary (SLMB) program, Medicare Part B premiums for those living between 100 and 120 percent of the federal poverty level will be covered by the program. For more information about both programs, call the national Medicare hot line at (800) MEDICARE (633-4227).

ACCESS TO HEALTH INSURANCE

CONTRACTUAL RIGHTS

An insurance policy is a contract between you (the insured) and your insurance company (the insurer). Your obligations under the contract are to pay your premiums on time and to provide your insurance company with the information it requests to process your claim. Your insurance company's obligations are to pay you benefits and provide other services as spelled out in the policy. If you meet your obligations, but your insurance company refuses to pay benefits (or perform another duty, such as renew your policy) in accordance with the terms of the policy, you may be able to sue your company for breach of contract. In addition to your contractual rights conferred by your insurance policy, you have other rights to health insurance under federal and state laws.

FEDERAL LAWS

No federal law guarantees a right to adequate health insurance. Four laws—the Health Insurance Portability and Accountability Act of 1996, COBRA, ERISA, and the Americans with Disabilities Act (ADA)—however, provide cancer survivors opportunities to keep health insurance they obtain at work, even after they are no longer employed. (See page 248 for an explanation of how the ADA applies to health insurance.)

THE HEALTH INSURANCE PORTABILITY AND ACCOUNTABILITY ACT OF 1996–The Health Insurance Portability and Accountability Act of 1996 (HIPAA) provides that no one can be denied health insurance because of a preexisting condition. They may, however, have a waiting period for preexisting conditions. State laws may offer more, but not fewer, benefits than those available under the federal HIPAA. While HIPAA is primarily a law for employer-sponsored group health plans, it also guarantees access to individual insurance to "eligible individuals."

A preexisting condition must relate to a condition for which medical advice, diagnosis, care, or treatment was recommended or received during the six-month period prior to an individual's enrollment date in the group health insurance plan. Furthermore, a preexisting condition exclusion may not last for more than 12 months (18 months for late enrollees) after an individual's enrollment date. This 12- or 18-month period must be reduced by the number of days of the individual's prior creditable coverage, excluding coverage before any break in coverage of 63 days or more. Simply stated, if you have a gap without health coverage for up to 63 days, you will not have a waiting period for preexisting conditions. If you have a gap without coverage of 64 days or more, you will have a one-year waiting period for preexisting conditions.

The Health Insurance Portability and Accountability Act does the following:

- Alleviates "job-lock" by allowing individuals who have been insured for at least 12 months to change to a new job without losing coverage, even if they previously have been diagnosed with cancer. In addition, for previously uninsured individuals, group plans cannot impose preexisting condition exclusions of more than 12 months for conditions for which medical advice, diagnosis, or treatment was received or recommended within the previous six months.
- Prevents group health plans from denying coverage based on health status factors such as current and past health, claims experience, medical history, and genetic information. Insurers may, however, uniformly exclude coverage for specific conditions and place lifetime caps on benefits.
- Increases insurance portability for people changing from a group policy to an individual one.
- Requires insurers of small groups to cover all interested small employers and to accept every eligible individual under the employer's plan who applies for coverage when first eligible.
- Requires health plans to renew coverage for groups and individuals in most cases.
- Establishes a demonstration project for medical savings accounts for small employers and self-employed individuals.
- Increases the tax deduction for health insurance expenses available to self-employed individuals.

The Act, however, does nothing to ensure the affordability of health insurance or to provide coverage to the millions of Americans who do not have health insurance.

COBRA–The Comprehensive Omnibus Budget Reconciliation Act (COBRA) requires employers to offer group medical coverage to employees and their dependents who otherwise would have lost their group coverage due to individual circumstances. Public and private employers with more than 20 employees are

---

"Questions and Answers: Recent Changes in Health Care Law" is available from the U.S. Department of Labor by calling 1-800-998-7542. The Web site is **www.dol.gov/ebsa**.

required to make continued insurance coverage available to employees who quit, are terminated, or work reduced hours. Some states require employers of fewer than 20 employees to provide similar benefits as COBRA. Check with your state insurance department to see if your state has a so-called mini-COBRA. Coverage must extend to surviving, divorced, or separated spouses, and to dependent children.

By allowing you to keep your group insurance coverage for a limited time, COBRA provides valuable time to shop for long-term coverage. Although you, and not your former employer, must pay for the continued coverage, the rate you pay may not exceed by more than 2 percent the rate set for your former coworkers. Continuation of coverage must be offered regardless of any health conditions, such as cancer.

Eligibility for the employee, spouse, and dependent child varies under COBRA. The employee becomes eligible if he or she loses group health coverage because of a reduction in hours or because of termination due to reasons other than gross employee misconduct. The spouse of an employee becomes eligible for any of four reasons:

1.   the death of a spouse;
2.   termination of a spouse's employment (for reasons other than gross misconduct) or reduction in a spouse's hours of employment;
3.   divorce or legal separation from a spouse; or
4.   a spouse becomes eligible for Medicare.

The dependent child of an employee becomes eligible for any of five reasons:
1.   the death of a parent;
2.   the termination of a parent's employment or reduction in a parent's hours;
3.   a parent's divorce or legal separation;
4.   a parent becomes eligible for Medicare; or
5.   a dependent ceases to be a "dependent child" under a specific group plan.

The continued coverage under COBRA must be identical to that offered to the families of your former coworkers. If your employment is terminated for any reason other than gross misconduct or if your hours are reduced, you and your dependents can continue coverage for up to 18 months. A qualified beneficiary who is determined to be disabled for Social Security purposes when he or she loses a job or works fewer hours can continue COBRA coverage for a total of 29 months. Your dependents can continue coverage for up to 36 months if their previous coverage will end because of any of the above reasons.

Continued coverage may be cut short in the following situations:
• your employer no longer provides group health insurance to any of its employees;
• your continuation coverage premium is not paid;

- you become covered under another group health plan; or
- you become eligible for Medicare.

The employee or family member must inform the group health plan administrator of a change in family status. The employer is responsible for notifying the group health plan of an employee's death, termination of employment, or reduction in hours. Employees and beneficiaries are given 60 days from the date they would lose coverage to decide whether to continue coverage.

COBRA is enforced by the Employee Benefits Security Administration of the U.S. Department of Labor. The first step to resolving a COBRA complaint is to try to work out a settlement with your employer. If no adequate solution can be reached, you should write the Department of Labor at Pension and Welfare Benefits Administration, U.S. Dept. of Labor, Room N-5658, 200 Constitution Ave. NW, Washington, DC 20210; (202) 523-8521. In certain cases, the Department of Labor may try to negotiate a solution before your case is filed in federal court. For more information about COBRA, link to www.dol.gov/dol/topic/health-plans/cobra.htm.

ERISA–Another federal law that may affect your coverage is the Employee Retirement and Income Security Act (ERISA). This federal law regulates employee-benefit or self-insured plans. See page 208 for a description of self-funded plans. Employee benefit plans are defined broadly. They include any plan designed to provide "medical, surgical, or hospital care benefits, or benefits in the event of sickness, accident, disability, death, or unemployment."

ERISA may provide a remedy to an employee who has been denied full participation in an employee benefit plan because of a cancer history. ERISA prohibits an employer from discriminating against an employee for the purpose of preventing him or her from collecting benefits under an employee benefit plan.

Some employers fear that a cancer survivor's participation in a group medical plan will drain benefit funds or increase the employer's insurance premiums. An employer may violate ERISA when, upon learning of a worker's cancer history, it dismisses that worker for the purpose of excluding him or her from a group health plan.

If an employer fires an employee for the purpose of cutting off the employee's benefits, regardless of whether the employee is considered disabled under the statute, the employer may be liable for a violation of ERISA. An employer also may violate ERISA by encouraging a person with a cancer history to retire as a "disabled" employee. Most benefit plans define disability narrowly to include only the most debilitating conditions. Individuals with a cancer history often do not fit under such a definition and should not be compelled to so label themselves.

Under certain circumstances, ERISA may provide grounds for a lawsuit to workers with a cancer history. ERISA covers both participants (employees) and beneficiaries (spouses and children). Thus, if the employee is fired because his or her child has cancer, the employee may be entitled to file a claim. ERISA, however, is inapplicable to many victims of employment discrimination, such as individuals who are denied a new job because of their medical status, employees who are subjected to differential treatment that does not affect their benefits, and employees whose compensation does not include benefits.

ERISA is enforced by the Employee Benefits Security Administration of the U.S. Department of Labor. The first step to secure your benefits is to file for all the benefits to which you are entitled under the plan. Your plan administrator must provide you a summary of the plan that tells you how the plan works, what benefits it provides, how they may be obtained or lost, and how you can enforce your rights under ERISA.

You must be notified within 90 days whether your claim for benefits is accepted or rejected. If you are not paid benefits to which you are entitled within 90 days, you may request a review of the denial, unless the plan administrator requests additional time to respond to your claim. You have at least 60 days from the date of denial to decide whether you will appeal the decision. If you do appeal and your claim is denied upon review, you must be told the reason for the denial and the plan rules upon which the decision was based.

WHO REGULATES YOUR INSURANCE POLICY

IF YOUR INSURER IS . . .	IT IS REGULATED BY . . .
Private company (for example, Blue Cross and Blue Shield, Aetna, U.S. Healthcare, etc.)	State Department of Insurance
HMO	Several state and federal agencies. Start with your State Department of Insurance or State Department of Health
Private employer or union self-insurance or self-financed plan	U.S. Department of Labor (Employee Benefits Security Administration)
Medicaid (sometimes called other names, for example "MediCal" in California)	State Department of Social Services
Medicare Supplemental Security Income Social Security Benefits	U.S. Social Security Administration
Veterans Benefits CHAMPUS	Department of Veterans Affairs

If you are still dissatisfied with the decision, you may file a complaint in federal court. You do not have to have an attorney to file a complaint in federal court, but the assistance of an attorney at this stage usually is helpful. The federal government does not have an informal administrative procedure to handle appeals from denial of benefits. Information about how to enforce your rights under ERISA may be obtained by writing the Department of Labor at Pension and Welfare Benefits Administration, U.S. Dept. of Labor, Room N-5658, 200 Constitution Ave. NW, Washington, DC 20210. For more information about ERISA, link to **www.dol.gov/dol/topic/health-plans/erisa.htm**.

STATE LAWS

Every state has an insurance commission or department that enforces state regulation of insurance companies. The commission determines what types of policies must be offered and when rates may be raised. States regulate insurance sold by insurance companies; they do not regulate self-insured employee benefit plans. State regulations cover all aspects of health insurance, including rates, policy conditions, termination or reinstatement of coverage, and the scope of coverage and benefits.

HEALTH INSURANCE FOR INDIVIDUALS AND DEPENDENTS

Insurance companies traditionally have avoided selling insurance to individuals for two reasons: they know individuals in need of their own insurance are more likely to be high risks (poor business), and administering many individual contracts requires a lot of time and labor of the insurer. As a result, finding insurance to purchase if you are looking to cover only yourself and your dependents can be difficult. Many states have laws to assure that individuals can purchase health insurance when they are barred from the marketplace due to their medical histories or other circumstances, or to ease the burden for people with preexisting conditions. State laws change frequently. Check with your state insurance department to determine all of your options and to learn how the laws and programs work in your state.

Your group plan may give you the right to convert to an individual plan. If you convert from a group to an individual policy, expect an increase in your premiums, and probably a reduction in your benefits.

High-risk pools require major insurers to participate in the plan and share the "risks" or costs of coverage for individuals in the pool. Risk pools usually provide a package of benefits with a choice of deductibles. Although the premiums are higher than those for individual insurance, most states impose a cap on the amount that can be charged. Most states also have a waiting period for individuals with a preexisting condition, during which you must wait for a period after the policy is issued until the policy will pay benefits. A waiting period of six months for preexisting conditions, such as cancer, is common. For example, if you are receiving cancer treatments in January and you join a high-risk pool with a six-month waiting period, some or all of your medical bills will not be covered by the plan until the following July. Some states, however, will waive the waiting period if you pay a specified premium surcharge. All aspects of these pools vary from state to state.

Most states have laws assuring the right of individuals leaving group coverage to convert their policy to an individual plan. These laws differ, so be sure you find out your rights and responsibilities before you convert your policy. Most importantly, conversion may not be your only, or best, option. A converted policy rarely resembles the group policy.

Open enrollment or guaranteed-issue programs assure that individuals can purchase health policies despite their medical histories or claims experience. The specific rules for these programs, such as exclusions for preexisting conditions, differ from state to state.

Some states have laws requiring carriers to limit preexisting waiting periods to a specified number of months following the effective date of coverage. These so-called portability laws require carriers to credit the time a person was covered by previous coverage in determining whether a preexisting condition waiting period has been satisfied. These laws, too, vary from state to state.

ADDITIONAL TIPS FOR PURCHASING HEALTH INSURANCE–Make sure any policy you purchase is guaranteed renewable. Be sure to read and understand the exclusions (some policies will refer to the exclusions as "omissions").

Study the definitions listed in the insurance plan pamphlet and make sure that you understand them—The company from whom you purchase a policy should be rated A or A+ by A.M. Best and Co., which rates all insurance companies. Best's annual directory is in the reference section of most public libraries and at **www.ambest.com/ratings.**

Be certain your agent and the agency with which you are dealing are both licensed by your state insurance department to sell health insurance—See pages 333–346 for a list of state insurance departments.

Never make a check payable to an individual agent—Checks should be made payable either to the agency or the insurance company.

Before signing the insurance application, make sure any preexisting conditions are listed on your application and that all information is correct—False information or misrepresentation of health conditions on your application may result in the denial of benefits or cancellation of your policy. If you find a mistake, ask the agent to complete a new application. If you find a mistake after the application has been forwarded to the insurance company, notify the insurance company in writing, with a copy of your letter to your insurance agent. If you apply for individual health insurance, most insurers do not ask any questions about your health because they must insure you, regardless of your health, as long as you can prove that you have been continuously insured for the last 12 or 18 months. See page 221 for a discussion of HIPAA.

If you are replacing an existing policy with a new one, do not cancel your current policy until you are sure that you have been approved by the new company and your coverage is in effect—Your new policy may have a waiting period for preexisting conditions if you cannot prove that you have been continuously insured for the last 12 or 18 months. You should understand completely the definition of a preexisting condition as stated by the company from which you are considering buying insurance. Do not drop your current policy until the waiting period for preexisting conditions under the new policy has expired.

Study your new policy carefully when it arrives—Many states have a law that allows you 10 to 30 days to examine a policy once it has been issued. If you return the policy during that time, you will get a full refund of any premiums you have paid. Take advantage of this time to study the new policy. A copy of your application will be included in the new policy, and you should check it again for errors. Your state insurance department can tell you how many days you have to review an individual policy in your state.

Check with the Medical Information Bureau (MIB) prior to applying for insurance to make sure the information they may have on file for you is accurate—The MIB is a Boston-based data bank that has medical and nonmedical information on millions of Americans to protect the insurance industry from fraud. An MIB report is comparable to a credit report. The MIB is a nonprofit association with hundreds of North American insurance industry members who share information through the data bank. They legally enter encoded information from insurance applications into the data bank and consult it when applications are pending before them.

You have the right to verify the information in your MIB file to ensure its accuracy. You can do so by contacting the Medical Information Bureau, Inc., P.O. Box 105—Essex Station, Boston, MA 02112; (617) 426-3660, **www.mib.com**.

Ask for a form to request disclosure of any information in your file. It also will tell you how you may correct any inaccurate information. MIB charges a small fee for this service.

Pay premiums quarterly rather than monthly, if you are paying your own premiums to save processing fees.

GETTING THE MOST OUT OF YOUR HEALTH INSURANCE

Cancer treatment often involves numerous bills from a variety of parties: the hospital, physicians (such as surgeons, anesthesiologists, oncologists, and radiologists), support services (such as nurses, social workers, nutritionists, and therapists), a radiology group, a pharmacy (drugs and medical supplies), and consumer businesses (for items such as wigs, breast inserts, and special clothing).

Keeping track of dozens of expenses, which can amount to tens or hundreds of thousands of dollars, can be confusing and exhausting. The key to collecting the maximum benefits to which you are entitled under your insurance policy is to keep accurate records of your medical expenses.

COLLECTING HEALTH INSURANCE BENEFITS

SUBMITTING CLAIMS—If you are using a network provider, you will make only a copayment and the provider will be responsible for submitting the balance of the claim to the insurer for reimbursement. Your responsibility ends with the copayment. However, if you are using an out-of-network provider, you are responsible for paying the bill and submitting the claim for reimbursement. Insurance will pay you directly for out-of-network claims in most cases. Be sure to attach an itemized bill to the claim form and mark the envelope "out-of-network claims."

If you are eligible for Medicare, the providers must, by law, submit the claims to Medicare on your behalf. Medicare will automatically forward your claim to some Medigap carriers, but not to all of them. Read your Medicare explanation of benefits carefully to see if Medicare forwarded your claim. If Medicare did not, you must make a copy of the explanation of Medicare benefits and mail it to your secondary insurer. In most cases, a claim form is not required, but you must put your Medigap policy number on the explanation of Medicare benefits. The same rules apply if you have secondary coverage through your former employer. Submit your claims in a timely fashion. Most insurance companies have a time limit for submitting claims. It could be one year from the date of service or it could be all of the preceding calendar year plus the current year. Make sure you know what your policy defines as the time limit.

Keep accurate records—This is essential to collecting maximum benefits. If you have a large number of bills, work on this chore frequently. Do not let the bills pile up for so many months that it becomes an unmanageable task. If you find this chore overwhelming and simply cannot figure out where to begin, you may be better off financially in the long run to hire a health claims processing service to do this for you.

Use an accountant's worksheet pad (available in your local stationery store)—Assign a number to each bill and apply that same number to each insurance explanation of benefits that you receive relative to that particular claim.

Make copies of all of your bills—Keep originals for follow-up unless your carrier is one of the few that insists on having the originals; in that case, keep very good copies for your records. Always submit the copy and keep the original for your records. Write the date you sent the claim on your original so you can follow up in five to six weeks.

Submit in the proper order—The patient's insurance is always primary, the spouse's is secondary.

WHY CLAIMS ARE REJECTED:
- Insurance identification number is incorrect on the claim.
- Information is incomplete on claim forms.
- Diagnosis is missing or incomplete; the diagnosis must always be consistent with the services offered. For example, if your doctor does a glucose tolerance test and the only diagnosis is breast cancer, insurance will not pay for the glucose tolerance test because it is not required for diagnosis of breast cancer. If the diagnoses are diabetes and breast cancer, insurance will pay for the glucose tolerance test.
- Date the services were provided is missing.
- First name of the patient is missing.
- Superbill is not legible.
- Reasons for multiple visits made in one day are not stated.
- Date is incorrect or the year is missing.
- Charges are not itemized.
- The insurance carrier wants additional information; be sure to study the explanation of benefits and send them what they want.

WHEN THE INSURER DOES NOT PAY ENOUGH OR DENIES YOUR CLAIM—*Send the claim back again*—When you send a claim back for review, it is not necessary to complete another claim form. Always send the explanation of benefits (EOB) with your notation written on it and a copy of the bill or whatever documentation is required.

Do not take "no" for an answer—Study the EOB form that comes with or without a check. Do not be satisfied with a greatly reduced amount of money for the claim.

Make sure that you are right—If your policy requires precertification, you or your health care provider must call a toll-free number before you are admitted to a hospital, or the policy will pay at a greatly reduced rate. It is your responsibility to tell your doctor to call the precertification number. Make sure you know whether your policy requires precertification. If yours is an emergency admission, you will have approximately 48 to 72 hours to report the admission. In extenuating circumstances, you may be able to get the insurer to pay at the normal rate, even though the precertification number was not called.

Make sure the total charges agree with the total amount of your bill—Do this by studying the EOB. Often, the insurer may forget to include one of the services rendered. When this happens, make a copy of the EOB and write on it exactly what happened. Then send the EOB and a copy of the actual bill back to the insurer.

Resubmit the claim and hope that a different claims examiner will process and pay it without question—Keep in mind that claims for durable medical equipment, prosthetic bras and implants, and chemotherapy wigs always require a copy of the prescription in addition to the bill.

Ask for a review of the denied claim—Simply write the following sentence on your EOB. "Please review—I think you should have paid more." If they still reject the claim, write on the EOB, "I would like to request a review of this denial of coverage by the peer review physicians." Do not take no for an answer. Often claims that are rejected the first time are paid the second time. You may have to send a rejected claim back for review five times before you finally get the answer you want.

If you have an HMO—If you are refused medical care, you have the right to appeal the decision made by your HMO. Your policy or benefits booklet should give you the phone number and instructions for filing an appeal. If your HMO still refuses to provide the medical care that you and a doctor believe you need, consider contacting your state health department, state insurance department, elected representative, or local media.

Always get the name of the customer service representative or claims examiner with whom you speak in a phone conversation—Keep a file on this particular claim, along with the date and the subject that was discussed. If you receive no response, as a final effort, you may have to write a letter to the general counsel of the insurance carrier explaining everything that has happened to date.

Be persistent!—If you are unable to resolve your claim with your insurance company, consider contacting
- The state or federal agency that regulates your insurance provider. (See page 225 for a chart that describes which agency regulates your insurance. See pages 333–346 for a list of state insurance departments.)
- A cancer advocacy or peer-support organization. Some organizations offer ombudsman programs to help survivors and their families maximize insurance reimbursement.
- An attorney. If your claim is not settled informally, consider filing a complaint in small-claims court or hiring an attorney to sue your insurance company.

COVERAGE OF INVESTIGATIONAL OR EXPERIMENTAL THERAPIES AND OFF-LABEL DRUGS

Cancer survivors who have health insurance may find some of their claims rejected because the insurance policy does not cover "experimental treatment." Unfortunately, what your doctor considers the best treatment for you may be considered "experimental" by your insurance company. For example, oncologists often use chemotherapy drugs to treat their patients for cancers other than the specific type of cancer indicated on the package insert. Although the Food and Drug Administration permits doctors to prescribe approved drugs for any use, some insurance companies and self-insured plans refuse to pay for chemotherapy that is used in a way not listed on the package insert. Many states have laws requiring insurers to cover these so-called "off-label uses" of anticancer drugs provided sufficient evidence of their usefulness against that type of cancer can be found in standard lists of drugs. Unfortunately, because these are state laws, self-insured plans need not comply.

The other major forms of cancer treatment that insurers may consider experimental are drugs and devices or procedures still under study and therefore not "standard" therapy. For example, bone marrow and peripheral stem cell transplants are procedures considered experimental as treatment for certain types of cancer and therefore often are not covered.

If you participate in a clinical trial to test a new treatment, your insurer may refuse to cover the patient care costs involving that trial. Although Medicare covers the routine care costs of clinical trials, many private insurers do not. These costs, which will include the hospital and physicians' bills, can be so expensive that patients are prevented from receiving the anti-cancer treatment their oncologist recommended for them.

If you are in this situation, appeal your insurer's decision, and with the help of your physician, exhaust every remedy, including possible legal action against your insurer. Many survivors have found that appeals reviewed by the medical department of the insurance company are overturned in their favor. Many states have passed a law mandating that all expenses related to experimental treatment must be covered by the health insurance plans.

Some survivors have found that they needed to involve an attorney before the insurer agreed to provide the coverage. Do not delay in seeking the help of an attorney. If you need treatment such as a bone marrow transplant, insurance company delay tactics can waste critical time. Sometimes it takes little more than a letter from an attorney to persuade the insurance company to "rethink" its position. Before you spend any money to retain an attorney, make sure he or she is experienced in handling these kinds of cases. See pages 264–266 for help in locating an attorney. Although every appeal is not successful, each appeal further encourages your insurance company to pay for the most current and promising treatment as determined by your physician.

LIFE INSURANCE AND "LIVING BENEFITS"

There have certainly been times when I have felt greater uncertainty about my long-term survival than I have at other times. In each of the last three autumns, I have wondered whether to plant the tulip and daffodil bulbs for the spring bloom or not to bother. Now again this past spring, a glory of living color rewarded me, and once again I have planted for next spring's blooming.

—Robert M. Mack, M.D., lung cancer survivor,
"Lessons from Living with Cancer," *New England Journal of Medicine,*
Vol. 311, No. 25, p. 1640, December 20, 1984.

LIFE INSURANCE

Life insurance provides two types of benefits: replacement of wages if a wage-earner dies and replacement of retirement income if a retired family member dies. Although most people agree that life insurance is practical protection in the event of unforeseen tragedy, many are confused about who needs life insurance and why. Insurance experts recommend buying life insurance when—

- you have young children (all adult wage earners in the family should be covered);
- you have a family without young children, and one spouse would suffer financial hardship if the other spouse died suddenly; or
- you are supporting an aged parent who depends on you for income.

When you apply for life insurance, your medical history becomes of vital interest to the insurance company. Very few insurers sell life insurance policies to "high risk" individuals.

Some companies market policies for people with serious health problems. Before buying such a policy, read it carefully. The benefits often are limited (you might have no coverage for the first two policy years), and these policies can be relatively expensive.

Although the questions asked on applications vary, common questions that affect the chance of cancer survivors securing life insurance include the following:

Have you been treated for cancer in the past twelve months?

Has any other insurance company ever rejected you, and if so, why?

You must answer these questions honestly. If you do not, and the company discovers the truth, it may cancel your policy or deny some or all of the benefits. If the company is suspicious about your medical history, it may check your file at the Medical Information Bureau. See page 228.

The company may ask you to submit to a medical exam, paid for by the company, so it can further evaluate your health. It may also conduct an investigation of your daily habits and medical history.

Once the company has collected the information it requires, it determines whether it will issue you life insurance, and if so, what rate it will charge you. Different companies have different systems for determining what your rate will be.

The following suggestions may increase the cancer survivor's ability to obtain adequate life insurance.

Try large companies that carefully grade the type and stage of cancer.

Obtain estimates from several companies—An efficient way to do this is to have an independent agent (one who does not work for a particular company) shop among the companies in your area to obtain the best possible plan for your needs. You may get a list of all licensed insurance brokers in your area from the State Insurance Department.

Consider a graded policy if you are unable to obtain a life insurance policy with full death benefits—If you die from cancer within the first few years of the policy (usually three years), a graded policy returns only your premium plus part of the face value of the policy to your beneficiaries. If you die after the waiting period has passed, the company will pay the full face value of the policy.

Try to obtain life insurance through a group plan—Many employers and organizations that offer group health insurance also offer group life insurance. The insurance company does not make an individual evaluation of the health of each plan member of a large group; however, your health may be considered if you participate in a plan with a small number of members (for example, if you are one of 30 workers). If your health is considered, you may be excluded from the plan, denied full benefits, or required to pay an extra premium.

Whether you will be able to buy life insurance and what rate you will pay will depend upon the type of cancer you have, when you were diagnosed, and your prognosis. When you apply for life insurance, you are rated and assigned a risk factor. If you are rated within a short time of being diagnosed with a malignancy, the company may decline to issue you a policy at all. If your prognosis improves, you may be issued a policy, but you may be charged an extra premium. The amount of this premium varies depending upon your individual medical history.

How do companies determine these figures? Large companies and reinsurers publish risk selection guides based on reports by their medical staffs. Underwriters then use these guides to evaluate your medical files and determine what policy, if any, it will issue you. Some companies, however, do not differentiate substantially between different types and stages of cancer.

LIVING BENEFITS–Life insurance can provide a needed source of cash to the terminally ill. The term "living benefits" is used to describe two separate methods for accessing most of the face value of your life insurance policy if you are terminally ill. While these benefits are beneficial to some, selling your life insurance is a decision to be made cautiously and with full knowledge of its advantages and disadvantages. You may wish to consult a personal financial planner, accountant, or lawyer to help you and your family determine if this is the best use of your life insurance funds.

The following are two basic methods for accessing living benefits.

1. "Accelerate" the death benefit of your policy through your insurer directly by purchasing a rider to your policy. Typically, you must have a life expectancy of six months or less, or be permanently confined to a nursing home. You can expect to receive approximately 80 percent of the face value of the policy through acceleration of your death benefit.

2. "Viaticating" your policy, or literally selling it to a third-party viatical settlement company. These companies typically pay 50 to 75 percent of the face value of your policy in exchange for designation of the company as beneficiary upon your death. The advantage of viaticating is that the companies' terms are more generous than riders on life insurance policies. You will be eligible to viaticate if your life expectancy is 24 months or less, thus providing a potential source of cash while you are still ambulatory and enjoying a good quality of life. Anticipate that the longer your life expectancy at the time you apply for viatication, the lower the cash award you will receive. Generally, you must keep paying premiums on the policy until your death even after you have viaticated.

Some important considerations before obtaining living benefits include the following:

Both accelerated benefits and viatical settlements currently qualify as income for tax purposes and for determination of eligibility for SSI and Medicaid—If you did not viaticate or accelerate, benefits paid to your beneficiary(ies) after your death would not subject them to income tax liability.

Any funds you receive while living means less money for your beneficiaries after you die—For this reason, you should carefully weigh the benefit of accessing living benefits.

Comparison shop—A wise consumer will do a lot of comparison shopping. Companies vary in their terms. Consider obtaining bids from at least six companies when considering viaticating. Know that past abuses of vulnerable consumers have occurred, leading to calls for state regulation of the viatical settlement industry.

Your life expectancy and other detailed medical information must be verified by your physician(s)—If you ask several firms to bid on your policy, they will all contact your doctor for verification. Inform your doctor's office that they may receive several requests so they are prepared.

Obtain professional advice if you encounter obstacles—Obtaining living benefits from a group life insurance policy can be more complex, but not impossible, because more parties are involved (such as employers and plan administrators).

When you viaticate, expect four to six weeks from the time you start the process until you receive payment.

Demand up front that the viatical settlement company whose bid you have accepted put the funds in a third-party escrow account.

Conclusion—When All Else Fails

Survivors often must overcome considerable obstacles to obtain and keep health, disability, and life insurance. If all of your attempts to secure insurance fail, talk with your doctor. Most doctors want to help you. Explain your financial status to your doctor and anyone else who will listen, such as the office manager or billing secretary. When the doctor knows your financial situation, he or she may be more apt to work with you.

Glossary of Insurance Terms

To maximize your benefits, you should have a clear understanding of the following health insurance and managed care jargon.

AGENT: An insurance company representative licensed by a state to sell insurance.

ASSIGNMENT: The transfer of one's rights to collect an amount payable under an insurance contract—assignment of benefits.

BASIC INSURANCE: Coverage of hospitalization costs only.

BENEFIT: The amount the insurance carrier pays.

BENEFIT PERIOD—MEDICARE: The period of time that begins the first day a person enters a hospital or skilled nursing facility and ends 60 days after discharge without being readmitted to either type of facility.

BROKER: An insurance solicitor, licensed by the state, who places business with a variety of insurance companies and who represents the buyer, not the company.

CARRIER: An insurance company that "writes" the insurance.

CATASTROPHIC INSURANCE: A type of limited health insurance designed to cover very high medical expenses. The deductibles are very high ($10,000 or above) and the premiums are low.

CARRY OVER: A provision in many major medical policies to avoid two deductibles if expenses are incurred toward the end of one calendar year, and illness continues into the new year. Usually October through December charges toward the deductible will count in the new year.

CERTIFICATE OF INSURANCE: Document given to employees to explain their group insurance benefits. In some cases it may be a benefits booklet.

COINSURANCE: The portion of the bill for which the insured is responsible.

COMMUNITY RATED: A method for determining premium amounts based on the claims experience of all covered individuals with the same coverage and the same insurer. It is the opposite of experience rated.

COMPREHENSIVE COVERAGE: Insurance is either comprehensive or limited. Comprehensive means broader coverage and/or higher indemnity payments than limited coverage.

CONVERSION: The exchange of one insurance policy providing temporary or group coverage for another individual policy—for example, when a person ceases working and an individual policy is issued to replace employer group coverage. No evidence of medical insurability is required.

COORDINATION OF BENEFITS: A group health policy provision designed to eliminate duplicate payments and provide the sequence in which coverage will apply when a person is insured under two contracts.

COPAYMENT: In managed care plans, the amount the insured must pay directly to the provider of the service. It is typically $5 to $15.

CPT-4-CURRENT PROCEDURE: Codes describing every procedure a provider can give a patient. Codes are used for billing purposes.

DEDUCTIBLE: The amount of money the insured must pay out of pocket before benefits begin. Deductibles are usually on a calendar year or policy year basis. Some policies have deductibles per diagnosis—the least desirable—or family deductibles. A policy may have a $250 deductible per individual with a $500 deductible per family. This means that when two individuals have each satisfied a $250 deductible, the remaining family members will not have to meet any deductible.

DIAGNOSIS RELATED GROUP (DRG): A system of paying hospitals based on the patient's diagnosis rather than on the total amount of service provided during his or her hospitalization.

ELIMINATION PERIOD: The first days of an illness that are not covered by insurance.

EVIDENCE OF INSURABILITY: Under medically underwritten insurance, this is proof of a person's physical condition or occupation determining his or her acceptance for insurance.

EXCLUSIONS: Specified illnesses, injuries, or conditions listed in the policy that are not covered. Experimental therapies, cosmetic surgery, and eyeglasses are common exclusions.

EXPERIENCE RATED: A method for determining premium amounts based on the claims experience of the contract holder (which is most often the employer group). It is the opposite of community rated.

EXPLANATION OF BENEFITS (EOB): One of these forms comes with or without an insurance check to explain what portion of the submitted bill was covered and why. If you have more than one policy covering you, this is your proof of what your primary coverage paid.

FEE-FOR-SERVICE: See indemnity insurance.

GUARANTEED ISSUE: Insurance carrier will issue the policy regardless of the health risk of the individual. In other words, no evidence of insurability is required.

HEALTH MAINTENANCE ORGANIZATION (HMO): The first and most traditional type of managed care plan. Like other types of managed care, HMOs are organizations that both finance health care (provide insurance) and provide the care by collecting fees in advance. HMOs employ or contract with many physicians and other providers from whom the enrollee may seek care.

HYBRID INSURANCE: See point-of-service plans.

ICD-9: Codes used in describing diagnoses referring to the International Classification of Diseases.

INDEMNITY INSURANCE: Traditional insurance that pays providers on a fee-for-service basis.

LIFETIME MAXIMUM: Total benefits that the insurance company will pay per individual over a lifetime.

MAJOR MEDICAL INSURANCE: Coverage of expenses excluding the hospital fee.

MANAGED CARE: Organizations that function as both insurer and provider of health care simultaneously. HMOs were the first type, but variations include preferred provider organizations and independent practice associations. HMOs tend to operate with stricter rules than their variations.

MEDICALLY NECESSARY: What the insurer (managed care or indemnity) determines was truly necessary care and will therefore cover.

OPEN ENROLLMENT: Insurance that is issued regardless of one's health status or risk, but may be limited to a certain period of the year.

PARTICIPATING PROVIDER: A health care provider who has joined a managed care plan and is willing to accept its contracts.

POINT-OF-SERVICE PLANS: Managed care plans that give the insured the option of seeing providers within the network and paying the copayment amount only, or seeing providers out of the network and getting reimbursed as you would under an indemnity policy. Although these plans are increasingly popular because they allow for choice of providers, the premiums are higher than plans that give you no coverage for providers outside the network.

PORTABILITY: Insurance that can be retained even if one leaves employment or the group plan.

PREEXISTING CONDITION: A health condition that existed before a policy was purchased. Companies' definitions of preexisting condition vary, but usually anything for which you have seen a doctor during the previous 12 months is a preexisting condition and will not be covered during the waiting period, which is typically six to twelve months after the effectiveness date of coverage.

PRIMARY CARE PROVIDER (PCP): Sometimes referred to as the gatekeeper, PCPs are nonspecialist physicians in many managed care plans that enrollees choose to serve as their coordinator for all the services they may need. PCPs must preapprove all referrals to specialists and use of services, including emergency room care.

PROVIDER: The supplier, physician, psychologist, pharmacist, or other health care professional providing a service to the insured.

PUBLIC HEALTH INSURANCE: Medicare or Medicaid.

REASONABLE AND CUSTOMARY (R&C): In medical insurance, an approach to benefits under which the policy agrees to pay the "reasonable and customary" charges for a service or procedure, rather than an agreed amount. "Customary" means the amount charged by a significant number of providers for a given service in a statistically similar geographical area. "Reasonable" means the usual or customary charge, whichever is less.

RELEASE OF INFORMATION: A form signed by the patient before information may be given out to an insurance company or third party.

RIDER: A legal document that modifies protection of a policy. It may either increase or decrease the payable benefits, or eliminate the condition entirely.

SCHEDULE OF BENEFITS: The list of benefits to which the insured is entitled.

SERVICE BENEFIT: An insurance benefit that fully pays for specific hospital or medical care services rendered.

STOP-LOSS: The point during a calendar year when your insurance policy pays 100 percent of costs for the remainder of the year. Thus, your out-of-pocket expenditures, or losses, stop. Most policies pay 80 percent and the individual pays 20 percent. If the policy has a $5,000 stop-loss point, 20 percent of that equals $1,000. This means that when you have spent $1,000 out of your pocket plus your deductible, the policy will pay 100 percent rather than 80 percent.

SUBSCRIBER: A person who holds an insurance policy. Also known as the enrollee, the insured, the certificate holder, or the policyholder.

SUPERBILL: An itemized billing statement given to the patient so that he or she may submit the claim directly to the insurance carrier.

THIRD-PARTY PAYER: An insurance carrier other than the doctor or patient that intervenes to pay hospital or medical bills.

UNDERWRITING: The process by which an insurance company determines whether and on what basis it will accept an application for insurance.

WAITING PERIOD: Time after the beginning of a policy date when benefits are not payable.

WAIVER: An agreement attached to a policy that exempts from coverage certain disabilities or injuries that are normally covered.

WAIVER OF PREMIUM: A provision included in some policies that exempts the insured from paying premiums if he or she is disabled during the life of the policy.

Chapter Thirteen

Working It Out

Your Employment Rights

by Barbara Hoffman, J.D.

Work on, My Medicine, work!

—William Shakespeare *(Othello)*

ORK FULFILLS A CRITICAL financial and emotional need for most cancer survivors. In addition to providing income and important benefits such as health insurance, employment can also be a source of self-esteem. Cancer, however, may create barriers to finding and keeping a job, wreaking havoc on your ability to pay your bills and insure your family.

Although an individual's risk for cancer increases with age, cancer often strikes working-age adults. Forty percent of all newly diagnosed survivors are between the ages of 20 and 64. The American Cancer Society estimates that approximately 80 percent of survivors who are employed at the time of diagnosis attempt to return to work. Personal factors such as age and type of cancer affect a survivor's ability to return to work. Many survivors are able to continue to perform their jobs, yet are denied the opportunity to work because of their cancer. Others may be unable or unwilling to perform their previous duties because of the severity of their illness. All survivors have the right to be treated as individuals at work and not as a stereotyped "cancer patient." Yet, in addition to waging a medical battle against cancer, some survivors face another struggle—obtaining and retaining employment.

This chapter describes how cancer affects survivors in the workplace; under what circumstances employment discrimination against survivors may be illegal; how you can avoid such discrimination; and what you can do when faced with such discrimination. This chapter also discusses vocational rehabilitation resources available to cancer survivors.

EMPLOYMENT DISCRIMINATION

About three o'clock or so I woke up in a total fright. I had been dreaming that I was wandering along the Beltway outside Washington trying to find the Raytheon plant that was located somewhere in those rolling hills. I was applying for a job after being turned down everywhere else. I had to find the plant to submit my resume, but I was hopelessly lost. My cancer had rendered me unemployable, and my family was going to be destitute.

—former U.S. Senator Paul Tsongas (*Heading Home,* Vintage: 1986)

EMPLOYMENT PROBLEMS FACED BY CANCER SURVIVORS

Until recently, cancer survivors faced many limits to job opportunities. Medical treatment often could not provide a length or quality of life necessary to work. Employers could discriminate against survivors without fear of being sued. Cancer survivors can now expect to live longer and better after diagnosis (see chapter 1). They also can enjoy the benefits of many new federal and state laws designed to protect their employment rights. Despite these medical and legal advances, many survivors still find that cancer creates barriers to obtaining and keeping employment.

Some employers and employees treat cancer survivors differently from other workers. Workplace problems most frequently reported by cancer survivors are dismissal, failure to hire, demotion, denial of promotion, undesirable transfer, denial of benefits, and hostility in the workplace. Although discrimination can be blatant and arbitrary, cancer-based discrimination is usually subtle and directed against an individual.

Job discrimination affects all cancer survivors, young and old, rich and poor. Nevertheless, some groups of survivors experience higher rates of discrimination than others. For example, studies suggest that blue-collar workers tend to encounter more problems obtaining and keeping a job than do white-collar workers. Survivors of childhood cancer confront different hurdles in the workplace from those faced by survivors diagnosed as adults. Although their employment rates differ little from the general population, survivors of childhood cancer report greater problems obtaining health, life, and disability insurance through work. They have slightly lower incomes and fewer opportunities in military careers than do other young adults. One study suggests that survivors who were diagnosed as young children faced less discrimination than those diagnosed as teenagers.

Adult cancer survivors who are denied job opportunities commonly experience stress and anxiety over economic insecurity, loss of independence, and reduced self-esteem. Many survivors who are able to keep their jobs find it difficult to change jobs, to advance, or to change their careers. Because cancer is often considered a preexisting condition, a new employer's health insurance policy may not cover cancer-related medical treatment for months or years after employment begins. Many survivors are unable to take the risk of working without health insurance coverage for cancer-related treatment. As a result, they face "job lock"; they remain in an undesirable job mainly to secure health insurance benefits for cancer treatment.

REASONS FOR EMPLOYMENT DISCRIMINATION

I lost my breast, not my brain.

—Mastectomy survivor in response to being fired from her job as a paralegal

Most employers treat cancer survivors fairly and legally. Some employers, however, erect unnecessary and sometimes illegal barriers to job opportunities for survivors. Most personnel decisions are driven by economic factors, not by charitable or personal considerations. Some employers face increased costs due to insurance expenses and lost productivity. Other employers worry about the psychological impact of an applicant's cancer history on other employees. Some employers fail to revise their personnel policies to comply with new laws. Employers who have updated personnel policies may not properly train their personnel managers to comply with these laws.

Although employers should evaluate cancer survivors on their individual qualifications for a job, some employers permit vague stereotypes and myths about cancer to color their decisions. For example, some people erroneously believe that cancer is contagious. The myth that cancer is contagious may result in physical and emotional isolation of survivors in the workplace. In California, one survivor who applied for a job with a medical emergency services company reported that he was asked by his interviewer, "Cancer, how did you catch that?" Another man reported that he "was transferred from his job in a hotel kitchen for fear that he might 'contaminate' the food." Other misconceptions about cancer, such as "cancer is always a death sentence" or "cancer renders workers unproductive," cause employers to treat cancer survivors differently from other workers. In fact, most cancer survivors who are employed at the time of diagnosis are able to return to work, often within a few weeks after starting treatment.

When Cancer-Based Discrimination Is Illegal

Under federal law and most state employment discrimination laws, an employer cannot treat a cancer survivor differently from other workers in job-related activities solely because he or she has been treated for cancer. You may be protected by these laws only if

- you are qualified for the job (you have the necessary skills, experience, and education), and you can do the essential duties of the job in question; and
- your employer treated you differently from other workers in job-related activities because of your cancer.

Federal Laws

Four federal laws provide some job protection to cancer survivors: the Americans with Disabilities Act, the Federal Rehabilitation Act, the Family and Medical Leave Act, and the Employee Retirement and Income Security Act.

The Americans with Disabilities Act (ADA)–*What the ADA Requires*—The Americans with Disabilities Act prohibits some types of job discrimination by employers, employment agencies, and labor unions against people who have or have had cancer. The ADA covers private employers with 15 or more employees, state and local governments, the legislative branch of the federal government, employment agencies, and labor unions. Regardless of whether your cancer is cured, is in remission, or is not responding to treatment, most cancers are considered a "disability" under the ADA.

The ADA prohibits employment discrimination against individuals who have a "disability," have a "record of a disability," or are "regarded as having a disability." A disability is a major health problem that substantially limits the ability to do everyday activities, such as drive a car or walk. Most cancer survivors, even those who do not consider themselves to be limited by their cancer, fit under at least one of these three groups. Thus, most cancer survivors are protected by the ADA from the time of diagnosis. You are covered by the ADA, for example, if:

- Your cancer currently substantially limits your ability to do everyday activities such as climbing stairs. A temporary, nonchronic impairment, such as a broken bone, usually is not considered a disability.
- At one time your cancer substantially limited your ability to do everyday activities, but no longer does. For example, during your treatment, you could not climb stairs, but now you can. The ADA protects most cancer survivors who have completed treatment because they have a "record of a disability."
- Your employer believes that your cancer substantially limits your ability to do everyday activities, even if you feel it does not.

Whether you are covered by the ADA is determined on a case-by-case basis. Most federal courts find that cancer survivors who are qualified for their jobs are covered by the ADA. For example, Claudia Berk was hired by Bates Advertising in 1980 as an advertising executive. She took time off for breast cancer treatment in 1993. After two and a half months of medical leave, Berk attempted to return to her position. At that time, she informed Bates that she could schedule her six to eight weeks of daily radiation treatments around her work schedule. After several months of negotiating with Berk about her work assignment, Bates fired her. Berk sued under the ADA. A New York federal court held that Berk's breast cancer was a disability under the ADA because it had substantially limited her in the past and because her breast cancer surgery created a "record of an impairment."

Some federal courts, however, have misapplied the ADA by placing cancer survivors in a catch-22 by concluding that a cancer survivor who is sufficiently healthy to work is not a person with a disability as defined by the ADA. For example, Phyllis Ellison was diagnosed with breast cancer in August 1993. After surgery, she had daily radiation treatments from mid-September through October 1993. Eager to continue to work, Ellison worked on a modified schedule until she felt back to normal by February 1994. On March 2, her employer, Software Spectrum, Inc., fired her. A Texas federal court dismissed Ellison's case and the appellate court affirmed. The appellate court concluded that Ellison could perform her job during and after her cancer treatment, and acknowledged that she experienced nausea, fatigue, swelling, inflammation, and pain resulting from her treatment. The appellate court ruled, however, that because Ellison could perform her essential job duties with accommodations, her cancer did not render her a "person with a disability." The court also ruled that her treatment history did not render her a person with a "record of an impairment." Finally, the appellate court held that Ellison's supervisor did not regard her as a person with a disability, despite her supervisor's insensitive and ignorant comments to her. When Ellison told her supervisor that she would need to change her working hours to accommodate her radiation treatments, "Logan expressed his irritation by suggesting that she get a mastectomy instead because her breasts were not worth saving." Moreover, when Ellison encountered a power outage at work when she returned from a radiation treatment and joined her co-workers in evacuating a dark building, "Logan laughed and said, 'Don't worry about it. Follow Phyllis . . . see, look over there. She's glowing.'"

Cancer survivors who never have been substantially limited in a major life activity may not be a "person with a disability" as defined by the ADA. Additionally, cancer survivors who, through medicine or other measures, can alleviate the limitations caused by cancer treatment may not have a disability as defined by the ADA.

The ADA prohibits discrimination in almost all job-related activities, including, but not limited to

- not hiring an applicant for a job or training program;
- firing a worker;
- providing unequal pay, working conditions, or benefits, such as pension, vacation time, and health insurance;
- punishing an employee for filing a discrimination complaint; or
- screening out disabled employees.

In most cases, a prospective employer may not ask you if you have ever had cancer. An employer has the right to know only if you are able to do the job at the time you apply for it. A prospective employer may not ask you about your health history, unless you have a visible disability and the employer could reasonably believe that it might affect your current ability to perform that job. A job offer may be contingent upon passing a relevant medical exam, provided that all prospective employees are subject to the same exam. An employer may ask you detailed questions about your health only after you have been offered a job.

Some people take genetic tests to determine whether they have an increased chance of getting certain cancers. Those who test positively may face discrimination because their employers may fear they will become ill, miss work, and raise insurance costs. Although the ADA does not specifically mention whether it prohibits discrimination based on genetic information, the Equal Employment Opportunity Commission (EEOC) recognizes that a healthy individual who has a genetic predisposition to a disease is "regarded" as disabled, and therefore is covered by the law. Thus, an employer may violate the ADA by discriminating against a person because he or she has a genetic marker for cancer. Additionally, the ADA does not prohibit employers from testing current employees for genetic information as long as the information is job-related and consistent with business necessity.

Federal employees specifically are protected from genetic-based discrimination by Executive Order. An Executive Order issued by President Clinton in 2000 prohibits federal departments and agencies from making employment decisions about civilian federal employees based on protected genetic information. The Order also prohibits federal employers from requiring genetic tests as a condition of being hired or receiving benefits.

Because the field of genetics is changing rapidly, so too are your related legal rights. For more information on genetics issues, contact:

Council for Responsible Genetics
5 Upland Road, Suite #3
Cambridge, MA 02140
(617) 868-0870
E-mail: crg@gene-watch.org
Web site: www.gene-watch.org

Your employer must keep your medical history in a file separate from your other personnel records. The only people entitled to see your medical file are supervisors who need to know whether you need an accommodation, emergency medical personnel, and government officials who enforce the ADA.

If you need extra time or help to do your job, the ADA requires an employer to provide you a *reasonable accommodation.* An *accommodation* is a change, such as in work hours or duties, to help you do your job during or after cancer treatment. For example, if you need to take time off for treatment, your employer may *accommodate* you by letting you work flexible hours until you finish treatment.

An employer does not have to make changes that would be an *undue hardship* on the business or other workers. Undue hardship refers to any accommodation that would be unduly costly, extensive, substantial, or disruptive, or that would fundamentally alter the nature or operation of the business. For example, if you have to miss a substantial amount of work time and your work cannot be performed by a temporary employee, your employer may be able to replace you. Additionally, in most circumstances, an employer does not have to provide an accommodation that would violate an established seniority system. Studies of employees with disabilities report that most employees can be accommodated with relatively simple and inexpensive solutions. Help creating accommodations is available from the Job Accommodation Network at (800) ADA-WORK.

An employer may fire or refuse to hire a cancer survivor under some circumstances. Because the law requires employers to treat all employees similarly, regardless of disability, an employer may fire a cancer survivor for legitimate reasons unrelated to his or her disability. For example, a Georgia sheriff's department hired Martin Smith in 1984 to work as an undercover investigator. Mr. Smith had a cancerous eye removed in 1993; however, he did not tell his supervisor that he had cancer. The following month, the department fired Mr. Smith because he had forged a magistrate's signature on a search warrant. A federal court ruled that the department did not violate the ADA because it had the right to fire any employee who forged a judge's signature and because it did not know at the time that Mr. Smith had cancer.

The ADA allows employers to establish attendance and leave policies that are uniformly applied to all employees, regardless of disability. Employers must grant leave to cancer survivors if other employees would be granted similar leave. They may be required to change leave policies as a reasonable accommodation. Employers are not obligated to provide additional paid leave, but accommodations may include leave flexibility and unpaid leave. Additionally, survivors have other rights to medical leave under the Family and Medical Leave Act (see page 252).

The ADA does not require employers to provide health insurance. When they choose to provide health insurance, however, they must do so fairly. For example, if your employer provides health insurance to all employees with jobs similar to yours, but does not provide you health insurance, the employer may be violating the ADA. The employer must prove that the failure to provide health insurance is based on legitimate actuarial data (statistics), or that the insurance plan would go broke or suffer a drastic increase in premiums, copayments, or deductibles. If your employer is a small business that can prove it is unable to obtain an insurance policy that will cover you, the employer may not have to provide you the same health benefits provided to your coworkers.

Most employment discrimination laws protect only the employee. The ADA offers protection more responsive to survivors' needs because it prohibits discrimination against family members, too. Employers may not discriminate against workers because of their relationship or association with a "disabled" person. Employers may not assume that your job performance would be affected by your need to care for a family member who has cancer. For example, employers may not treat you differently because they assume that you would use excessive leave to care for your spouse who has cancer. Additionally, employers that provide health insurance benefits to dependents of employees may not decrease benefits to an employee solely because that employee has a dependent who has cancer. State laws, however, do not protect you if an employer treats you differently because a family member has cancer (see pages 253–256 for a discussion of state employment discrimination laws).

How the ADA is enforced—If you believe you have been treated differently by an employer covered by the Americans with Disabilities Act because of your cancer history, you must file a complaint with the U.S. Equal Employment Opportunity Commission (EEOC) to enforce your rights. You must file a complaint within 180 days of when you learned of the discriminatory act. Although you do not have to hire an attorney to file the complaint for you, an experienced attorney can help you evaluate your chances of obtaining the remedy you desire and can draft the complaint in a way to best represent your claim.

The EEOC will appoint an investigator to evaluate your claim. If the EEOC determines that your rights may have been violated, it will attempt to settle the dispute. If no settlement is reached, the EEOC may sue on your behalf or may grant you the right to file your own lawsuit in federal court. Most ADA complaints are resolved at the administrative level and do not proceed to court.

Your complaint should be filed with the closest regional EEOC office. To be linked with your regional EEOC office and to obtain information about how to file a complaint, call the EEOC Public Information System at (800) 669-4000. You can obtain publications from the EEOC that explain the ADA and how to enforce your rights under the law by calling (800) 669-EEOC (3362). For other general information and publications about the ADA, contact the Disability and Business Technical Assistance Center at (800) 949-4232. You can link to the EEOC at **www.eeoc.gov**.

If you can prove you are qualified for a job but have been discriminated against because of your cancer history, you may be entitled to back pay and benefits, injunctive relief such as reinstatement, equitable monetary damages, and attorney's fees. The Americans with Disabilities Act allows an award for compensatory or punitive damages up to $300,000 for intentional discrimination. Intentional discrimination, however, is difficult to prove. These damages are not available against state or local governments or against a private employer who made a "good faith" effort to accommodate you. You have fewer remedies if you work for a state employee. A federal court can order a state employer to hire or accommodate you, but it cannot order a state to pay you money damages.

Roughly 2 percent of all complaints filed under the ADA claim cancer-based discrimination. Indeed, the first employment discrimination case under the ADA to reach a jury was brought by a cancer survivor. Charles Wessel was fired by AIC Security Investigations, an Illinois security company, when the company's owner learned that the cancer in Wessel's lung had spread to his brain. A federal jury found that Wessel's employer violated the ADA because Wessel was able to perform his job as executive director when he was fired. Wessel was ultimately awarded $50,000 in compensatory damages (one year's salary) and $150,000 in punitive damages. An Illinois federal court found that punitive damages were appropriate because Wessel's employer intentionally fired an excellent worker because he was dying.

THE FEDERAL REHABILITATION ACT—*What the Rehabilitation Act requires*—Prior to the passage of the Americans with Disabilities Act in 1990, the Federal Rehabilitation Act was the only federal law that prohibited cancer-based employment discrimination. The Rehabilitation Act bans public employers and private employers that receive public funds from discriminating on the basis of a disability. The following employees continue to be covered by the Rehabilitation Act, but not by the ADA:

- Employees of the executive branch of the federal government (covered by Section 501 of the Rehabilitation Act).
- Employees of employers that receive federal contracts and have fewer than 15 workers (covered by Section 503 of the Rehabilitation Act).
- Employees of employers that receive federal financial assistance and have fewer than 15 workers (covered by Section 504 of the Rehabilitation Act).

For example, small companies that receive federal grants for research and development, physicians in small groups that receive Medicare Part B funds, and small health agencies that receive Medicaid payments may be subject to the Rehabilitation Act but not to the ADA. The military does not have to obey either the ADA or the Federal Rehabilitation Act, although retired military personnel and civilian employees of the Department of Defense are protected.

Like the ADA, the Rehabilitation Act protects cancer survivors, regardless of extent of disability. The Rehabilitation Act protects only qualified workers and requires employers to provide reasonable accommodations.

The U.S. Department of Labor regulations that enforce the Rehabilitation Act recognize that people with a cancer history often experience employment discrimination by employers and coworkers based on misconceptions about their illness long after they are fully recovered. The regulations explain that someone who has a history of a medical impairment is covered by the law because "the attitude of employers, supervisors, and coworkers toward that previous impairment may result in an individual experiencing difficulty in securing, retaining, or advancing in employment. The mentally restored, those who have had heart attacks or cancer often experience such difficulty."

> By amending the definition of "handicapped individual" to include not only those who are actually impaired, but also those who are regarded as impaired and who, as a result, are substantially limited in major life activity, Congress acknowledged that society's accumulated myths and fears about disability and disease are as handicapping as are the physical limitations that flow from actual impairment. Few aspects of a handicap give rise to the same level of public fear and misapprehension as contagiousness. Even those who suffer or have recovered from such noninfectious diseases as epilepsy or cancer have faced discrimination based on the irrational fear that they might be contagious.
>
> —U.S. Supreme Court Justice William Brennan
> *Arline v. School Board of Nassau County* (1987)

How the Rehabilitation Act is enforced—Cancer survivors have won lawsuits under the Federal Rehabilitation Act. In 1988, a federal court agreed that the Rehabilitation Act protected healthy cancer survivors from employment discrimination.

The Houston Fire Department had a policy against hiring anyone with a history of lymphoma, regardless of whether the survivor was ill or in complete remission. Walter Ritchie, who had been successfully treated for lymphoma in 1981, applied in 1985 for a position as a fire cadet. Although Mr. Ritchie passed all of the required tests, the city refused to hire him solely because of his cancer history. A federal court found that the city violated Mr. Ritchie's rights under the Rehabilitation Act by assuming that his cancer history made him unfit for the job. The court required the city to hire Mr. Ritchie and to consider applicants based on their individual abilities, not irrelevant medical histories.

To enforce your rights as a federal employee (Section 501), you must file a complaint with the government within 30 days of the job action against you. To enforce your rights against an employer that has a federal contract of more than $10,000 (Section 503), you must file a complaint within 180 days with your local office of the U.S. Department of Labor, Office of Federal Contract Compliance Programs. To enforce your rights against an employer that receives federal funds (Section 504), you have up to 180 days to file a lawsuit in federal court or a complaint with the federal agency that provided federal funds to your employer. Remedies under Section 504 of the Federal Rehabilitation Act include, but are not limited to, back pay, reinstatement, and attorney's fees, but do not include punitive damages.

FEDERAL REHABILITATION ACT INFORMATION

Section 503 (employer is a federal contractor)
Department of Labor
Office of Federal Contract Compliance Programs
(888) 37-OFCCP
www.dol.gov/esa/ofccp
Answers questions about Section 503 and provides assistance filing a complaint.

Section 504 (employer receives federal funds)
Department of Justice
Civil Rights Division
Disability Rights Section - NYAV
950 Pennsylvania Avenue NW
Washington, DC 20035
www.usdoj.gov/crt/drs/drshome.htm
(800) 514-0301
Information on how to file a 504 complaint with the appropriate agency.

THE FAMILY AND MEDICAL LEAVE ACT (FMLA)—In 1993, Congress enacted the Family and Medical Leave Act to provide job security to workers who must attend to the serious medical needs of themselves or their dependents. The Family and Medical Leave Act requires employers with 50 or more employees to provide up to 12 weeks of unpaid, job-protected leave for family members who need time off to address their own serious illness or to care for a seriously ill child, parent, spouse, or a healthy newborn or newly adopted child. An employee must have worked at least 25 hours per week for one year to be covered. The law allows companies to exempt their highest paid workers. Employees may enforce their rights by filing a lawsuit within two years of any alleged discrimination.

The Family and Medical Leave Act affects cancer survivors in the following ways:

- provides 12 weeks of unpaid leave during any 12-month period;
- requires employers to continue to provide benefits—including health insurance—during the leave period;
- requires employers to restore employees to the same or equivalent position at the end of the leave period;
- allows leave to care for a spouse, child, or parent who has a "serious health condition";
- allows leave because a serious health condition renders the employee "unable to perform the functions of the position";
- allows an intermittent or reduced work schedule when "medically necessary" (under some circumstances, an employer may transfer the employee to a position with equivalent pay and benefits to accommodate the new work schedule);
- requires employees to make reasonable efforts to schedule foreseeable medical care so as to not to unduly disrupt the workplace;
- requires employees to give employers 30 days notice of foreseeable medical leave or as much notice as is practicable;
- allows employers to require employees to provide certification of medical needs and allows employers to seek a second opinion (at employer's expense) to corroborate medical need;
- permits employers to provide more generous leave provisions than those required by the Family and Medical Leave Act; and
- allows employees to "stack" leave under the Family and Medical Leave Act with leave allowable under state medical leave law.

You have up to two years (three for "willful violations") to file a lawsuit in federal court or to file a complaint with the Employment Standards Administration, Wage and Hour Division of the U.S. Department of Labor. Check your local telephone book under "United States Government" for your regional office of the Wage and Hour Division.

For more information on the Family and Medical Leave Act, contact:

National Partnership for Women & Families
1875 Connecticut Ave., NW Suite 650
Washington, DC 20009
(202) 986-2600
www.nationalpartnership.org

THE EMPLOYEE RETIREMENT AND INCOME SECURITY ACT (ERISA)—The
Employee Retirement and Income Security Act may provide a remedy to an
employee who has been denied full participation in an employee benefit plan
because of a cancer history. ERISA prohibits an employer from discriminating
against an employee for the purpose of preventing him or her from collecting benefits under an employee benefit plan. All employers who offer benefit packages
to their employees are subject to ERISA. For a more complete description of
ERISA, see Chapter 12.

STATE LAWS

STATE EMPLOYMENT DISCRIMINATION LAWS–Most employers have to comply with
federal and state employment discrimination laws. Cancer survivors who face discrimination by employers not covered by federal law must turn to state laws for
relief. Every state has a law that regulates, to some extent, employment discrimination against people with disabilities. The application of these laws to cancer-
based discrimination varies widely.

Many state laws have been amended to parallel the requirements of the ADA.
Most state laws cover cancer survivors because they prohibit job discrimination
against persons who
- have a disability;
- have a record of a disability; or
- are regarded by others as having a disability.

State and federal laws define "disability" in a variety of ways. For example, you
may have a "disability" under the ADA, yet not have a "disability" as defined by
your state law or by the Social Security Act.

All states except Alabama and Mississippi have laws that prohibit discrimination against people with disabilities in public and private employment. Alabama
and Mississippi laws, which have not been amended since the 1970s, cover only
state employees. Several states, such as New Jersey, cover all employers regardless
of the number of employees. The laws in most states, however, cover only
employers with a minimum number of employees.

In states that do not protect individuals with a record of a disability or those
who are regarded by others as having a disability, you actually must be disabled

by your cancer to be protected by the law. A few states, such as California and Vermont, expressly prohibit discrimination against cancer survivors.

Cancer survivors have brought successful employment discrimination cases in state courts. For example, Renee Engel was fired from her job as a financial analyst with the Seattle Fire Department after she was diagnosed with ovarian cancer in 1990. She filed a lawsuit in state court in 1992 to reclaim lost wages, five years of lost seniority, health care benefits, vacation, sick leave, and retirement. A jury unanimously ruled in her favor and ordered the city of Seattle to pay her $264,000 for economic damage, back pay, lost benefits, and pain and suffering. The judge also ordered the city of Seattle to pay her attorneys' fees ($58,000).

Any type of employer, including a law firm, may violate state laws regarding cancer survivors' rights. For four years, Jane Karuschkat worked as a capable and loyal legal secretary for a small New York law firm. Then in 1992, she was diagnosed with stage III invasive breast cancer. In an effort to minimize the impact of her illness on her coworkers, Ms. Karuschkat scheduled medical appointments during lunch hours, after work, or on weekends. She even returned to work full-time only ten days after having a mastectomy. Less than two months after her diagnosis, Jessel Rothman, the attorney who owned the law firm, told her that she was fired because he could not "afford" to keep her. At that time, she still had not used all of her vacation and sick days.

Ms. Karuschkat sued her employer in state court for violating the New York Human Rights Act. After a lengthy trial, the State Division of Human Rights ruled in 1996 that Mr. Rothman illegally fired Ms. Karuschkat solely because she had breast cancer, and that he failed to provide her reasonable accommodation (flextime for chemotherapy treatments—one Monday a month for six months). The court ordered Mr. Rothman to pay her $34,679.50 in back pay, $50,000 for emotional distress, pain, suffering and humiliation, and to stop discriminating against his employees based on their disabilities.

Although state discrimination laws vary substantially, they all share one thing in common with the federal law: only "qualified" workers are entitled to relief. For example, a federal court ruled that a nursing home could force Carol Klein, a licensed physical therapist, to retire in 1990 while she was being treated for colon cancer that had metastasized to her brain and lung. The U.S. Court of Appeals for the Sixth Circuit found that Ms. Klein was not "qualified" to perform her job at the time she resigned because she was unable to perform the "essential functions" of the job, even with reasonable accommodations. The court held that the nursing home did not violate Ms. Klein's rights under either Ohio law or the Federal Rehabilitation Act.

Most state laws prohibit discrimination in "terms and conditions of employment," such as salary, benefits, duties, and promotional opportunities. Some state laws, like the federal ADA, require employers to provide reasonable accommodations for an employee's disability. The most protective laws prohibit employers from asking about your medical history until after they offer you a job.

The type of remedy to which you may be entitled depends not only on the state where you work, but on where your complaint is resolved (state agency or state court). Most states offer some or all of the following remedies:

- An order requiring the employer to "cease and desist" discriminatory activity.
- An offer for a position that you were denied.
- Reinstatement if you were fired or demoted.
- Back pay.
- Lost benefits (such as insurance and seniority).
- Money to compensate you for your injury.
- The costs of filing the complaint (court and attorney's fees).

Most states have a state agency that enforces the state's fair employment practices law. Some states permit you to file a lawsuit in state court to enforce your rights. Others require you to file a complaint with the state agency before or instead of going to court. Under most state laws, you have up to 180 days from the time you learn of the action against you to file a complaint with your state enforcement agency.

More information about the laws in your state is available from

- your state division on civil rights or human rights commission;
- an attorney who is experienced in job discrimination cases;
- the EEOC Public Information System at (800) 669-4000, for help locating the appropriate state enforcement agency.

Although each state has different procedures, most state agencies will handle a complaint using the following four steps:

1. An investigator will accept a complaint signed by you if you believe an employer has violated your rights under the state antidiscrimination law.
2. The investigator will ask the employer to present his or her side of the story.
3. If the investigator decides that you did not state a claim under the law, he or she will dismiss your case. If the investigator decides that you may have a legitimate claim against the employer, he or she will try to get you and the employer to reach a fair settlement. Most complaints are resolved at this stage.
4. If you and the employer cannot come to an agreement, the investigator may recommend that your case be heard by a judge. Most states allow you or your employer to appeal an unfavorable decision to a court or to a higher level in the state agency.

For example, the New York State Division of Human Rights ruled that a medical institute violated a cancer survivor's rights under the New York Human Rights Law, which prohibits discrimination based on disability. Lisa Goldsmith, M.D., applied for admission in 1976 to the New York Psychoanalytic Institute.

Three committees had to approve her admission. Two of the committees found that Dr. Goldsmith was highly qualified and gave her excellent evaluations. The third committee rejected her application because of her cancer history. Dr. Goldsmith had been treated for Hodgkin's disease, but had been in remission since April 1974. The Institute allowed reapplications, but turned Dr. Goldsmith down again in 1978.

Dr. Goldsmith filed a complaint with the New York Human Rights Division. The Division found that the Institute's actions were unlawful because they were based solely on Dr. Goldsmith's cancer history.

The Institute appealed the decision to state court. The Appellate Division of the New York Supreme Court affirmed the Division's decision. The court reasoned that the Institute denied a qualified applicant like Dr. Goldsmith the opportunity to enjoy a full and productive life after her cancer experience.

Idaho, Louisiana, and a number of states that have an enforcement agency allow you to enforce the law yourself by filing a lawsuit in state court. You should consult with a private attorney and a state agency before you act. Each state has different rules regarding when you may file a lawsuit in state court. Choosing where to file a complaint (state agency or court) involves a number of factors (such as which forum is likely to provide the swiftest solution, what remedies are available, and whether you can maintain an agency complaint and a lawsuit simultaneously). As under federal law, you do not have to hire an attorney to file a state law employment discrimination complaint for you. An experienced attorney, however, can help you evaluate your chances of obtaining the remedy you desire and can draft the complaint in a way to best represent your claim.

STATE MEDICAL LEAVE LAWS–Some employers give their employees paid or unpaid medical leave. Employees who do not receive medical leave as a job benefit may have a right to medical leave under state law. Check with your human resources department to learn whether your employer provides leave and what steps you must take to get it.

Many states have leave laws similar to the federal Family and Medical Leave Act in that they guarantee employees in the private sector unpaid leave for pregnancy, childbirth, and the adoption of a child. Some state laws provide employees with medical leave to address a serious illness, such as cancer. Several states provide coverage more extensive than the federal law.

State medical leave laws vary widely in the following ways:
- how long an employee can take leave
- which employees may take leave (most states require an employee to have worked for a minimum period of time)
- which employers must provide leave (a few states have leave laws that apply to employers of fewer than 50 employees)

- the definition of a "family member" for whose illness an employee may take family medical leave
- the type of illness that entitles an employee to medical leave
- how much notice an employee must give prior to taking leave
- whether an employee continues to receive benefits while on leave and who pays for them
- how the law is enforced (by state agency or through private lawsuit)

Contact your state civil rights enforcement agency for more information on how to enforce your rights under your state medical leave law. For further information on state family leave laws, contact the National Partnership for Women and Families at **www.nationalpartnership.org.**

STATE LAWS GOVERNING ACCESS TO YOUR EMPLOYMENT RECORDS—Employers are entitled to collect all medical information about you necessary to ensure that you are qualified for your job and for health insurance purposes. This may include information about your cancer history. A few states have laws that specify what information an employer may keep in your personnel file. In general, employers may disclose information about your medical history only to persons with a legitimate need to know for a legitimate business reason. Many cancer survivors, however, find that their medical history was revealed improperly by their employer or coworkers to other employees, prospective employers, insurance agents, and creditors.

You can take several steps to decrease the chance your cancer history will be revealed. If you tell your employer or coworkers about your medical history, be specific about whether you want the information to remain private. Ask your doctors, nurses, and social workers not to disclose your medical history to anyone without your written permission. If your employer reveals your cancer history without your permission, you may have a claim for invasion of privacy. See page 47 for more information about your medical records and privacy rights.

HOW TO AVOID EMPLOYMENT DISCRIMINATION

Lawsuits are neither the only nor usually the best way to fight employment discrimination. State and federal antidiscrimination laws help cancer survivors in two ways. First, they discourage discrimination. Second, they offer remedies when discrimination does occur. These laws, however, should be used as a last resort because they can be costly and time consuming, and they may not result in a fair solution.

The first step is to try to avoid discrimination. If that fails, the next step is to attempt a reasonable settlement with the employer. If informal efforts fail, however, a lawsuit may be the most effective next step. The most constructive efforts against cancer-based discrimination are those that eliminate opportunities for discrimination in the first place. The following are some steps that cancer survivors can take to lessen the chance of encountering employment discrimination.

DO NOT VOLUNTEER THE INFORMATION THAT YOU HAVE OR HAVE HAD CANCER UNLESS IT DIRECTLY AFFECTS YOUR QUALIFICATIONS FOR A JOB–An employer has the right—under accepted business practices and most state and federal laws—to know only if you can perform the essential duties of the job. Unless it directly affects your ability to do that job, you have no obligation to disclose your medical history any more than any other personal or confidential information. Few jobs, for example, require a woman to have two breasts or a man to have a prostate gland.

DO NOT LIE ON A JOB OR INSURANCE APPLICATION–If you are hired and your employer later learns that you lied, you may legally be fired for your dishonesty. Insurance companies may refuse to pay benefits or may cancel your coverage. Federal and state laws that prohibit employment discrimination do not guarantee that all employers will refrain from illegally asking survivors about their cancer histories or about gaps in their education or employment. If you are asked a question that you think is illegal, give an honest (and perhaps indirect) answer that emphasizes your current abilities to do the job.

KEEP IN MIND YOUR LEGAL RIGHTS–For example, under the Americans with Disabilities Act, an employer may not ask about your medical history, require you to take a medical examination, or request medical records from your doctor before making a conditional job offer. Once an employer has made a conditional job offer, the employer can require you to submit to a medical examination only if it is required of all other applicants for the job. The medical examination may consider only your ability to perform safely the essential duties of that job.

KEEP THE FOCUS ON YOUR CURRENT ABILITY TO DO THE JOB IN QUESTION–Employers may not ask how often you were absent from past jobs, but they can ask if you can meet the employer's current attendance requirements.

If a job interviewer asks you an illegal question, such as "Have you ever had cancer?" one way to respond is, "That's a very interesting question. I'm a little curious. How does that question relate to the job for which I'm interviewing?" This puts the burden back on the interviewer to ask you only about your current qualifications.

If a written questionnaire asks an illegal question about your medical history, you could respond, "I am presently fit to perform the duties of the job for which I am applying," or "I currently have no medical condition that would interfere with my ability to perform the duties of the job for which I am applying."

If you believe it is necessary or desirable to discuss your cancer history, do so in a way that keeps the focus on your current abilities. You should tell an interviewer what you can do (skills and experience), will do (why you want to work there), and how you will fit in with that workplace.

APPLY ONLY FOR JOBS THAT YOU ARE ABLE TO DO–An employer may reject you for a job for which you are not qualified, regardless of your medical history.

IF YOU HAVE TO EXPLAIN A LONG PERIOD OF UNEMPLOYMENT DURING CANCER TREATMENT, IF POSSIBLE, EXPLAIN IT IN A WAY THAT SHOWS YOUR ILLNESS IS PAST, AND THAT YOU ARE IN GOOD HEALTH AND ARE EXPECTED TO REMAIN HEALTHY–One way to deemphasize a gap in your school or work history because of cancer treatment is to organize your resume by experience and skills, instead of by date. Time off between jobs has become commonplace. With corporate downsizing and untraditional career paths, employers now are less likely to assume that a long period of unemployment is related to a serious illness.

OFFER YOUR EMPLOYER A LETTER FROM YOUR DOCTOR THAT EXPLAINS YOUR CURRENT HEALTH STATUS, PROGNOSIS, AND ABILITY TO PERFORM THE ESSENTIAL DUTIES OF THE JOB FOR WHICH YOU ARE APPLYING–Be prepared to educate the interviewer about your cancer and why cancer often does not result in death or disability.

ASK A JOB COUNSELOR FOR HELP WITH RESUME PREPARATION AND JOB INTERVIEWING SKILLS–Practice answers to expected questions such as "Why did you miss a year of work?" or "Why did you leave your last job?" Answers to these questions must be honest, but should stress your current qualifications for the job and not past problems, if any, resulting from your cancer experience.

IF YOU ARE INTERVIEWING FOR A JOB, DO NOT ASK ABOUT HEALTH INSURANCE UNTIL AFTER YOU HAVE BEEN GIVEN A JOB OFFER–Then ask to see the "benefits package." Once you have been offered a job, but prior to accepting it, review it to make sure it meets your needs.

IF POSSIBLE LOOK FOR JOBS WITH STATE OR LOCAL GOVERNMENTS OR LARGE EMPLOYERS (50+ EMPLOYEES)–They are less likely than small employers to discriminate. Large employers are subject to more federal and state laws than are small employers. Because large employers have a large pool of employees participating in group health insurance, their insurance costs are less likely to be affected by the medical expenses of one employee. Do not rule out small employers, however. One study found that smaller employers tended to provide a family-type atmosphere and were more likely to offer flexible work schedules (1995 study of 422 cancer patients at the M.D. Anderson Cancer Center in Houston, Texas).

DO NOT DISCRIMINATE AGAINST YOURSELF BY ASSUMING THAT YOU HAVE A DISABILITY–Although cancer treatment leaves some survivors with serious physical or mental disabilities, many survivors are capable of performing the same duties and activities that they did prior to diagnosis. With the help of your medical team, make an honest assessment of your abilities compared with the mental and physical demands of the job.

How to Enforce Your Legal Rights

Cancer survivors have numerous options to enforce their legal rights. If you suspect that you are being treated differently at work because of your cancer history, consider an informal solution before leaping into a lawsuit.

If you face discrimination, consider the following suggestions.

Consider Using Your Employer's Policies and Procedures for Resolving Employment Issues Informally

–All state and local government employers are required to have a grievance procedure and a designated compliance officer for civil rights violations of persons with disabilities. Many private employers have formal grievance procedures.

Tell Your Employer That You Are Aware of Your Legal Rights and Would Rather Resolve the Issues Openly and Honestly Than File a Lawsuit

–Be careful of what you say during discussions so that your employer will not use something you say to hurt your claim should your discussions fail to resolve the problem.

Timothy Calonita, the late New York attorney, advocate, and Hodgkin's disease survivor, counseled one survivor through a potential job problem without having to resort to a lawsuit. Another Hodgkin's disease survivor, who was eight months pregnant, took time off from her job at a bank for cancer treatment. After having a healthy baby, she returned to her workplace seeking reinstatement. The bank manager told her that he had no openings, but that another branch several hours away in a less desirable neighborhood could hire her. Instead of taking the less desirable position or immediately filing a legal complaint, the survivor made an appointment with the regional manager of the bank. She brought with her newspaper articles about employment discrimination against cancer survivors. She then praised the regional manager, thanking him for continuing her employment at the bank and for not responding to her cancer like those employers vilified in the newspaper articles. The end result: the regional manager promoted her to a position in her old branch.

If You Need to Be Accommodated in Some Way to Help You Work, Such As Flexible Working Hours to Keep Doctor's Appointments, Suggest Several Alternatives to Your Employer

–The following situation suggests one possible reaction to employment discrimination.

You must receive chemotherapy one day a week. Your doctor will give you Friday afternoon appointments. You inform your boss who says, "I'm sorry, but I'll have to let you go because your job demands that you work at least forty hours per week."

One way to respond is, "My doctor and I believe I am able to continue working. Because I can stay at work until 1:00 P.M. on Fridays, I would be pleased to work an extra hour or two Mondays through Thursdays to make up the missed time. My doctor anticipates that I will need chemotherapy for only _____ weeks, so I should be back to my regular schedule by _____. I understand that the state human rights law protects my right to work if I am able to continue to perform my job despite my illness."

If your employer offers to accommodate you, do not turn down the offer lightly. Such an offer may be in the employer's favor if the case ends up before a judge. The Job Accommodation Network, a free service of the President's Committee on Employment of People with Disabilities, helps employers fashion accommodations for employees with disabilities. Call (800) ADA-WORK for more information.

EDUCATE EMPLOYERS AND COWORKERS WHO MIGHT BELIEVE THAT PEOPLE CANNOT SURVIVE CANCER OR REMAIN PRODUCTIVE WORKERS—You might, for example, give your employer a letter from your doctor explaining the type of cancer you have or have had, and why you are able to work. More than 9 million Americans are cancer survivors, so there is a good chance that some of your coworkers may have had cancer and are now valued employees.

ASK A MEMBER OF YOUR HEALTH-CARE TEAM TO WRITE OR CALL YOUR EMPLOYER TO OFFER TO MEDIATE THE CONFLICT, AND SUGGEST WAYS FOR YOUR EMPLOYER TO ACCOMMODATE YOU.

SEEK SUPPORT FROM YOUR COWORKERS—They have an interest in protecting themselves from future discrimination.

Despite good personal advocacy, sometimes informal solutions fail. Cancer survivors should then take the following steps to preserve their rights to seek a legal remedy:

KEEP CAREFULLY WRITTEN RECORDS OF ALL RELEVANT EVENTS AT WORK—In a lawsuit, positive performance evaluations or good attendance records show that you were qualified for the job. Other events, however, may be evidence that your employer violated your rights, such as, for example, if your employer moves you from a job that has much public interaction to a job that has little interaction with the public after you experience hair loss from chemotherapy. Keep complete notes of telephone calls and meetings (including dates, times, and attendees), letters, and the names and addresses of witnesses. Make written notes as events occur instead of trying to recall the events weeks or months later.

PAUSE BEFORE YOU SUE—Carefully evaluate your goals. Do you want your job back, a change in working conditions, certain benefits, a written apology, or something else? Consider the positive and negative aspects of a lawsuit. Potential positive aspects include getting a job and monetary damages, protecting your rights, and tearing down barriers for other survivors. Potential negative aspects include long court battles with no guarantee of victory (cases can drag on for many years and employers win more often than do employees), legal fees and expenses, stress, a hostile relationship between you and the people you sue (including your employer and former coworkers), and a reputation in your field as a troublemaker.

CONSIDER AN INFORMAL SETTLEMENT OF YOUR COMPLAINT—Someone, such as a union representative, a human resources or personnel officer of your company, or a social worker, may be able to assist as a mediator. Your state or federal representative or local media may help persuade your employer to treat you fairly. Keep in mind that the first step most government agencies and companies take when they receive a complaint is to try to resolve the dispute without a costly trial.

OBSERVE FILING DEADLINES SO THAT YOU DO NOT LOSE YOUR OPTION TO FILE A COMPLAINT UNDER STATE OR FEDERAL LAW—You have 180 days from the date of an action against you to file a complaint under federal law with the U.S. Equal Employment Opportunity Commission. If you work for the federal government, you have only 45 days to begin counseling with an equal employment opportunity counselor. Under most state laws, you have 180 days to file a complaint with the state agency. If you file a complaint and later change your mind, you can drop the lawsuit at any time.

If you decide to file a complaint with an agency or in state court, the following suggestions may ease your legal journey:

YOU ARE YOUR BEST ADVOCATE—Federal and state agencies, as well as federal and state courts, handle thousands of cases annually. Litigation can drag on for years. If you have a case in the system, periodically follow up on the status of your case with a letter or telephone call, either personally or through your lawyer. Educate your lawyer and the agency or court about your type of cancer and your specific abilities. The more your attorney knows about you, the better he or she can help you.

CHOOSE THE AGENCY MOST RESPONSIVE TO YOU—In some situations, a single act may support a claim of discrimination under more than one law. For example, a cancer survivor who is denied a job by an employer in New York City may have a claim under the New York Human Rights Law (state), the New York City Law on Human Rights (city), and the Americans with Disabilities Act (federal).

If you have a choice of remedies, you may file a complaint with each relevant enforcement agency. One agency may "stay" (not act on) your claim until another agency issues a decision. You may always drop a complaint at any time once you determine which agency is most responsive to your claim. Factors to consider when choosing a resource include the types of remedies available, how quickly the agency responds to complaints (ask them how long the process usually takes), and which office is most convenient to you.

BE PREPARED TO ENDURE THE NUMEROUS STAGES OF LITIGATION–If you file a lawsuit, you have the initial burden of "stating a claim under the law." In other words, you must allege facts that, if true, would entitle you to win your lawsuit unless your employer had a legitimate defense. "Stating a claim under the law" does not mean you automatically win. It does mean, however, that you have alleged sufficient facts to have your day in court. To state a claim that your employer violated the law, you must produce facts that show each of the following:

- You have a cancer history, or your employer mistakenly thought you had cancer, that substantially limited a major life activity.
- You were qualified for the job.
- You were denied the position, fired, or treated unfairly despite your qualifications.
- The employer sought to fill or filled the position with someone who did not have a disability or was not regarded as being disabled.

As an example, the following facts would state a claim under the Americans with Disabilities Act:

- You have breast cancer (you have a physical impairment that substantially limits a major life activity).
- You have twenty years' experience as an office manager of a company with twenty employees and you always received good performance evaluations (you are qualified for your job).
- You took three weeks off for breast cancer surgery and can receive follow-up treatments without affecting your work schedule (you are able to perform the duties of your job).
- Your company fired you the day you returned to work because it did not want the risk of having to hire a temporary worker should you become unable to work in the future (discrimination because of speculative fear of future disability).

The following scenario would not state a claim under the ADA:

- You work as a receptionist for a company with 13 employees (employer too small to be subject to the ADA).
- You have a laryngectomy and learn esophageal speech, and your employer transfers you to a lower paying job after receiving customer complaints that they cannot understand you (you are unable to perform reasonably the essential duties of a receptionist).

Once you have stated a claim, the burden then shifts to the employer to raise a legitimate defense. The most common defenses are as follows:

- You were not qualified for the job.
- We looked at your qualifications, not your cancer history.
- We are reorganizing and dismissed everyone in your department.

If the employer raises a defense, the burden shifts back to you to show that its defense is a pretext to hide the truth.

Most lawsuits, like agency investigations, are either settled or dismissed. If you do go to trial and win your lawsuit, a federal or state judge may order your employer to reinstate you and to compensate you for your harm, including back pay, and your attorney's fees.

BE PREPARED FOR ANY RESULT—Even if your legal rights were violated, there is no guarantee that a public agency or court will provide you a fair remedy. Sometimes a well-financed employer can wear you down financially and emotionally with seemingly endless motions and appeals. A trained job counselor, social worker, nurse, or clergy may help you deal with the personal issues that result from employment discrimination resulting from your cancer history.

CHOOSE A LAWYER WHO HAS EXPERIENCE IN EMPLOYMENT DISCRIMINATION—You do not have to have a lawyer to represent you before an enforcement agency or court. However, someone who is represented by a lawyer experienced in job discrimination, especially the legal rights of people with disabilities, is more likely to meet with success.

FINDING A LAWYER

You can receive help in finding a lawyer experienced in employment discrimination by contacting the following groups:

YOUR LOCAL BAR ASSOCIATION—Most county and state bar associations have a lawyer referral service that provides the names of lawyers in your area who have experience in job discrimination. Many can also refer you to a local public interest law center. Look in the telephone book under "State" and "County" listings, as well as under "Lawyer Referral Services," "Legal Services," and "Attorneys" and "Lawyers."

YOUR REGIONAL EEOC OFFICE—Some EEOC offices provide attorney referrals.

LOCAL ORGANIZATIONS THAT PROVIDE CANCER SURVIVORS SUPPORT AND SERVICES—Some local cancer organizations and hospitals keep a list of lawyers who represent cancer survivors in job discrimination cases.

NATIONAL CANCER ORGANIZATIONS

The National Coalition for Cancer Survivorship
1010 Wayne Avenue, Seventh Floor
Silver Spring, MD 20910
(877) 622-7937

E-mail: info@canceradvocacy.org
Web site: www.canceradvocacy.org
NCCS provides publications, answers to questions about employment rights, and assistance in locating legal resources.

American Cancer Society (ACS)
(800) ACS-2345
www.cancer.org
Services vary widely from county to county. Some ACS units may be able to help you find a lawyer.

CancerCare, Inc.
275 Seventh Avenue
New York, NY 10001
(800) 813-HOPE
E-mail: info@cancercare.org
Web site: www.cancercare.org
CancerCare provides assistance by oncology social workers, including answers to questions about employment rights and assistance locating legal resources.

The Childhood Cancer Ombudsman Program
874 Monument Drive
Montross, VA 22520
(804) 493-7127 (fax)
E-mail: gpmonaco@rivnet.net
Since 1970, the CCOP has helped solve problems for families, patients, and adult cancer survivors. Services include analysis of cases involving access and discrimination issues in health care, insurance, employment, and education, by Ombudsmen volunteers from medicine, genetics, rehabilitation, ethics, education, psychology, social work, and law.

Medical Care Ombudsman Volunteer Program
Medical Care Management Corporation
5272 River Road, Suite 650
Bethesda, MD 20816-1405
(301) 652-1818
E-mail: mcman@mcman.com
Web site: www.mcman.com
Initiated in 1991, the MCOVP addresses health care access issues that may involve insurance, discrimination, and underlying employment issues. Expert medical analysis may assist in resolving these issues. As a community service for patients with diseases such as, but not limited to, cancer, MCOVP will review,

at no charge, as many medical cases as its panel of over 500 medical experts affiliated with over 100 academic medical centers can accommodate, when physicians
have recommended a high-technology or high-risk procedure or complicated
medical care. To obtain an expert review, you must complete a "request for volunteer assistance," available from the above address.

NATIONAL ATTORNEY REFERRAL ORGANIZATIONS

National Employment Lawyers Association
44 Montgomery Street
San Francisco, CA 94104
www.nela.org

The NELA is a national, nonprofit, professional membership organization of
lawyers who represent workers in employment disputes. To obtain a list of lawyers
in your area, send a self-addressed stamped envelope to NELA with a brief note
that gives the city and state where you are seeking a lawyer. Do not send a long
explanation of your question or any supporting papers.

LOCAL PUBLIC INTEREST LAW CENTERS AND DISABILITY RIGHTS ORGANIZA-
TIONS—Many large cities have public interest law centers that can recommend attorneys with experience in civil rights litigation. Some organizations that advocate on
behalf of individuals with disabilities, such as Protection and Advocacy agencies and
law school clinical programs, may offer legal referrals in your community.

WORKERS' COMPENSATION LAWS

Workers' compensation laws provide fixed income and medical expenses to
employees or their dependents in case of employment-related accidents and illness. The purpose of workers' compensation laws is to compensate, without the
complexities of litigation, workers who are injured on the job. In short, workers'
compensation offers no-fault health benefits.

Workers' compensation laws are commonly applied to cases where an employee
is hurt in an accident at work. Workers who contract occupational cancers (for
example, miners, shipyard workers, and nuclear power plant employees) may be
entitled to workers' compensation. In some cases, workers have recovered benefits
where an injury at work aggravated a preexisting cancerous condition. However,
because the cause of cancer often is unknown, cancer is not generally considered
an injury caused by work. In most cases, you must obtain expert medical testi-
mony to show that your work caused or aggravated your cancer.

Workers benefit from these laws because, to collect compensation, they do not
have to prove that their employer negligently harmed them. Employers are strictly
liable to their workers who are hurt on the job. Employers benefit because they
agree to pay a fixed benefit to an injured employee in return for protection from

being sued. Workers' compensation is the only remedy the worker is entitled to receive. A worker who accepts workers' compensation benefits for one injury may not then sue his or her employer for causing that injury.

Workers' compensation laws are state laws. State laws vary as to the amount of compensation, the types of employment covered, and the duration of benefits. Federal employees are covered by a separate law, the Federal Employees Compensation Act. For information about the law in your state, contact your state Department of Labor or Workers' Compensation Division (look under "State Government" in your telephone book).

UNEMPLOYMENT DISABILITY LAWS

Some states provide for unemployment disability benefits for people who are unable to work because of illness or injury unrelated to their jobs. The worker and his or her physician must usually fill out a form provided by the employer to receive disability benefits. Benefits (some percentage of the weekly wage) are paid until the disability ends or a fixed period of time has passed. State laws do not guarantee that a worker may return to his or her job. An employer may replace the worker for any legitimate business reason. For information about the law in your state, contact the state Department of Labor or Unemployment Division.

VOCATIONAL REHABILITATION

Some cancer survivors, especially those who were physically disabled by their treatment, may benefit from vocational rehabilitation services offered by public and private agencies. Vocational rehabilitation services help people whose disabilities make it hard to find or keep a job. Depending on the agency, services may include financial assistance, job training and counseling, and the provision of special equipment.

One important way in which rehabilitation services help cancer survivors is to suggest job accommodations. A job accommodation is a change in the job or workplace that fairly balances the worker's abilities with the employer's needs.

Cancer survivors can benefit from many types of job accommodations, including flexible work hours to accommodate medical treatments; "borrowing" sick days from future years; changing job duties (such as reducing lifting); redesigning the equipment used to perform a job; and retraining a worker for a new skill.

For example, an accommodation for a survivor whose larynx has been removed may include speech therapy and electronic speech aids. Vocational rehabilitation may be appropriate for survivors at different stages of work, including those who are entering the job market for the first time, entering the job market after retraining, or those unable to perform the duties of the previous job.

Resources are available to help your employer create an appropriate accommodation. The Job Accommodation Network, a free service of the federal Office of Disability Employment Policy, was established in 1984 to provide information on practical job accommodations (see page 269 for the address and telephone number). The Network has a toll-free number to reach a consultant who can suggest appropriate accommodations for a particular situation. Any company, regardless of size, may call the Network whenever it has a disabled employee whom it wants to promote, help return to work from injury or illness, help perform a present job more easily, or hire for a vacant job.

STATE VOCATIONAL REHABILITATION RESOURCES

Every state has a vocational rehabilitation agency that provides direct services to individuals. You are covered by the agency in the state where you live, not where you work.

The Federal Rehabilitation Act requires state rehabilitation agencies to provide the following minimum services:
- evaluation of your rehabilitation potential;
- counseling and guidance;
- placement services; and
- rehabilitation engineering services if you need physical accommodations, such as a special piece of equipment (the agency is not required to provide you the equipment, but it must help determine what type of equipment would assist you).

In addition to these minimum services, many states offer additional services, such as transportation and special equipment.

You can find your state rehabilitation agency in the telephone directory under one of the following state departments: Labor, Human Resources, Public Welfare, Human Services, or Education. In addition, some states have independent rehabilitation commissions, listed under "Vocational Rehabilitation Services" or "Rehabilitation Services."

FEDERAL VOCATIONAL REHABILITATION RESOURCES

Although the federal Rehabilitation Services Administration does not provide direct services, it is responsible for ensuring that each state agency complies with federal law. If you believe your state agency is unreasonably denying you rehabilitation services, you may file a complaint with

U.S. Department of Education
Rehabilitation Services Administration
Office of the Commissioner
Office of Special Education and Rehabilitation Services

330 C Street, S.W.
Washington, DC 20202
(202) 732-1282
www.ed.gov/about/offices/list/osers/index.html?src=oc

For help in creating an accommodation, your employer may contact

Job Accommodation Network
Office of Disability Employment Policy
P.O. Box 6080
Morgantown, WV 26506-6080
(800) JAN-PCEH (526-7234)
www.jan.wvu.edu

You may choose between filing a lawsuit in court or filing a complaint with the Employment Standards Administration, Wage and Hour Division of the U.S. Department of Labor. Check your local telephone book under "United States Government" for your regional office of the Wage and Hour Division. Most complaints filed with the Wage and Hour Division are resolved informally.

CONCLUSION

Unlike the cancer survivors of a generation ago, survivors today have expanding job opportunities. Not only has the quality of life after cancer treatment improved, but now state and federal laws require employers to treat survivors based on their individual abilities and not their cancer histories. No longer can employers assume that cancer survivors are unproductive liabilities to be avoided or dismissed. Survivors should be aware of their legal rights—and be willing to advocate for themselves and others—so they can protect their right to be treated with fairness and dignity at work.

Chapter Fourteen

Legal and Financial Concerns

by Barbara Hoffman, J.D.

Financial Costs and Resources

The Expenses of Cancer Treatment

When I had to give up my Empress Club card with Canada Airlines International, I felt like a spectator watching life from the outside. The loss of the club card, a symbol of my success as a salesman, symbolized my loss of full participation in life.

—a multiple myeloma survivor

CANCER CAN HAVE A DEVASTATING financial impact on survivors and their families. Two types of expenses are associated with cancer care: (1) direct medical costs and (2) related nonmedical expenses.

Direct medical costs are those resulting from cancer treatment, such as physician's fees, hospital expenses, and pharmacy bills. Most of these expenses are covered by basic health insurance plans. The extent of your direct medical costs depends on the type of cancer, the extent of insurance coverage, and the community where you are treated.

Everyone recognizes that medical care for a serious illness can be quite expensive. Few people, however, are prepared for the nonmedical costs of illness until they are faced with mounting bills. Most nonmedical costs related to cancer care are not covered by health insurance. Depending on the extent of your insurance policy, you may have to pay for such nonmedical items as transportation to and from treatment, childcare, a nurse's aide, a housekeeper, a counselor, or treatment-related consumer products, such as wigs or prostheses. In addition, many survivors find that their insurance premiums are increased and sometimes insurance is discontinued after diagnosis.

Cancer can have an especially harmful financial impact on those survivors who are not employed, do not have adequate health insurance, or do not have savings or other financial resources. The cost of cancer care is particularly high for those who require expensive long-term care, including long stays in a hospital, rehabilitation, or care in a nursing home.

As survivors' costs are increasing, their income is often decreasing. Survivors who are unable to work or those who face employment discrimination may experience a loss of income and insurance benefits. As a result, many cancer survivors must dip into their savings or borrow money to pay for cancer care.

If the costs of cancer care far exceed your resources, you may want to contact a financial counselor to help you plan a budget. Look in the telephone directory under "consumer credit counseling services" for a nonprofit service that can help you manage your bills. A nonprofit service is likely to provide free or inexpensive assistance; a for-profit company will charge you a fee for its services.

If you cannot locate a nonprofit service in your community, contact the National Foundation for Consumer Credit, Inc. (NFCC) for the name of a credit counseling service in your area.

National Foundation for Consumer Credit
(800) 388-2227
www.nfcc.org

The NFCC is a nonprofit umbrella membership organization of more than four hundred nonprofit consumer credit counseling services. The NFCC provides confidential financial counseling for people having trouble managing their bills. No one is turned away because of inability to pay.

PRIVATE SOURCES OF FINANCIAL SUPPORT

A number of organizations provide financial support for the costs of direct medical care and related expenses. Organizations such as CancerCare, Inc., some units or divisions of the American Cancer Society, and the Leukemia and Lymphoma Society provide assistance such as free transportation to and from treatment when a volunteer is available. Cancer screening programs, meals, and lending libraries of wigs, hospital beds, wheelchairs, and other products may be available. Some organizations offer stipends to families who cannot pay their bills.

The type and amount of financial help available varies from community to community. To learn what is available in your community, contact
- the social work department of your hospital
- the person in your doctor's office who handles billing
- national and community cancer organizations
- pharmaceutical companies that offer free drugs to patients
- public community health clinics and public hospitals
- community service organizations
- religious organizations
- social and fraternal organizations
- your labor union
- your local congressional representative's office
- your local public assistance office

See pages 349–353 for a list of organizations that provide financial assistance.

PUBLIC SOURCES OF FINANCIAL SUPPORT

PUBLIC HOSPITALS–Most states have hospitals that provide free medical care. The federal government gives some hospitals money for building costs through a program called Hill-Burton. These hospitals must provide certain services to people who cannot pay for their care, but these funds are generally available on a first-come, first-served basis and are often depleted by the end of a given fiscal year. For more information and a list of hospitals in your area that receive Hill-Burton funding, contact the U.S. Department of Health and Human Services, Office of Special Programs, (800) 638-0742, **www.hrsa.gov/osp/dfcr/obtain/CONSFAQ.htm**.

Additionally, many public hospitals provide free medical care to people who do not have insurance. Those hospitals that are linked to university or medical center cancer programs may be able to offer a wide range of cancer treatment and other services.

SOCIAL SECURITY BENEFITS–One source of federal financial assistance is Social Security. The Social Security Act creates several programs for providing financial assistance to qualified individuals. These programs include disability insurance benefits, unemployment compensation, and supplemental security income for the disabled. The following section describes each of the major Social Security programs. For more information about these programs, contact the Social Security Administration's toll-free hotline at (800) 772-1213.

Retirement Benefits—To be eligible for retirement benefits, you need not be disabled or poor. All that is required is that you be of a certain age and have paid into the Social Security system for a specified number of quarters. Under certain circumstances, children of retirees may receive additional benefits.

Spouses', Survivors', and Dependents' Benefits—A widow, a widower, a surviving divorced spouse, and a child or parent of a person who was entitled to Social Security benefits may directly receive those benefits if certain conditions are met.

Supplemental Security Income (SSI) Benefits—The SSI program is designed to provide income to people with income below the federal minimum level and who are 65 or older or blind or disabled. Eligibility is determined by need, not by whether you paid into Social Security as an employee. Although SSI payments can be quite small, in many states an individual receiving SSI benefits will automatically be eligible for Medicaid and may also receive a state supplemental payment.

Disability Insurance Benefits—Disability benefits are designed to provide income to people who are unable to work because of a disability. You are entitled to receive disability benefits while you are disabled before the age of 65 if
  • you have enough Social Security earnings to be insured for disability;
  • you apply for benefits;

- you have a physical or mental disability that prevents you from doing any substantial gainful work;
- the disability is expected to last, or has lasted, at least 12 months, or is expected to result in death; and
- you have been disabled for five consecutive months.

In some cases, spouses of disabled claimants are also entitled to benefits.

The amount of disability benefits is based on a sliding scale determined by elaborate and frequently changing formulas based on your age and past earnings. An employed person may not collect benefits. Workers may not receive both workers' compensation and Social Security disability for the same illness. The medical records of individuals who apply for Social Security disability benefits are evaluated according to regulations issued by the Social Security Administration. Individuals who are denied benefits may appeal to an administrative law judge.

To determine whether your cancer is a disability under the law, the Social Security Administration considers the type of cancer you have, the extent of metastasis, and your response to treatment. Small localized tumors that respond to therapy usually are not considered impairments. For example, early-stage prostate cancer that is successfully treated with surgery is not considered a severe impairment. Cancer that has spread beyond regional lymph nodes, however, usually is considered a severe impairment. Otherwise, your diagnosis is evaluated on a case-by-case basis.

To apply for disability benefits, you must obtain a form from your local Social Security Administration Office (look in the telephone directory under "United States Government, Department of Health and Human Services"). You can apply by mail or telephone if you are physically unable to go to the Social Security office. Apply as soon as you become disabled because you must wait five months after you file before you begin receiving payments.

After determining that you are eligible financially, the Social Security Administration gives your application to the state disability agency to determine, according to a complex formula, whether you are disabled under the law. If you are denied benefits, you may appeal to a federal administrative law judge. The judge will hold a hearing to consider all of the evidence. If you are found to be disabled (but not permanently disabled), your case will be reviewed at least once every three years. When your condition improves and you are able to return to work, benefits will be discontinued.

VETERANS' BENEFITS–The Department of Veterans Affairs (VA) offers a variety of benefits to veterans. Although most disability benefits apply to veterans whose disability is service-connected—which cancer seldom is—some benefits are available to cancer survivor veterans.

Depending on when you served, your age, and your income, you may be eligible for a non-service-connected pension. An additional allowance may be paid if you are in a nursing home, if you need a home aid, or if you are housebound because of your illness.

Hospital care in VA facilities is provided to veterans who meet certain conditions, such as those who are eligible for Medicaid, have a VA pension, or have a limited income. Care is also provided to veterans who need care related to exposure to cancer-causing substances (including dioxin, Agent Orange, and radiation). Outpatient care and medical equipment are also available at VA facilities under certain circumstances.

The Department of Veterans Affairs offers a variety of other benefits to qualified veterans, including life insurance, burial benefits, a death pension to dependents if the veteran's death is non-service-connected, and civil service preference certificates for government employment.

For more information, look in the telephone directory under "United States Government, Department of Veterans Affairs," for the number to reach a VA representative. Toll-free telephone service is available in all 50 states. If you are a beneficiary or policyholder, call the VA Insurance Service, (800) 669-8477, at any time for information about your insurance coverage or (877) 222-VETS to enroll in a VA health benefits program.

DEDUCTING MEDICAL EXPENSES FROM YOUR TAXES—Part of the money you spend on medical care for yourself, your spouse, and your dependents may be itemized as deductions for federal income tax purposes. Keep track of physicians' fees, costs of prescription drugs, dental expenses, home nursing fees, hospital bills, medical insurance premiums that you (not your employer) paid, laboratory bills, and transportation and lodging expenses if you sought medical care away from your home.

At the end of the calendar year, add up all of your medical expenses. From this number, you must then subtract 7.5 percent of your gross income. You may deduct the balance from your income subject to federal income tax.

For example, if your gross income was $20,000, and you had $10,000 in medical expenses, you could claim a tax deduction of $8,500 for your medical expenses.

$$\begin{array}{r} \text{Total medical expenses} \quad \$10,000 \\ \underline{- \text{ 7.5 percent of gross income} \quad - \; 1,500} \text{ (7.5 percent of \$20,000)} \\ \text{Medical deduction} \quad \$8,500 \end{array}$$

The Internal Revenue Service (IRS) has a number of free publications that describe deductions related to health care. An IRS counselor also will answer your questions about tax regulations over the telephone. You can reach the Internal Revenue Service at (800) 829-1040 (for information) or (800) 829-3676 (for publications).

Of the scores of free publications available from the IRS, the following are of particular relevance to the tax concerns of cancer survivors:

Publication 502 *Medical and Dental Expenses*
Publication 503 *Child and Dependent Care Expenses*
Publication 524 *Credit for the Elderly or the Disabled*
Publication 525 *Taxable and Nontaxable Income*
Publication 529 *Miscellaneous Deductions*
Publication 554 *Tax Information for Older Americans*
Publication 559 *Survivors, Executors, and Administrators*
Publication 721 *Tax Guide to U.S. Civil Service Retirement Benefits*
Publication 907 *Tax Highlights for Persons with Disabilities*

PLANNING YOUR PERSONAL AND FINANCIAL FUTURE

The anticipation of death has made it essential for me to give thought to emotional and practical preparations for my children, my mother, my helpmate and partner, and other important people in my life. I have a sense of great satisfaction in having arranged for such practical matters as wills, death benefits, trust funds, and a retirement plan. For the most part, this activity has been associated not with a sense of impending doom or imminent death but with a sense that making these arrangements now frees me from future concern.

—Robert M. Mack, M.D., lung cancer survivor,
"Lessons from Living with Cancer," *New England Journal
of Medicine,* Vol. 311, No. 25 (December 24, 1984), 1640.

Personal and financial planning for the future is important to ensure that your desires for yourself and your property are carried out according to your intentions. Although you may have only limited control over the progress of your disease, with proper planning, you can affect how decisions concerning your medical care and property will be made even after you become incapable of doing so yourself.

PERSONAL PLANNING: ADVANCE HEALTH DIRECTIVES

A cancer experience often means complicated choices among a variety of complex medical decisions. For one of every two survivors, cancer means facing the reality of death. Because it is your life, you should be the ultimate decision maker about whether to continue medical treatment. Most physicians are trained to provide all reasonable life-sustaining treatment. Because cancer may leave you physically or mentally incapable of expressing your preferences, you should express your desires in advance.

Every state has laws recognizing advance health directives. Advance directives are signed legal documents that inform your family and physicians of your choices for future medical care, including whether you want to stop or not even start life-sustaining treatment. A properly signed and witnessed directive acts as a contract between you and your physician. Your physician must honor your instructions or transfer you to the care of another doctor who will follow your directive. If you have not expressed your desires in advance, your doctors, after talking with your close relatives, will use their best judgment to choose medical care in your best interests. The two most recognized types of advance health directives are a durable power of attorney for health care and a living will.

Durable Power of Attorney for Health Care—A durable power of attorney is a legal document that lets you appoint someone to speak for you. It allows you to transfer your legal right to make health decisions to someone you choose as your "agent" or "proxy." Durable means that your agent can make decisions for you only when you become unable to do so yourself. You can give any adult your power of attorney. Your agent need not be an attorney; most people choose a close family member or friend.

Preparing a durable power of attorney is the best way to ensure that you receive the type of medical care you want. You can specify any type of medical care. Doctors can prolong life in many ways, including with surgery, drugs, respirators, tube feeding, IV fluids, and kidney dialysis. The more specific you are, the more likely you will receive the care you would have chosen. You should give detailed instructions concerning
- whether and under what conditions you should receive life-sustaining treatment;
- whether and under what conditions you should have a "do not resuscitate" (DNR) order;
- whether and under what conditions you should receive pain medications, artificial nutrition and hydration, or surgery;
- your preference for where you want to receive treatment (hospital, hospice, or home);
- general language that covers unanticipated events in your health, finances, or available medical treatment; and
- the names and addresses of the persons you have chosen as your agents.

Avoid vague words such as "hopeless," "extreme," and "heroic." Be specific when using words such as "terminal" or "irreversible." You may consider your cancer terminal if your physician tells you that you are unlikely to live for more than two years; your physician may consider your cancer terminal only when you are within days of death.

Living Will—A living will is a statement that tells your family and your doctor that you do not want your life prolonged by medical procedures if you are near death without any chance for recovery. Similar to your right to refuse medical treatment, you have the right to state in advance of being incapacitated that you do not want to be kept alive by certain procedures.

A living will is not as effective as a durable power of attorney because it simply expresses your preferences to your physicians. Your physician may struggle with medical, legal, ethical, and personal values that conflict with your living will if medical circumstances or pressures from family members intervene. Your doctor and family may not want to "lose" you, even though you may prefer to die with dignity. A durable power of attorney gives legal authority to a person—not a piece of paper—someone you know and trust to act in your place. Your agent can serve as your advocate to ensure that your wishes are carried out.

How to Make Your Future Health Care Choices—The best way to influence future medical decisions is to complete the types of health care directives recognized by your state and to discuss your decisions with your family and doctors to make sure they will honor your wishes. Most states recognize both a durable power of attorney and a living will. These laws vary widely as to when and how you may express future medical decisions, how old you must be, and how the law is enforced.

You do not need an attorney to make a durable power of attorney or a living will. Most states provide a form to complete and have signed by witnesses. You can identify your own end-of-life issues by using *Five Wishes,* an easy-to-use legal document offered by the organization Aging with Dignity. *Five Wishes* helps you plan your end-of-life care by identifying interventions you do and do not want. It helps you identify

- The person you want to make care decisions for you when you cannot.
- The kind of medical treatment you want or do not want.
- How comfortable you want to be.
- How you want people to treat you.
- What you want your loved ones to know.

Five Wishes meets the legal requirements under the health decision laws of most states and the District of Columbia. Even in states where it is not legally recognized, it can serve as a guide to help you discuss your end-of-life choices with your family and doctor. *Five Wishes* is available in English, Spanish, and Vietnamese from:

Aging with Dignity
P.O. Box 1661
Tallahassee, FL 32303-1661
(888) 5WISHES (594-7437)
www.agingwithdignity.org

You also can obtain a copy of an advance directive form from an attorney, local library, or Partnership for Caring. Partnership for Caring is a national, nonprofit organization devoted to raising consumer expectations for excellent end-of-life care and increasing demand for such care. It provides information on advance health directives, including information about state laws and model forms.

Partnership for Caring: America's Voices for the Dying
1620 Eye Street NW, Suite 202
Washington, DC 20006
800-989-9455
Web site: **www.partnershipforcaring.org**
E-mail: **pfc@partnershipforcaring.org**

Choose as a proxy someone you are confident will be willing and able to carry out your wishes. You may wish to appoint two proxies, the second to make decisions if the first is unable to do so. Critical medical decisions, such as withdrawing life support equipment, are very difficult. They should be entrusted only to those family members or friends who would make the same decision that you would make about your treatment.

To keep your advance health directive current, you should review it regularly, and write your initials and the date you reviewed it on the document. If you change your mind about an instruction, write in your new instruction, initial and date it. If you decide not to have a directive any more, destroy each copy.

Make sure that the people who will be involved in your medical care have a copy of your health care directives. Give a copy to your doctor to keep in his or her files. Discuss your decision with your doctor and ask him or her to continue to be your advocate even if another doctor will be treating you. Keep another copy with your personal papers (not in a bank safety deposit box), so that others can find it if necessary. Place a card in your wallet that states you have a health care directive and where it can be found.

Your Right to Refuse Medical Treatment

In 1990, the U.S. Supreme Court ruled that individuals have the right to control their own medical care. Nancy Cruzan, 30, was admitted to a Missouri hospital after suffering permanent brain damage resulting from a car accident. Once her physicians concluded that she was in a persistent vegetative state from which she would not recover, her parents asked the hospital to discontinue artificial food and water. The hospital did not want to end treatment and ultimately allow Ms. Cruzan to die because she was incapable of expressing her own wishes.

The Supreme Court ruled that physicians must follow "clear and convincing evidence" of an individual's wishes concerning medical care. Such preferences include the right to die, even if close family members object to withholding life-sustaining treatment. The Supreme Court sent the case back to state court. The state court found clear and convincing evidence that, prior to her death, Ms. Cruzan clearly had expressed her desire not to receive life-sustaining treatment under the circumstances she faced. The court ordered the hospital to withhold treatment. Ms. Cruzan died thirteen days later.

To ensure that your doctors and family respect your wishes, provide written "clear and convincing evidence" of your desires in the form of an advance health directive. Record your desires before you begin treatment. The Patient Self-Determination Act requires all facilities that receive Medicare or Medicaid, such as hospitals or nursing homes, to discuss health care directives with newly admitted patients. The law also requires the facility to record your health care directives as part of your medical records.

FINANCIAL PLANNING: PLANNING FOR YOUR PROPERTY

TRADITIONAL WILLS—A traditional will is a written document that states how you would like your property to be distributed when you die. Contemplating writing a will may cause anxiety, as few people are comfortable thinking about their own death. It is essential however, if you want to control how your property is distributed after your death.

A traditional will is one way for you to ensure that your decisions about your property and family are respected. Even the most simple will should perform three tasks:

1. Explain how your property should be distributed.
2. Appoint someone to take care of your minor and/or disabled children.
3. Appoint an executor (the person you choose to make sure the instructions in your will are followed).

If you die without a valid will, your state will distribute your property according to state probate laws. The result may or may not be the same result you intended. State probate laws are designed to promote fairness and predictability in estate management. They are not designed to protect your family's long-term financial needs after your death.

Before you prepare a will, complete the following steps to ensure that your will reflects your carefully considered intentions:

- Discuss long-term financial needs with all family members.
- Make a list of your property (major items such as house, car, insurance policies, heirlooms).
- Decide who ("beneficiaries") you want to receive what.
- If you have minor and/or disabled children, decide who you want to be responsible for their care and ask that person if he or she is willing to serve as your children's "testamentary guardian."
- Select your will's executor and ask that person if he or she is willing to be responsible for distributing your assets.

You may write your own will; however, your will is more likely to withstand any legal challenge if it is prepared by an attorney. Your state or local bar association can help you locate an attorney with experience in drafting wills. If your will is challenged and declared invalid, the state may disregard your intentions and distribute your property according to its probate laws. The money you save in writing your own will while you are alive may be lost several times over in court battles over your will after your death.

Each state has laws that establish formalities a will must meet to ensure that your wishes are enforced. For example, some states require that two adults witness you sign the will, while other states require three witnesses. Some states recognize a handwritten will, while other states require that it be typed.

Every state requires, at a minimum, the following three elements to recognize a will as valid:

1. If you are preparing a will, you must be capable of making decisions about your property. You must understand what the purpose of the will is, know the nature of your property, know the beneficiaries you name, and be acting of your own free will.
2. Your will must be witnessed by "disinterested witnesses." These are adults who do not stand to gain by your death and who are not named in your will as a beneficiary, executor, or trustee.
3. You must sign and date the will in the presence of the disinterested witnesses. You must also make it known to them that you intend the document to serve as your will and that you are signing it without coercion.

After you prepare a will, you must make certain it remains safe and reflects your current wishes. Give a copy of your will to your attorney and keep a copy for yourself. Because your safety deposit box may be sealed temporarily after your death, an attorney's office is the safest place to keep a will. Also, review your will every few years to determine whether it reflects your current intentions and assets. If you decide to change your will, have an attorney make the changes or write a new will to ensure that your new, and not old, instructions are followed.

TRUSTS AND ESTATES—A trust is a fiduciary relationship in which one party (the trustee) holds title to property for the benefit of another party (the beneficiary). Several different types of trusts accomplish different purposes. Trusts legally may shield your assets to keep you qualified for government benefits such as Social Security and Medicaid. For example, one way to avoid having to "spend down" your money (reduce your assets) to qualify for Medicaid is to give your money to a family member or friend in the form of a trust. Under the terms of such a trust, the family member or friend agrees to spend the money on your care.

By establishing a trust, you may appoint a "trustee" to use his or her discretion in making all decisions about your assets. You also may restrict the types of decisions the trustee may make. Some trusts take effect only once you become disabled, while others transfer decision-making powers to a trustee as soon as you sign the documents. You should choose as your trustee someone who is able to make competent financial decisions regarding tasks such as operating your business, borrowing money, managing real estate, and filing your tax returns.

Trusts can be quite complex. They must comply with state laws, and they have a variety of tax consequences. You should contact an attorney to help you draft a trust to be certain that it will accomplish the purpose you intend. A power of attorney is less complicated and expensive than a trust. A trust, however, is more flexible than a power of attorney.

POWER OF ATTORNEY—Just as you may authorize an agent to make health care decisions for you, you may grant another person the right to make financial decisions for you by granting a "power of attorney." This is a simple and inexpensive procedure in which you select another person (your "agent") to act in your place and on your behalf.

When you give a power of attorney to your agent, you permit him or her to manage your assets, such as your bank accounts, stocks, and house. Many cancer survivors can relieve themselves of the burden of paying bills and making financial decisions by granting that authority to a responsible person.

Granting or revoking a power of attorney involves the power to manage your property and must comply with state laws to be valid. You should, therefore, consult with an attorney to prepare the documents that will express your intentions and be accepted by banks and other institutions.

OTHER LEGAL CONCERNS OF CANCER SURVIVORS

MEDICAL MALPRACTICE

Most physicians, hospitals, and other health care providers give survivors quality cancer treatment that meets professional standards. Health care providers have every incentive, from personal to financial, to provide you with quality cancer treatment. In a small number of situations, however, medical care falls below professional standards. In such situations, a cancer survivor may have a claim for medical malpractice.

The most common medical malpractice claim is the "failure to diagnose," and the most common of these failures is the failure to diagnose cancer. Cancer survivors sue members of their treatment team for mistakes during diagnosis, surgery, chemotherapy, and radiation treatment.

For example, Regina Rieger was being treated in Maryland and the District of Columbia for abdominal pain. Although she had a positive hemoccult test and she told her physicians that she had an extensive history of colon cancer in her family, her doctors did not find any cancer. After several months of treatment, Ms. Rieger moved to Mississippi. The same day that she moved, a Mississippi doctor diagnosed her with colon cancer. She had surgery and substantial cancer treatment in Mississippi.

Ms. Rieger sued her previous doctors for failing to diagnose her colon cancer earlier. In 1994, a jury found that her doctors had breached their professional standard of care. A court awarded Ms. Rieger $350,000 for pain and suffering and $18,200 for economic damages.

A patient's claim may be weakened and damages reduced if he or she contributes to the malpractice by failing to follow a doctor's reasonable advice or instructions. For example, Ann Claudet was a patient of Dr. Raymond Weyrich, a Louisiana plastic surgeon. He examined her breasts on a number of occasions. Although he eventually detected a lump in her breast, he did not believe it was cancer. More than once, Ms. Claudet expressed concern to Dr. Weyrich about the lump, but he told her that there was no cause for alarm. Although Dr. Weyrich advised her to return for a follow-up visit in three months, she waited over one year to return. Subsequently, a biopsy revealed breast cancer.

In 1995, a Louisiana jury found that Dr. Weyrich was liable for malpractice for failing to diagnose Ms. Claudet's breast cancer. The harm resulting from the delay in diagnosis, and resulting delay in treatment, substantially decreased the probability that Ms. Claudet would survive (from 75 percent to 42 percent). The jury also found that Ms. Claudet was at fault for 30 percent of her harm because she failed to follow Dr. Weyrich's advice for follow-up care. The jury determined that Ms. Claudet should be awarded $600,000 for pain and suffering, $180,000 for future lost wages, and $30,000 for future cost of insurance premiums. Because Louisiana law, like many state laws, placed a cap on damages, Ms. Claudet could not recover all of the damages.

If a delay in diagnosis is reasonable, however, it is not grounds for malpractice. On March 28, 1978, Margherita Henning's doctor examined her for a lump in her breast. He took a mammogram and found no visible difference from the mammogram he took in 1976. He told Ms. Henning to observe the lump and return immediately if she noticed any changes. He told her to return in a month if she noticed no changes. Ms. Henning found no changes and returned to her doctor's office on May 8, 1978. At that time, her doctor suspected a change in the lump and scheduled a biopsy. When the biopsy revealed early breast cancer, her doctor referred her to two oncologists. Ms. Henning's treatment was unsuccessful and she died. A New Mexico court held that her doctor met the duty of skill, knowledge, and care that he owed Ms. Henning under the circumstances, that he diagnosed her breast cancer at the earliest possible stage, and that the one-month delay had no effect on her outcome.

RESPONSIBILITY OF CARE–Anyone who provides you medical care has some responsibility for the quality of that care. Hospitals are responsible for their employees, and under some circumstances, for physicians who have admitting privileges. Physicians are responsible for their own work, as well as that of their employees.

All doctors and caregivers have a duty to give their patients reasonable professional medical care, which means that your doctor must act with the minimum level of skill and learning common to other doctors in his or her community and field of expertise. A specialist in one field is measured against other specialists in that same field.

What is "reasonable" depends on professional standards determined by state laws, accrediting agencies, professional societies, hospital rules, expert opinions, and common medical practice. Examples of unreasonable care include the following:

- Your doctor negligently delayed diagnosing your cancer and the delay significantly changed your prognosis and/or treatment.
- Your surgeon failed to remove all malignant tumors that reasonably could be expected to be removed by a surgeon.
- You were harmed by inappropriate radiation therapy or chemotherapy that was given at a frequency, dose, or time considered not medically professional.
- Your doctor prescribed the wrong medication or you were given the wrong amount of medication.
- Your doctor failed to perform an important test that most other similarly situated doctors would consider essential. For example, your mother and grandmother had breast cancer, and you discover a suspicious lump in your breast, but your doctor decides to wait a few months without performing any diagnostic tests.
- Your doctor was grossly negligent in treating you. For example, he stated that he was an expert in treating your type of cancer, when in fact, you were his first cancer patient.
- Your doctor erroneously and negligently diagnosed a malignancy when in fact none existed, and consequently you were subjected to needless worry or treatment.

Your doctor does not have a duty to guarantee a particular result or to provide you with the most up-to-date form of treatment. Although many patients are unhappy with the outcome of their treatment, very few have a legitimate malpractice claim against their doctor.

BRINGING A MALPRACTICE CASE—Malpractice suits are controlled by state law. Every state sets a statute of limitations, a deadline by which you may file a lawsuit. In most states, you must file a lawsuit within two or three years from either when you were actually injured or when you learned of your injury. A few states provide you only one year to file a lawsuit, and a few others provide more than three years.

You cannot sue your doctor simply because he or she makes an error in judgment. To bring a malpractice claim against your doctor, you must show three things:

1. Your doctor treated you for a medical condition.
2. You were harmed by your doctor's treatment.
3. Your doctor did not exercise reasonable professional care.

Your doctor's treatment must actually have caused your injury. It need not have been the only cause of your injury, but it must have been a substantial factor. In determining the cause of your injury, a court will consider if you contributed to your injury, for example, by smoking or failing to follow your doctor's instructions. Even if you would have died from your cancer regardless of your doctor's mistakes, your family may have a claim for malpractice if your doctor negligently hastened your death.

Like most lawsuits, most malpractice cases are either settled or dismissed. Few result in a trial. If you win a malpractice case, you may be entitled to an award that restores you or your family, at least financially, to the condition you would be in if your doctor had not made a mistake. For example, you may win lost wages, reimbursement for medical expenses, and an award for "pain and suffering." The types and amounts of damages available are determined by state law. If you are considering a lawsuit, consult with an attorney who has experience in medical malpractice cases. Your local or state bar association may be able to provide you a referral.

ACCESS TO FINANCIAL CREDIT

Before the 1990s, cancer survivors occasionally faced discrimination in applying for credit, such as educational loans and mortgages. The Americans with Disabilities Act (ADA), passed in 1990, prohibits this type of discrimination.

Title III of the ADA provides that "[n]o individual shall be discriminated against on the basis of disability in the full and equal enjoyment of goods, services, facilities, privileges, advantages, or accommodation of any place of public accommodation by any person who owns, leases (or leases to), or operates a place of public accommodation." Banks and other financial institutions are "public accommodations." Cancer survivors are protected as individuals with a disability (see pages 244–251 for a discussion of how the ADA covers cancer survivors).

A cancer survivor may not be denied a loan or other financial service solely because of his or her cancer history. A financial institution must consider whether its credit policies screen out individuals with disabilities or unreasonably impede access to credit. A financial institution has the burden of proving that its credit policy is necessary as a sound business practice.

You can file a lawsuit in federal court to enforce Title III of the ADA. The only remedy available through a private lawsuit, however, is an injunction (an order to stop the discriminatory practice). You also may file a complaint with the U.S. Department of Justice, which is authorized to bring lawsuits in cases of general public importance or where a "pattern or practice" of discrimination may exist.

In these cases, the Justice Department may seek monetary damages and civil penalties. For more information on how to enforce your rights under Title III of the ADA, contact the

United States Department of Justice
Civil Rights Division
950 Pennsylvania Ave. NW
Disability Rights Section—NYAV
Washington, DC 20530
(800) 514-0301
www.ada.gov

ADOPTING A CHILD

Some children and young adults who are treated for cancer face fertility problems as a result of their cancer or treatment. See Chapter 4 for a discussion of how cancer treatment can affect fertility. Adoption is one alternative for survivors who want children. Survivors should be well prepared before trying to adopt a child because some cancer survivors face barriers to adopting solely related to their cancer experience.

Domestic and international adoptions can be arranged through private and public licensed adoption agencies or through attorneys. Adoption laws are regulated by state, federal, and when appropriate, international laws.

All prospective adoptive parents must have a preadoptive home study completed by a licensed adoption agency. The home study includes a medical exam by the prospective parents' physician. The physician also must complete a medical report that describes your current health status and history of chronic illness. You should answer all questions in an honest, detailed, and positive manner. An agency is most likely to accept a physician's evaluation if it is sufficiently detailed to present an accurate picture of your current health and prognosis.

Adoption agencies may not discriminate against cancer survivors solely because of their cancer histories. Because adoption agencies are "public accommodations" under Title III of the Americans with Disabilities Act, they may not prohibit all cancer survivors from adopting. Agencies must consider survivors on an individual basis and evaluate their health as they would other applicants.

An adoption agency may not screen out individuals with disabilities or unreasonably burden the adoption process. It must prove that its criteria are necessary to ensure appropriate adoptions. Because the right to equal treatment by an adoption agency is provided by Title III of the ADA, the enforcement procedures are the same as described on pages 244 to 251.

Shop carefully for an adoption agency, physician, and attorney who understand the medical and emotional impact of your cancer history. They should work together as your advocates to secure your right to adopt.

For information on infertility, contact:

RESOLVE: The National Infertility Association
1310 Broadway
Somerville, MA 02144-1731
(888) 623-0744
E-mail: resolveinc@aol.com
Web site: www.resolve.org

RESOLVE is a nonprofit organization that provides support and information to people who experience infertility and to increase awareness of infertility issues through public education and advocacy.

For information on adoption, contact:

National Adoption Information Clearinghouse
330 C Street, SW
Washington, DC 20447
(703) 352-3488 or (888) 385-3206
E-mail: naic@calib.com
Web site: http://naic.acf.hhs.gov

NAIC is a clearinghouse of information under the U.S. Department of Health and Human Services, Administration for Children and Families.

National Council for Adoption
225 N. Washington Street
Alexandria, VA 22314-2561
(703) 299-6633
E-mail: info@ncfa-usa.org
Web site: www.ncfa-usa.org

NCFA is a nonprofit organization that provides information and public education, advocacy for families, and assistance with choosing an adoption agency or attorney.

Part Four

Taking Care of Yourself

Chapter Fifteen

Cancer Survivorship

Defining Our Destiny

by Susan Leigh, R.N., B.S.N.

Survival, quite simply, begins when you are told you have cancer . . . and continues for the rest of your life.

—Fitzhugh Mullan

*S*URVIVORSHIP IN RELATION TO cancer is a relatively new concept. Not long ago, these words seemed mutually exclusive because a cancer diagnosis meant almost certain death. Thankfully, recent advances in technology, science, and the delivery of therapy have changed forever the way we think about cancer. We even have created new terminology for how we talk about cancer. The concept of *survivorship* is part of this new terminology.

Survivorship begins at diagnosis and continues through and beyond treatment. It is dynamic, not static. It is not limited to a single state of health (cured) or time frame (five years). Survivorship permeates every aspect of your life after diagnosis.

Approximately 9 million people are living today with a history of cancer. Roughly half have survived five years or more. This growing population is witnessing dramatic changes—both scientific and social—that are helping to dispel myths about cancer and its treatment, redefine the language and stages of survival, and promote an evolution from passive patienthood to proactive survivorship.

CANCER MYTHS

. . . if it was not fatal, it was not cancer

—Susan Sontag, *Illness As Metaphor*

A HISTORICAL PERSPECTIVE

Historically, attitudes about cancer were frequently defined by myths and fears of the unknown, and paralleled the effectiveness of available treatments. Until we know what causes all cancers and how they can be treated effectively, a cancer diagnosis may continue to be viewed as a death sentence, instilling dread and masquerading as a ruthless, secretive assailant. Even though recent advances in science and medical technology have increased our chances for surviving many types of cancer, the often paralyzing fear of dying from the disease remains a major part of our culture.

When the biology of a disease is not understood, myth and speculation are apt to define the sickness. For example, cancer continues to be identified, incorrectly, as one fatal disease, with overly simplistic ideas about its causes and treatment. Some people believe that stress caused their cancer rather than genetic predisposition, dangerous health habits, or environmental carcinogens. Others mistakenly believe that all cancer treatment causes hair loss and severe nausea and vomiting. In fact, different treatments cause different side effects, individual reactions to therapy differ, and effective therapies to counteract adverse problems are available.

Paired with these myths are other misunderstandings about cancer. In centuries past, cancer was thought to be caused by emotional resignation and hopelessness. Even recently, attempts to identify cancer personalities became a popular trend. Theories evolved suggesting that too many negative thoughts or repressed feelings caused cancer. This pop psychology often oversimplifies what causes cancer and blames the sick individual for having done something wrong, thus adding to the already overwhelming trauma. For many survivors, though, a more comforting or supportive view of being diagnosed with cancer is one attributed to Elisabeth Kübler-Ross: "My responsibility for my cancer does not mean I caused my cancer. It means I choose how I work with what has happened."

Although the blanket paranoia surrounding cancer is gradually diminishing, the disease continues to harbor elements of fear, stigma, shunning, discrimination, and withdrawal of support. Not all myths are rooted in the individual, though. The health care system, too, is full of myths, misunderstandings, and major changes.

HEALTH CARE MYTHS

As medical researchers and clinicians focus primarily on curing disease and saving lives, survivors tend to focus on both the quantity and quality of their lives. This concern about quality, both in individual priorities and in our health delivery system, is rapidly dispelling more myths about health care. Two of these myths include (1) the all-powerful role of the physician and (2) the healing environment within our hospitals.

Doctors historically held all power and control in managing patients. Recently, that tide has dramatically shifted as the bureaucracy of managed care has created a businesslike atmosphere in hospitals and outpatient clinics. Where all decisions concerning patient care were once made by physicians, many are now controlled by financing and regulatory agencies. Physicians, nurses, and support staff spend increasingly more time on administrative matters, which leaves less time for patient care. People wait longer for appointments, have fewer choices of providers, and incur greater out-of-pocket expenses. The system is definitely changing, and not always for the better.

In response to these changes, a new type of health care consumer is emerging. Survivors are assertive in asking questions, gathering information, finding resources, and making decisions. As decision-making powers shift, relationships with the health care team either can be enhanced or strained, depending upon the circumstances and personalities involved. Subsequently, both survivors and physicians need good communication skills to effectively use their time together and to agree on a treatment plan.

The Cancer Survival Toolbox, a free audio program, helps survivors develop the skills needed to negotiate this changing system. The Toolbox provides guidance on communicating, finding information, making decisions, solving problems, negotiating, and standing up for your rights. It also addresses the needs of older survivors and caregivers, and finding ways to pay for care. For a free copy of the Cancer Survival Toolbox, contact:

National Coalition for Cancer Survivorship
(877) TOOLS4U (866-5748)
www.cancersurvivaltoolbox.org

What has happened to the healing environment in our hospitals and clinics? Diagnosis-related groups (DRGs), ambulatory patient classifications (APCs), cost containment, utilization reviews, quality assurance, and an overwhelming amount of paperwork have complicated and dehumanized care. While the old system allowed unlimited stays in the hospital and actually encouraged passivity and invalidism, the new system has gone to the other extreme. To reduce expenses, hospitals discharge patients as quickly as possible and relegate complicated cancer treatments to outpatient clinics. Survivors, then, return home sooner and sicker. The home, rather than the hospital, has become the healing environment. In many cases this change is an improvement over the hospital environment. But it also can mean that greater responsibility for care and recovery is placed on the survivor, family members, or other caregivers, often without adequate preparation and support. Subsequently, these changing social trends are forcing once passive patients to become more proactive survivors, and thus are fueling a consumer-driven survivorship movement.

ORIGINS OF THE CANCER SURVIVORSHIP MOVEMENT

The cancer survivorship movement gradually grew out of the collective efforts of individuals and groups who recognized the multiple dimensions of life after cancer, and then identified the unmet needs of survivors within their own communities. The heart and soul of this grassroots movement began with persons who either struggled through their own cancer experience or cared for people with cancer, and who wanted to make the journey a little easier for those who would follow.

As the specialty of oncology emerged, the cancer patients' agenda was often set by health care providers, especially physicians. Some support programs even required physician referrals. Doctors decided what cancer-related information and programs were appropriate for their patients. Thus, survivors' experiences varied widely from community to community. Support groups were often facilitated by nurses who had little training in group process, but who recognized the need for psychosocial care. Social workers were rare and overworked. Yet as survivors lived longer and the survivor population grew, so did the need for supportive groups and organizations that would address issues often overlooked or minimized by the health care community.

Eventually, survivors realized they were more than their diagnoses. Living longer and being free of disease were no longer the only standards of success. Survivors also were concerned about psychological and spiritual well-being, social and vocational problems, and economic, legal, and end-of-life issues. Concern about the quality of their lives gave rise to a proliferation of support groups, hotlines, educational materials, and patient networks that were created by the very people who needed these resources. By combining the passion, energies, and needs of survivors with the expertise of oncology professionals, the survivorship movement took root.

Survivors themselves recognized the need to coordinate the independent and diverse nature of this expanding movement. In October 1986, 22 individuals who shared an interest in cancer survival gathered in Albuquerque, New Mexico, at the invitation of Catherine Logan-Carrillo, Fitzhugh Mullan, M.D., and Edith Lenneberg. As founder and executive director of Living Through Cancer (currently People Living Through Cancer), Ms. Logan-Carrillo brought a personal, local, and grassroots expertise to the meeting. As a physician in the Public Health Service, Dr. Mullan contributed a national and political perspective along with personal experience. As a founding member of the Ostomy Association, Ms. Lenneberg brought the experience of uniting mutual aid groups into a national organization. All shared a vision of unifying the divergent activities around the country, and thus strengthening a fragmented survivorship movement.

Many of the participants in this initial meeting had personal histories of cancer, as well as experience providing a wide variety of services to cancer survivors and their families. At the time, no method or structure existed to link groups, share educational materials, raise awareness, or stimulate the development of survivorship-related programs and research. While the Candlelighters Childhood Cancer Foundation provided an excellent network for children with cancer and their families, no organized group advocated for the overall concerns of adult cancer survivors in medicine, science, economics, and politics.

In response to the need for a national network to coordinate widespread and diverse activities, to create a comprehensive clearinghouse for survivorship materials, to promote the study of survivorship, and to advocate for cancer survivors on a national level, the meeting participants founded the National Coalition for Cancer Survivorship (NCCS).

The Semantics of Survivorship

A Medical Approach

When cancer was considered incurable, the term "survivor" applied to the family members whose loved one died from the disease. For years, health professionals and insurance companies used the word "survivor" this way. By the 1960s, the promise for surviving cancer began to change dramatically. Treatment for Hodgkin's disease and childhood leukemias offered the first major glimpse of controlling—maybe even curing—specific cancers. Combinations of chemotherapy and radiation therapy, added to traditional surgery, elevated our expectations about surviving cancer.

Once potentially curative therapy became a reality, doctors selected the five-year mark as a measure of success—either five years from the date of diagnosis or from the end of treatment. If cancer did not return within this time frame, the patient would graduate to survivor status and hopefully regain a normal life expectancy.

Although doctors now seldom use the five-year mark for measuring survival, medical professionals still tend to describe "patients" as anyone receiving therapy, and "survivors" as former patients who are not under treatment. This distinction makes sense to many who are delivering care, who require parameters for scientific study, or who need more specific categories for care. Others—specifically certain survivors—have been less comfortable with these labels. In recognizing that survivors should have the freedom to choose their own identity, the National Coalition for Cancer Survivorship embraced a broad definition of a cancer survivor: "From the time of its discovery and for the balance of life, an individual diagnosed with cancer is a survivor."

A Consumer Approach

. . . always a survivor, sometimes a patient, never a victim.

—Wendy Harpham, M.D., author and cancer survivor

Many people who have had cancer feel that survivorship extends far beyond the restrictions of time and treatment. Some people remain alive for over five years but are not cured of their disease. They may require long-term maintenance therapy, or they may periodically change types of treatment. Others experience late recurrences, are diagnosed with second malignancies, develop delayed effects of treatment, or may, in fact, be dying. Meanwhile, they are doing the best that they can to live as well as they can. If survival is considered a process rather than an end point, these people surely are survivors.

Whether on or off treatment, cured or not cured, people who have had cancer now describe themselves in multiple ways. Cancer survivors choose words that are powerful *(veterans, activists, warriors, advocates)*; existential *(blessed, triumpher, victor, thriver)*; and pragmatic *(former patient, graduate, consumer, customer)*. While all of these labels seem confusing and cause many heated discussions among survivors themselves, many people agree with the author Ross Gray in *Persons with Cancer Speak Out,* that "the act of defining is an act of power." Survivors found a voice in rejecting victimization, accepting responsibility, and discovering their power.

SEASONS OF SURVIVAL

Fitzhugh Mullan was the first to describe survivorship as "the act of living on . . . a dynamic concept with no artificial boundaries." Barbara Carter, an oncology nurse and early NCCS board member, further defined this theme as a process of "going through," suggesting movement through phases. With these models, the concept of survivorship can be viewed as a continual, ongoing process rather than a stage or outcome of survival. Survivorship, then, would begin at the moment of diagnosis and continue for the remainder of life. It is not just about long-term survival, which is how the medical profession generally defines it, but rather it is the ever-changing process or experience of living with, through, and beyond cancer.

Cancer survivors have different issues depending upon their individual circumstances and where they are along their cancer journey. In the classic article *Seasons of Survival: Reflections of a Physician with Cancer,* Fitzhugh Mullan was the first to propose a model of survival comprising different and somewhat distinct stages. He called these stages, or seasons, acute, extended, and permanent.

ACUTE STAGE

During treatment, there is an elegant economy to our thoughts. There is no reason to worry about the future. We may not have one.

—Glenna Halvorson-Boyd and Lisa Hunter, *Dancing in Limbo: Making Sense of Life after Cancer*

The acute (or immediate) stage of survival begins at the time of your diagnostic work-up and continues through the initial courses of surgery, chemotherapy, radiation, or other therapies. Most people refer to you as a patient during this stage, when the primary focus is on physical survival.

Usually, without any prior training, you are required to make sophisticated medical decisions at a time when you feel vulnerable, afraid, and pressured. You often do not understand the scientific basis for selecting one therapy over another, and may not feel confident in your ability to make these important decisions. Because of your inexperience or lack of understanding, you may rely on your physicians to decide your course of therapy. You may, however, seek more information or learn how to communicate more effectively to better understand your choices.

Supportive services are most available during diagnosis and treatment. Access to the medical team, counselors, patient support networks, resource libraries, hotlines, and family support systems can help you navigate through this stage. The picture can change dramatically, however, once treatment ends.

EXTENDED STAGE

I was no longer actively engaged in 'cancer combat,' and a dreadful fear engulfed me: when would the other shoe drop?

—Glenna Halvorson-Boyd and Lisa Hunter, *Dancing in Limbo:*
Making Sense of Life after Cancer

There had been no formal exit from sick to well, no instruction sheet on what to do next with my life. Cancer was my 'trial by fire.' In surviving it, I had learned many precious lessons. Perhaps one of the most important: Staying alive is just the initial challenge; living with the consequences of the disease and therapy becomes a lifelong responsibility.

—Carolyn Runowicz and Donna Haupt, *To Be Alive:*
A Woman's Guide to a Full Life after Cancer

If your disease responds during the initial course of therapy, you will move into the extended (or intermediate) stage of survival. This stage often is described as watchful waiting, limbo, or remission as you monitor your body for signs that the disease has returned.

Uncertainty about the future prevails as medical-based support systems are no longer readily available. Meanwhile, recovery means dealing with the physical, emotional, and social after-effects of treatment. Physically, you may continue to deal with lingering side effects, such as fatigue, pain, and neuropathy (numbness). Emotionally, you probably harbor fears about cancer recurrence or feel anxious about the future. Socially, you may have problems relating to family and friends, or experience problems, and even discrimination, when returning to work. Although no longer a patient, you may not feel entirely healthy either. It may be difficult feeling like a survivor. Ambiguity defines this stage as you often find yourself afloat in a mixture of joy and fear—you are happy to be alive and finished with treatments, yet afraid of what the future may hold.

During this transitional stage, many survivors need continued support. Community and peer networks often replace institutional support during this stage. Recovery entails regaining both physical and psychological stamina. A new sense of "normal" gradually replaces what was normal to you before your diagnosis.

PERMANENT STAGE

With cancer, people confront death. With survival, they feel an urgency to reexamine how they live the rest of their lives.

—Glenna Halvorson-Boyd and Lisa Hunter, *Dancing in Limbo:*
Making Sense of Life after Cancer

A certain level of trust and comfort gradually returns as you enter the permanent (or long-term) stage of survival. The permanent stage of survival is roughly equivalent to cure or sustained remission. While most survivors experience a gradual evolution from a state of "surviving to thriving," a small number of them must deal with chronic, debilitating, or delayed effects of therapy. As a long-term survivor, you may have no physical evidence of disease and appear to have recovered fully. You never forget, however, the life-threatening experience of having survived cancer. The metaphor of the Damocles syndrome illustrates the anxiety of living under a sword that is dangling by a thread, never knowing if or when it might drop.

Another major problem many long-term survivors experience is a lack of guidelines for the best long-term medical care. Unlike adult survivors, childhood cancer survivors are carefully followed by their doctors to identify potential problems and to provide early interventions. Adults, on the other hand, often feel burdened by what some call the "glorification of recovery"—you are praised for overcoming adversity, yet are made to feel ungrateful if you have continued complaints. The appearance of health can actually hamper the identification of real problems as no one wants to believe that something may be wrong. Medical personnel often think that recovery from a once-fatal illness should be reward enough. This feeling that people who survive cancer treatment should simply get on with their lives also is frequently reflected in interactions with family and friends:

> One of the hardest aspects of completing treatment is that the average observer seems to expect you to feel only relief and joy. The average person does not recognize the stress of completing therapy. You may keep your fears and anxieties to yourself to avoid sounding ungrateful or pathologically depressed. Surviving your personal challenge of cancer can be very lonely.
>
> —Wendy Harpham, M.D., *After Cancer: A Guide to Your New Life*

Even long-term survivors who are cancer-free face a risk for new cancers, treatment-related complications, insurance and employment problems, and continued psychological trauma from surviving a life-threatening experience. As the population of cancer survivors increases, the medical community must address long-term survival issues. Survivors need access to appropriate specialists to resolve these medical and psychosocial problems.

Years ago, people with cancer would not question their physicians' orders, request second opinions, seek medical information, talk to others in similar situations, or band together politically. Fortunately, both medical and social changes have created more intelligent, inquisitive, and responsible health-care consumers. Survivors develop publications, resource networks, and support programs; provide expert advice about quality-of-life issues; and build community-based resource centers that meet the specific and unique needs of their own communities. Today, survivors across the country are more proactive and outspoken by advocating for:

- policy changes in science, medicine, and politics (for example, the National Coalition for Cancer Survivorship helped to create the Office of Cancer Survivorship in the National Cancer Institute);
- cancer therapies that are effective, accessible, and affordable;
- medical insurance that is affordable, obtainable, and portable;
- employment opportunities that are free of discrimination;
- access to continued medical care with doctors who understand the special needs of long-term survivors;
- mental health therapists who understand the psychological trauma of individuals and families who face a life-threatening illness;
- community-based peer support networks that connect newly diagnosed survivors and their family members to the veterans who have "been there";
- research that is focused on prevention of secondary cancers, late effects of therapy, and chronic illness;
- a growing acceptance of complementary and alternative medicine (CAM), or integrative medicine, in cancer care; and
- education that promotes health, wellness, and advocacy skills.

Survivors and their caregivers, both personal and professional, have laid the groundwork for survivorship. One of their greatest gifts to today's survivors is knowledge, for knowledge is power. No cancer journey is easy. But with information, understanding, support, and resources, cancer survivors are dispelling myths and improving the quality of their lives with, through, and beyond cancer.

Chapter Sixteen

Survivors as Advocates

by Ellen Stovall and
Elizabeth J. Clark, Ph.D., M.S.W.

I have always felt good about my ability to be an advocate for others—for my friends, my family, and for people I don't even know—but when I was diagnosed with cancer, something happened that I would have never expected: I didn't know how to advocate for myself. And even if I had known how, I didn't know what words to use or how to use them. Suddenly, and without any warning, it was as though I were a child but without the blessed innocence that comes with childhood. Like the neophyte child, I had no more than a crude language to use when I spoke. And when I did speak, it was in a primitive way, as if my voice were frozen and stuck—trapped in my throat by a paralyzing fear that I'd never be able to speak up for myself. Would I . . . could I . . . ever find my own voice?

—Remarks by a cancer survivor to medical students

*A*S YOU WERE GROWING UP, you learned behaviors that gave you a feeling of security when dealing with life's ordinary circumstances. Among these behaviors were resourcefulness and communication, problem-solving, and negotiation skills. You have used these and other skills in practical ways throughout your life. A cancer diagnosis, however, may reduce these skills.

Experts in psychosocial behavior generally agree that your capacity to be self-reliant, to advocate for yourself, and to move forward is temporarily diminished by a cancer diagnosis. They also agree that these skills will reemerge at some point during your cancer experience. When you are in the initial stages of cancer, however, little comfort is derived from hearing that this reduced coping capacity is temporary, predictable, normal, expected, and even natural. Accustomed to being effective, resourceful, and reasonable, nothing about this altered state seems remotely normal or natural. You are in a state of suspended animation. It is as though you are teetering on a high wire—dangling—in a freefall and without a net.

You may be overcome with a fear of having cancer. Fear can paralyze you and keep you from moving forward in a reasonable fashion. Given the magnitude of the consequences—life, quality of life, death—moving forward is essential, but you may not know how to do so. Dr. Martin Luther King Jr. called this decision/indecision phenomenon a "paralysis of analysis."

While the necessity to act in the wake of a cancer diagnosis cannot be overstated, resist the tendency to react to each challenge with the same urgency. A fundamental key to achieving effective self-advocacy is to determine a deliberate plan and measurable goals. This plan should begin with seeking information and developing a clear way to communicate with those who can help you most: your health care team, your family and friends, and other cancer survivors. In summary, you need to become your own best advocate.

CANCER SURVIVORS CAN ADVOCATE FOR THEMSELVES

When diagnosed with cancer, one of the first things that you can do to advocate for yourself is to recognize that you are not alone. The National Coalition for Cancer Survivorship's definition of a cancer survivor is "anyone with a diagnosis of cancer, whether newly diagnosed or in remission or with recurrence or terminal cancer." Millions of people have been where you are and are surviving. They have experienced the unwelcome intrusion of cancer into their lives and have had many of the same reactions.

Just like the survivor quoted at the beginning of this chapter, you may feel that you cannot advocate for yourself. Yet, advocacy is "active support on behalf of something." When you begin to act on behalf of yourself, even if not at your peak level, you are involved in self-advocacy.

Through feeling empowered to act on their own behalf, survivors can meet most of their needs on a personal level, and can communicate these needs to their family, friends, and caregivers. An example of self-advocacy is when you seek a second opinion because you have doubts about your diagnosis or treatment plan. Rather than doing nothing about your doubts or worrying about what your doctor will think about your asking for a second opinion, you actively do something in your own interest. Self-advocacy can help you cope with cancer in many ways:

- Advocacy gives you some stability and a feeling of regaining some control of your life.
- Advocacy is confidence building in the way it helps you face challenges that seem insurmountable.
- Advocacy is a way of reaching out to others. It can be as simple as asking your doctor or nurse for the name of someone to talk with who has survived your particular type of cancer.
- Advocacy can improve your quality of life.
- Self-advocacy may turn feeling hopeless and helpless into feeling hopeful.

EMPOWERED SURVIVORS

Noted author and cancer survivor Natalie Davis Spingarn referred to a *new breed of cancer survivors.* As Susan Leigh pointed out in the previous chapter, these *empowered* survivors symbolize an evolution in medical practice—from the passive patient model to one that encourages patient participation in making the important decisions that will affect both the length and quality of life.

These survivors generally believe in equality in relationships and view their caregivers as partners in their health care. In hospital clinics and physicians' waiting rooms, you can observe survivors who are more outwardly comfortable with self-advocacy. They are equipped with pencil and paper or tape recorders, and are frequently accompanied by a family member or friend. They spend little time in denial or deferred decision making. Rather, they turn their fear and anxieties into energies directed toward obtaining up-to-date information, and becoming more adept at communicating, problem solving, and negotiating.

You may have little control over many factors that affect your cancer experience: your personality, degree of wellness or illness, education, economic status, social skills, age, and access to care. No matter what your life circumstances, however, self-advocacy will make it easier for you to make decisions about your care that will enhance your quality of life.

You Can Learn Self-Advocacy

You may not feel that you can identify with the profile of an "active patient." You may think that you lack self-advocacy skills, yet these skills can be learned. The remainder of this chapter outlines ways that will help you become a more effective advocate—first for yourself and then for others.

Advocacy skills can be obtained in a variety of ways. One way is through peer support or self-help groups. These groups can provide education about cancer, can help to normalize the cancer experience, and can give you a wealth of tips to navigate the health care system and find information. They also can provide an opportunity for assertiveness training through role playing and other exercises.

Four skills are essential to cancer advocacy. When used during your diagnosis and treatment, these skills can contribute significantly to your overall well-being and healing.

Information-Seeking Skills

You will need facts about the diagnosis, available treatment options, treatment side effects, and coping strategies, all of which are discussed in previous chapters. Being an informed consumer is the key to cancer survivorship and provides the best foundation for the other three self-advocacy skills.

Communication Skills

Learning communication skills so that you can be a better advocate for yourself with your doctor will be helpful only if both you and your doctor assume equal responsibility for your care. Most oncologists respect the active patient model and encourage patients to be very involved in planning their care.

A virtual glut of books, magazine, booklets, and Web sites promote effective communication. A booklet written especially for communication about cancer is available from the NCCS. Entitled *Teamwork: A Cancer Patient's Guide to Talking with Your Doctor,* the booklet includes the following practical suggestions:

- Prepare questions before your doctor's appointment and write them down.
- Ask for information in familiar terms (doctors frequently, and unintentionally, lapse into "doctor-speak," using words like "dyspepsia" and "alopecia" to describe loss of appetite and hair loss).
- Make sure you understand what you heard by rephrasing the doctor's responses.
- Take notes or tape record the discussion.
- Ask who in the doctor's office you can call if you have more questions after you leave.

If you feel accomplished in basic communication skills, you may want to explore other areas to enhance your skill level. These include developing better listening techniques, identifying nonverbal cues, getting assertiveness training, and learning new methods of problem-solving and negotiation.

PROBLEM-SOLVING SKILLS

Cancer presents one of life's biggest challenges because it is a predicament that has few clear-cut solutions. As such, it requires deliberate and strategic decision making. If you laid the groundwork during the information-gathering phase of your illness, you probably have lots of information and options to consider. You need to learn how to think through this maze of data, how to sort the information, and how to develop an action plan.

Think about problem-solving techniques that you have used during other crises in your life. Do they apply when dealing with cancer-related problems? Some people do "pro and con" lists or "if X, then Y" lists for sorting out options. Others talk with people whose opinions they respect and then act on consensus. Still others seek and use expert advice. Do not forget that other cancer survivors are also experts because they may have had similar problems. Their ideas, suggestions, and attitudes may be especially helpful.

NEGOTIATION SKILLS

We use negotiation and bargaining skills in our everyday life. At its simplest, a conversation with a friend about where to have dinner or what movie to see can involve negotiation. More difficult are situations where serious conflicts arise when parties hold different values or opinions about a situation or a problem. Effective negotiation relies on good communication, resourcefulness, keeping an open mind, and knowing your options.

A cancer diagnosis may present situations that require specific and deliberate negotiation and conflict resolution skills. For example, problems related to insurance and employment may be complex and not easily resolved. While these situations may be difficult, practical ways to deal with them often exist. Finding solutions may be as simple as reading about your rights. In cases that are not as easily managed, or where the relationship between the conflicted parties has broken down, a mediator, patient advocate, or legal counsel may be necessary.

CANCER SURVIVORS AS ADVOCATES FOR OTHERS

Whether at age 20 or 80, cancer is a life-transforming—life-awakening—experience. Many survivors want to "give something back" in gratitude for their own recovery or for the help that they have received. The cancer survivorship movement relies on this model of peer support—the veteran helping the rookie—to convey the wisdom of what has been learned from one's own experience to help another.

For example, when people learn you have had cancer, they may call you and ask you to speak to a family member or friend who has been diagnosed recently. If you are comfortable speaking on a personal level, talking with the newly diagnosed cancer survivor can be an act of advocacy.

Suggestions for other ways to use your personal experience to help others include:
- starting a support group in your community;
- volunteering for a local organization's hot line or cancer information line;
- speaking about your cancer experience to community organizations and civic groups;
- making sure your library has a variety of up-to-date resources on cancer, especially those that were helpful to you when you were seeking information;
- speaking to medical students, nurses, social workers, hospital staff, and employers and employees about your cancer experience; and
- telling your story publicly to the media or the legislature to help change public opinion and public policy about cancer. In other words, get the message out.

NATIONAL CANCER ADVOCACY

A growing number of cancer survivors and their supporters, family, and friends participate in national cancer advocacy. The high visibility of well-known people who identify themselves as cancer survivors—most notably, world-class athletes like hockey player Wayne Gretzky and multiple Tour de France winner Lance Armstrong—have heightened the public's awareness of cancer survivorship. Lance Armstrong stands out more than most because he is as much identified as a cancer survivor as he is a world-class cyclist. He started the Lance Armstrong Foundation to support research into cancer survivorship after he was treated for testicular cancer. National events like the Susan G. Komen Foundation's Race for the Cure™ and the Avon Breast Cancer 3-Day Events publicize efforts to find a cure for breast cancer. The active lobbying by the consumer-driven, grassroots-based National Breast Cancer Coalition (NBCC) is arguably the most successful and focused effort for eradicating breast cancer nationwide.

Even with this heightened attention to cancer through celebrity and mass media runs/walks and marketing campaigns, only a small fraction of the more than 9 million cancer survivors in this country involve themselves in public issues related to cancer. Those who have chosen to either start an organization or to participate in one that supports research and heath policy matters find their advocacy a rewarding, though challenging, exercise.

A CASE EXAMPLE OF SURVIVOR-LED ADVOCACY

The National Coalition for Cancer Survivorship (NCCS) is very proud of the role it has played in working with the cancer community to focus from the survivor's perspective on health policy matters that affect cancer survivors and their families. NCCS has always distinguished this kind of advocacy as different from, but complementary to, that of the large voluntary health agencies and professional societies with which NCCS works. This advocacy is a relatively new phenomenon that began in earnest during the mid-1980s, emerging from patient-centered, patient-driven organizations, as distinguished from advocacy from provider-centered and provider-governed organizations. It is NCCS's vision of advocacy that led to the formation of the Cancer Leadership Council (CLC).

CANCER LEADERSHIP COUNCIL

The Cancer Leadership Council (CLC) first met in 1993 when NCCS convened a group of eight like-minded organizations to develop a consensus statement on health care reform. At that time, the CLC focused on initiatives that would guarantee cancer survivors access to high-quality care provided by cancer specialists. Since 1993, the CLC has grown to 29 groups that work on patient-centered policy issues that affect quality cancer care.

One of the CLC's first victories was helping persuade Medicare to pay for the routine patient care costs for beneficiaries participating in clinical trials. The CLC continues to tackle cancer survivors' quality-of-life issues—access to care, patients' rights, cancer research funding, clinical trials, reimbursement, FDA reform, genetic testing, pain management, privacy, genetic nondiscrimination, and care at the end of life.

The CLC offers a place where patient advocates not only sit at the table—they built the table. And at the CLC table, patient advocates analyze, evaluate, discuss, understand, and ultimately develop strategies to influence public policies that will affect cancer survivors' lives. Because political victories, such as Medicare coverage of clinical trials, can be short-lived, the CLC continues to represent the needs of cancer survivors and their families in Washington. NCCS's work at the Cancer Leadership Council is proof that together survivors can change the public policies that affect the quality of every cancer survivor's life.

CONCLUSION

With communication comes understanding and clarity; with understanding, fear diminishes; in the absence of fear, hope emerges; and in the presence of hope, anything is possible.

—Ellen Stovall

While the cancer experience is not unique, each individual's experience with cancer is his or her own. The models for self-advocacy exist in the footprints of the millions of survivors who have gone before who are now able to network with their fellow survivors to assist them in resolving the isolating effects of cancer. The wealth of information found in the experiences of veteran survivors can be indispensable to the newly diagnosed. The footprints of the myriad of national survivor-led organizations can inspire hope for a future where the voice of survivors will play a much larger role in setting the health policies that will affect their lives. The experiences of these individuals and the organizations that advocate on their behalf are a powerful resource for self-advocacy and public interest advocacy.

Chapter Seventeen

Resources

by Barbara Hoffman, J.D.

C ANCER SURVIVORS, health professionals, and public agencies have developed thousands of resources to help cancer survivors gather information and obtain help. National and local organizations provide answers to questions and support services to cancer survivors. This chapter describes many helpful resources and explains how to determine which resource is appropriate for you.

FINDING AND USING CANCER RESOURCES

LOCATING CANCER RESOURCES

National and local organizations can provide information and assistance on medical issues (such as treatment options, clinical trials, and treatment-related issues), peer and professional support services, home health care, hospice services, rehabilitation (physical, occupational, and vocational), financial assistance, housing, transportation services, employment and insurance rights, and individual and national advocacy. Before you contact a resource, make a list of the information you are seeking. Write down the answers you receive, such as telephone numbers or referrals to another organization. Keep the information in a folder or notebook because you are likely to need some of it at different times throughout your cancer experience.

Cancer survivors can find a wide variety of resources in many ways:

Professionals who provide your cancer treatment. The doctors, nurses, social workers, and other health professionals who provide your medical care should know your specific needs, as well as the appropriate local resources. If you received treatment at a hospital, ask to speak with someone in the social work, home care, or discharge planning department.

National cancer organizations. Most national cancer organizations have publications, online resources, links to local organizations, and staff who can answer individual questions.

Local cancer organizations. Local cancer organizations provide a variety of individual services and information about local resources.

Public agencies. Public agencies may provide financial help, transportation, senior services, and civil rights enforcement.

Libraries. Most public libraries, as well as patient libraries in cancer centers, can help you find resources. Ask a librarian for assistance in finding print and online resources.

Online. Every cancer-related issue is addressed somewhere on the Internet. See below for a discussion of evaluating cancer-related information on the Internet.

How Do You Know You Are Getting Reliable Information?

Thousands of books, pamphlets, articles, radio and television shows, and Web sites offer information about cancer. How do you know whether the source is providing you with accurate, current, and unbiased information? Note the source of the information. Public sources, such as the National Cancer Institute, and established *nonprofit* national cancer organizations, such as the National Coalition for Cancer Survivorship, American Cancer Society, and CancerCare, provide accurate and timely information, as well as links to other sources of reliable information. Consider whether the source has a for-profit agenda, such as the sale of a particular cancer treatment, to determine whether it provides unbiased information.

The date of the information is particularly important. Cancer diagnoses, treatments, and prognoses change significantly over time. Related issues, such as insurance and employment rights, access to quality cancer care, support services, and community resources, also change from year to year. Check the publication date on the material you read, including this book. The more current it is, the more reliable it is.

When you find information through the Internet, the National Cancer Institute suggests asking 10 questions to decide whether the site you are using provides reliable and accurate information:

1. *Who runs the site?* A Web site should identify the organization or individual who runs the site.

2. *What is the purpose of the site?* Is the purpose of the site to provide unbiased information or to promote a particular organization, product, treatment, or service?

3. *What is the source of the information?* The site should identify the original source of the information.

4. *What supports the information?* If the information is presented as fact, it should be supported by a reference to professional literature, such as a medical journal. Without such support, the information may be merely opinion or advice.

5. *How is the information selected?* Does the site have an editorial board of experts?

6. *How current is the information?* Information, especially medical and legal information, should be very current. Each major page of the site should state when it was last updated.

7. *How does the site choose links to other sites?* Most Web sites have a policy on what links they will post. For example, many medical sites do not link to other sites. Many nonprofit national cancer organizations provide links to nonprofit sites, and some commercial sites link to any site that asks or pays for a link.

8. *Who pays for the site?* The last three letters of the site's address is one way to identify who pays to produce the site, and thus help you learn the purpose of the site. The most common source identifiers are:

> .gov—government agency
> .org—nonprofit organization
> .com—commercial company
> .edu—university

9. *What information about you does the site collect and why?* Web sites routinely track the paths visitors take through its sites to determine what pages are being used. Many Web sites, however, ask you to "subscribe" or "become a member." The site may seek this information to charge you a user fee, to gather information for research or marketing purposes, or to tailor the information it provides you to your special needs. Carefully read the site's privacy policy before you give any personal information to a Web site.

10. *How does the site manage interactions with visitors?* The site should provide a way for you to ask questions or seek assistance using the site.

Answers to most of these 10 questions should be provided by the site. Look under "About this Site" or "Mission Statement" or e-mail the site with your questions.

Resources

These resources are provided for informational purposes only. NCCS, the editors, and authors are not responsible for the information provided by the organizations listed. The medical information you may receive should not be used for self-diagnosis or instead of consulting with health professionals. For medical questions, please talk with your doctor.

Medical Information about Cancer

Public Agencies
The National Cancer Institute's Cancer Information Service
Building 31, Room 10A16
9000 Rockville Pike
Bethesda, MD 20892
(800) 422-6237 [(800)-4-CANCER]
(800) 332-8615 (TTY for deaf and hard-of-hearing callers)
www.cancer.gov

The National Cancer Institute's (NCI) Cancer Information Service provides a national telephone service that answers questions and sends publications on most cancer-related topics, including clinical trials. In addition to the Cancer Information Service, NCI's Office of Cancer Survivorship funds research on survivorship issues and supports public education programs on cancer survivorship. NCI's CancerFax provides information on cancer treatment screening, prevention, genetics, complementary and alternative medicine, and supportive care. Call (800) 624-2511 or (301) 402-5874 and follow the recorded instructions.

National Institutes of Health
National Center for Complementary and Alternative Medicine
P.O. Box 7923
Gaithersburg, MD 20898-7923
(888) 644-6226
www.nccam.nih.gov

Promotes research and provides information on complementary and alternative medicine.

Food and Drug Administration
Medwatch
(888) INFO-FDA (463-6332)
www.fda.gov/medwatch/index.html

Food and Drug Administration program that provides timely safety information on the drugs and other medical products regulated by the FDA.

NCI-DESIGNATED CANCER CENTERS

The NCI-designated Cancer Centers are 61 research-oriented institutions across America that NCI recognizes for scientific excellence and for their extensive resources focused on cancer and cancer-related problems. Three types of Cancer Centers are recognized:
- "Cancer centers" conduct basic scientific research (i.e., laboratory studies) into how and why cancer originates and develops.
- "Clinical cancer centers" conduct both basic scientific research and clinical research, including cancer clinical trials. Clinical centers may have programs in cancer prevention, control and population research and many also have outreach, education and information activities.
- "Comprehensive cancer centers" have broad programs involving and integrating all three major areas of research: basic scientific research; clinical research and prevention; control and population research. They offer an extensive range of trials, and have significant activities in outreach, education and information.

WEST
California
USC/Norris Comprehensive Cancer Center
Los Angeles, CA
(800) 872-2273
http://ccnt.hsc.usc.edu

Jonsson Comprehensive Cancer Center at UCLA
Los Angeles, CA
(310) 825-5268
www.cancer.mednet.ucla.edu

City of Hope Comprehensive Cancer Center
Duarte, CA
(800) 826-4673
www.cityofhope.org

Chao Family Comprehensive Cancer Center
University of California/Irvine
Orange, CA
(714) 456-8200
www.ucihs.uci.edu/cancer

University of California, Davis Cancer Center
Davis, CA
(800) 362-5566
www.ucdmc.ucdavis.edu/cancer

University of California, San Diego Cancer Center
La Jolla, CA
(858) 534-7600
http://cancer.ucsd.edu

University of California, San Francisco Cancer Center
San Francisco, CA
(800) 888-8664
http://cc.ucsf.edu

MID-ATLANTIC
District of Columbia
Lombardi Cancer Center
Georgetown University Medical Center
Washington, DC

(202) 444-4000
http://lombardi.georgetown.edu

Maryland
The Sidney Kimmel Comprehensive Cancer Center
Johns Hopkins Oncology Center
Baltimore, MD
(410) 955-8964
www.hopkinskimmel/cancercenter.org

New Jersey
The Cancer Institute of New Jersey
Robert Wood Johnson Medical School
New Brunswick, NJ
(732) 235-2465
www.cinj.org

New York
Albert Einstein Cancer Center
Yeshiva University
Bronx, NY
(718) 430-2302
www.aecom.yu.edu/cancer

Herbert Irving Comprehensive Cancer Center
Columbia University
New York, NY
(212) 305-8602
www.ccc.columbia.edu

New York University Cancer Institute
New York, NY
(212) 263-3551
www.med.nyu.edu/nyuci

Memorial Sloan-Kettering Cancer Center
New York, NY
(212) 639-2000
www.mskcc.org

Roswell Park Cancer Institute
Buffalo, NY
(877) 275-7724
www.roswellpark.org

Pennsylvania
Fox Chase Cancer Center
Philadelphia, PA
(888) 369-2427
www.fccc.edu

Kimmel Cancer Center—Thomas Jefferson University
Philadelphia, PA
(215) 503-4500
www.kimmelcancercenter.org

University of Pennsylvania Abramson Cancer Center
Philadelphia, PA
(215) 349-8382
www.penncancer.com

University of Pittsburgh Cancer Institute
Pittsburgh, PA
(412) 647-2811
www.upmccancercenters.com

MIDWEST
Illinois
The Robert H. Lurie Comprehensive Cancer Center
Northwestern University
Chicago, IL
(312) 908-5250
www.lurie.nwu.edu

University of Chicago Cancer Research Center
Chicago, IL
(888) 824-0200
www-uccrc.uchicago.edu

Indiana
Indiana University Cancer Center
Indianapolis, IN
(888) 600-4822
www.iucc.iu.edu

Iowa
Holden Comprehensive Cancer Center
University of Iowa

Iowa City, IA
(800) 237-1225
www.uihealthcare.com

Michigan
Barbara Ann Karmanos Cancer Institute
Wayne State University
Detroit, MI
(800) 527-6266
www.karmanos.org

University of Michigan Comprehensive Cancer Center
Ann Arbor, MI
(800) 865-1125
www.cancer.med.umich.edu

Minnesota
Mayo Clinic Cancer Center
Rochester, MN
(507) 284-2111
www.mayoclinic.org/cancercenter

University of Minnesota Cancer Center
Minneapolis, MN
(612) 624-8484
www.cancer.umn.edu

Missouri
Siteman Cancer Center
Washington University School of Medicine
St. Louis, MO
(314) 747-7222
(800) 600-3606
www.siteman.wustl.edu

Ohio
OSU Comprehensive Cancer Center
Columbus, OH
(800) 293-5066
www.jamesline.com

Ireland Cancer Center—University Hospitals of Cleveland
Cleveland, OH

(800) 641-2422
www.irelandcancercenter.org

Wisconsin
University of Wisconsin Comprehensive Cancer Center
Madison, WI
(800) 622-8922
www.cancer.wisc.edu

New England
Connecticut
Yale Comprehensive Cancer Center
Yale University School of Medicine
New Haven, CT
(203) 785-4095
www.infomed.yale.edu/ycc

Massachusetts
Dana-Farber Cancer Institute
Boston, MA
(617) 632-3000
(866) 408-3324
www.dana-farber.net

New Hampshire
Norris Cotton Cancer Center
Lebanon, NH
(800) 639-6918
www.dartmouth.edu/dms/nccc

Vermont
Vermont Cancer Center
University of Vermont College of Medicine
Burlington, VT
(802) 656-4414
www.vermontcancer.org

Northwest and Central Plains
Colorado
University of Colorado Cancer Center
Denver, CO
(800) 473-2288
www.uccc.info

Eppley Cancer Center
University of Nebraska Medical Center

Omaha, NE
(402) 559-4000
(800) 999-5465 (Cancer HelpLink)
www.unmc.edu/cancercenter

Oregon
OHSU Cancer Institute
Oregon Health and Science University
Portland, OR
(503) 494-1617
www.ohsuhealth.com/ohsu-cancer

Utah
Huntsman Cancer Institute
University of Utah
Salt Lake City, UT
(877) 585-0303
www.hci.utah.edu

Washington
Fred Hutchinson Cancer Research Center
Seattle, WA
(206) 667-5000
www.fhcrc.org

SOUTHEAST
Alabama
Birmingham Comprehensive Cancer Center
University of Alabama
Birmingham, AL
(800) 822-0933
www.ccc.uab.edu

Florida
H. Lee Moffitt Cancer Center and Research Institute
University of South Florida
Tampa, FL
(888) MOFFITT (663-3488)
www.moffitt.usf.edu

North Carolina
Comprehensive Cancer Center of Wake Forest University
Winston-Salem, NC

(336) 716-4464
www1.wfubmc.edu/cancer

Duke Comprehensive Cancer Center
Durham, NC
(888) ASK-DUKE (275-3853)
www.cancer.duke.edu

UNC Lineberger Comprehensive Cancer Center
University of North Carolina
Chapel Hill, NC
(919) 966-3036
http://cancer.med.unc.edu

Tennessee
St. Jude's Children's Research Hospital
Memphis, TN
(901) 495-3300
www.stjude.org

Vanderbilt-Ingram Cancer Center
Vanderbilt University
Nashville, TN
(800) 811-8480
www.vanderbiltcancer.org

Virginia
The Cancer Center
University of Virginia Health System
Charlottesville, VA
(800) 223-9173
www.healthsystem.virginia.edu/internet/cancer

Massey Cancer Center
Virginia Commonwealth University
Richmond, VA
(804) 828-0450
www.vcu.edu/mcc

SOUTHWEST
Arizona
Arizona Cancer Center
University of Arizona

Tucson, AZ
(800) 622-2673
www.azcc.arizona.edu

Hawaii
Cancer Research Center of Hawaii
University of Hawaii at Manoa
Honolulu, HI
(808) 586-3010
www.hawaii.edu/crch

Texas
MD Anderson Cancer Center
University of Texas
Houston, TX
(800) 392-1611
www.mdanderson.org

San Antonio Cancer Institute
San Antonio, TX
(210) 616-5590
www.ccc.saci.org

NONPROFIT ORGANIZATIONS

American Cancer Society
1599 Clifton Road NE
Atlanta, GA 30329-4251
(800) ACS-2345
www.cancer.org
   Provides publications, counseling, financial assistance, and public education
programs.

Cancer Care
275 Seventh Avenue
New York, NY 10001
(800) 813-HOPE or (212) 302-2400
www.cancercare.org
   Staffed by oncology social workers and other professionals; provides counseling, education, referrals, publications, and financial assistance.

National Coalition for Cancer Survivorship
1010 Wayne Avenue, Suite 770
Silver Spring, MD 20910

(877) 622-7937
www.canceradvocacy.org
   NCCS is the only survivor-led organization working on behalf of all cancer survivors. NCCS's mission is to advocate for quality cancer care for all Americans. NCCS provides educational resources and publications, and leads national advocacy efforts on behalf of survivors and those who care for them.

PROFESSIONAL MEDICAL SOCIETIES

American Board of Medical Specialties
1007 Church Street, Suite 404
Evanston, IL 60201-5913
(866) 275-2267
www.abms.org/which.asp
   The American Board of Medical Specialties (ABMS) publishes a list of board-certified physicians. The *Official ABMS Directory of Board Certified Medical Specialists* lists doctors' names along with their specialty and their educational background. This resource is available in most public libraries and on the Internet at www.abms.org/newsearch.asp.

American College of Surgeons
Office of Public Information
633 North Saint Clair Street
Chicago, IL 60611-3211
(312) 202-5000
http://web.facs.org
   The ACOS accredits cancer programs at hospitals and other treatment facilities. More than 1,400 programs in the United States have been designated by the ACOS as Approved Cancer Programs.

American Medical Association
515 North State Street
Chicago, IL 60610
(312) 464-5000
www.ama-assn.org
   The American Medical Association (AMA) provides an online service called AMA Physician Select that offers basic professional information on virtually every licensed physician in the United States and its possessions. The database can be searched by doctor's name or by medical specialty. The AMA Physician Select service is located at http://www.ama-assn.org/aps/amahg.htm on the Internet.

American Society of Clinical Oncology
1900 Duke Street, Suite 200
Alexandria, VA 22314

(703) 299-0150
www.asco.org

The American Society of Clinical Oncology (ASCO) provides an online list of doctors who are members of ASCO. The member database has the names and affiliations of over 15,000 oncologists worldwide. It can be searched by doctor's name, institution's name, location, and/or type of board certification. ASCO offers a Web site that helps patients and families find accurate, reliable, and oncologist-approved information about cancer at www.peoplelivingwithcancer.org.

Association of Oncology Social Work
1211 Locust Street
Philadelphia, PA 19107
(215) 599-6093
www.aosw.org

AOSW is an organization of oncology social workers and others who work on behalf of cancer survivors.

Joint Commission on Accreditation of Healthcare Organizations
One Renaissance Boulevard
Oakbrook Terrace, IL 60181-4294
(630) 792-5800
www.jcaho.org

The JCAHO is an independent, not-for-profit organization that evaluates and accredits health care organizations and programs in the United States. It also offers information for the general public about choosing a treatment facility. The JCAHO offers an online Quality Check service that patients can use to determine whether a specific facility has been accredited by the JCAHO and to view the organization's performance reports.

National Committee for Quality Assurance
2000 L Street, NW
Suite 500
Washington, DC 20036
(202) 955-3500
www.ncqa.org

The NCQA is a nonprofit organization that evaluates and accredits health care organizations and provides report cards on health plan performance.

Oncology Nursing Society
125 Enterprise Drive
Pittsburgh, PA 15275-1214

(866) 257-4ONS (4667)
www.ons.org

ONS is a national organization of more than 25,000 registered nurses who work with persons who have cancer. Web site has a special section for patient information and educational resources.

CLINICAL TRIALS

The following provide information about clinical trials for cancer treatment.

National Cancer Institute Clinical Trials
(800) 422-6897
www.cancer.gov

Acurian
(866) 566-5966
www.acurian.com/patient

Centerwatch
(617) 856-5900
www.centerwatch.com

Cycle of Hope
www.cycleofhope.org

Emerging Med
(877) 601-8601
www.emergingmed.com

HopeLink
(650) 373-7300
www.hopelink.com

National Coalition for Cancer Cooperative Groups
www.trialcheck.org

Oncolink Clinical Trials
www.oncolink.upenn.edu

LONG-TERM SURVIVORSHIP INFORMATION

Association of Cancer Online Resources (ACOR)
www.acor.org

Collection of online communities designed to provide timely and accurate information in a supportive environment. Sponsors listservs for long-term survivors.

National Cancer Institute's Office of Cancer Survivorship
6130 Executive Boulevard Room 4089A
Bethesda, MD 20892-7397
(301) 402-2964
http://dccps.nci.nih.gov/ocs
   Funds research on survivorship issues and supports public education programs
on cancer survivorship. OCS's Web site has a section on follow-up medical care
after treatment, including a list of long-term follow-up clinics at http://dccps.nci.
nih.gov/ocs/follow.html.

CHILDHOOD CANCER SURVIVORS

Candlelighters Childhood Cancer Foundation
P.O. Box 498
Kensington, MD 20895
(800) 366-2223
www.candlelighters.org
   Provides support and information to families of children with cancer and to
adult survivors of childhood cancer.

Childhood Cancer Center
www.patientcenters.com/childcancer
   Provides printed information about childhood cancer, including *Childhood
Cancer Survivors: A Practical Guide to Your Future* (O'Reilly, 2000), a practical and
comprehensive book by Nancy Keene, Wendy Hobbie, and Kathy Ruccione.

Foundation for the Children's Oncology Group
(800) 458-6223
www.nccf.org
   The Foundation for the Children's Oncology Group funds pediatric cancer
research, and promotes education and advocacy for children with cancer.

Pediatric Oncology Resource Center
www.acor.org/ped-onc/
   Provides information and resources for families and friends of children who
have or had childhood cancer.

RELATED HEALTH AND SUPPORT RESOURCES

CAREGIVER INFORMATION
Caregiver Media Group
6365 Taft Street, Suite 3006
Hollywood, FL 33024
(800) 829-2734
www.caregiver.com

Provides an online newsletter, workshops, audiotapes, and information about caregivers and the work force, caregiver tips, etc.

Family Caregiver Alliance
690 Market Street, Suite 600
San Francisco, CA 94104
(800) 445-8106
www.caregiver.org
Provides a clearinghouse that covers current medical, social, public policy, and caregiving issues related to adult brain impairments, including tumors. Provides online support group, online caregiver consultation, fact sheets, reading lists, etc., for adults.

National Family Caregivers Association
10400 Connecticut Avenue, #500
Kensington, MD 20895-3944
(800) 896-3650
www.nfcacares.org
Advocates on behalf of caregivers. Services include education, information, support, validation, public awareness, and advocacy.

Well Spouse Foundation
63 West Main Street, Suite H
Freehold, NJ 07728
(800) 838-0879
www.wellspouse.org
Provides a bimonthly newsletter, pamphlets, mutual aid support groups in many areas, letter-writing support groups, annual conference, and regional and weekend meetings around the country.

COMPLEMENTARY AND ALTERNATIVE MEDICINE AND SYMPTOM MANAGEMENT

Alternative Medicine Foundation
P.O. Box 60016
Potomac, MD 20859-0016
(301) 340-1960
www.AMFoundation.org
Nonprofit organization designed to provide responsible and reliable information about complementary and alternative medicines to the public and to health professionals.

ConsumerLab.com
333 Mamaroneck Avenue

White Plains, NY 10605
(914) 722-9149
www.consumerlab.com

Provides independent test results and information to help consumers and health care professionals evaluate health, wellness, and nutrition products.

FERTILITY, SEXUALITY, AND GENETIC INFORMATION

Adoptive Families of America (AFA)
2309 Como Avenue
St. Paul, MN 55108
(800) 372-3300
www.adoptivefam.org

Provides education, links, and publications on pre- and post-adoption topics.

Alliance of Genetic Support Groups
4301 Connecticut Avenue NW #404
Washington, DC 20008
(800) 336-GENE or (202) 966-5557
www.geneticalliance.org

Nonprofit coalition of support groups, professionals, and consumers dedicated to promoting the interests of children, adults, and families with or at risk for genetic disorders. Specializes in linking people interested in genetic conditions with organizations that provide support and information.

American Academy of Adoption Attorneys
P.O. Box 33053
Washington, DC 20033
(202) 832-2222
www.adoptionattorneys.org

Provides referrals to adoption attorneys.

American Association of Sex Educators, Counselors, and Therapists
P.O. Box 5488
Richmond, VA 23220-0488
www.aasect.org

Provides referrals to a certified sexuality educator, counselor, or therapist in your area.

American Infertility Association
666 Fifth Avenue, Suite 278
New York, NY
(718) 621-5083
www.americaninfertility.org

Provides publications, resources, and information on peer networking and support groups.

American Society for Reproductive Medicine
1209 Montgomery Highway
Birmingham, AL 35216-2809
(205) 978-5000
www.asrm.org
Nonprofit organization devoted to advancing knowledge and expertise in reproductive medicine.

FertileHope
P.O. Box 624
New York, NY 10014
(888) 994-HOPE
www.fertilehope.org
Nonprofit organization dedicated to helping cancer survivors faced with infertility. Offers publications, resources, and financial assistance.

National Adoption Information Clearinghouse
330 C Street, SW
Washington, DC 20447
(703) 352-3488 or (888) 385-3206
http://naic.acf.hhs.gov
NAIC is a clearinghouse of information under the U.S. Department of Health and Human Services, Administration for Children and Families.

National Council for Adoption
225 N. Washington Street
Alexandria, VA 22314-2561
(703) 299-6633
www.ncfa-usa.org
NCFA is a nonprofit organization that provides information and public education, advocacy for families, and assistance with choosing an adoption agency or attorney.

National Infertility Network Exchange
P.O. Box 204
East Meadow, NY 11554
(516) 794-5772
www.nine-infertility.org
Nonprofit organization that offers peer support for infertile couples, referral to appropriate professionals, and educational materials.

National Society of Genetic Counselors
233 Canterbury Drive
Wallingford, PA 19086
(610) 872-7608
www.nsgc.org
   Provides referrals to local genetic counseling services.

RESOLVE: The National Infertility Association
1310 Broadway
Somerville, MA 02144
(888) 623-0744
www.resolve.org
   Provides timely, compassionate support and information through advocacy and public education to individuals who are experiencing infertility issues.

HOSPICE AND END-OF-LIFE INFORMATION

Aging with Dignity
P.O. Box 1661
Tallahassee, FL 32303-1661
(888) 5WISHES (594-7437)
www.agingwithdignity.org
   Provides documents to help plan end-of-life care.

Hospice Association of America
228 Seventh Street, SE
Washington, DC 20003
(202) 546-4759
www.nahc.org/haa/home.html
   HAA provides facts and statistics about hospice programs, and the publication *Information about Hospice: A Consumer's Guide.* This guide offers information about the advantages and financial aspects of hospice, how to select quality hospice care that is best suited for a patient's needs, and state resources available to patients.

Hospice Education Institute
119 Westbrook Road
Essex, CT 06426-1510
(860) 767-1620/(800) 331-1620
www.hospiceworld.org
   The Hospice Education Institute offers information and referrals on various hospice programs around the country and provides regional seminars on hospice care throughout the United States. Comments or suggestions about hospice programs are also welcomed from health professionals and hospice volunteers.

Hospice Foundation of America
2001 S Street, NW, #300
Washington, DC 20009
(800) 854-3402
www.hospicefoundation.org
Nonprofit organization that promotes hospice care. Works to educate professionals and families on caregiving, terminal illness, loss, and bereavement.

National Hospice and Palliative Care Organization
1700 Diagonal Road, Suite 625
Alexandria, VA 22314
(800) 658-8898 (Helpline)
(703) 837-1500
www.nhpco.org
NHPCO is an association of programs that provide hospice and palliative care. It offers discussion groups, publications, information about how to find a hospice, and information about the financial aspects of hospice. Some Spanish-language publications are available, and staff are able to answer calls in Spanish.

Partnership for Caring: America's Voices for the Dying
1620 Eye Street, NW, Suite 202
Washington, DC 20006
(800) 989-9455
www.partnershipforcaring.org
Offers information on end-of-life issues, including advance directives and state laws.

Viatical Association of America
800 Mayfair Circle
Orlando, FL 32803
(800) 842-9811
www.viatical.org
Provides a list of viatical companies that will buy your life insurance policies under certain conditions.

MINORITY AND SPECIAL POPULATIONS

Intercultural Cancer Council (ICC)
6655 Travis, Suite 322
Houston, TX 77030-1312
(713) 798-4617
www.iccnetwork.org
Promotes policies, programs, partnerships, and research to eliminate the unequal burden of cancer among racial and ethnic minorities and medically underserved populations.

Mary-Helen Mautner Project for Lesbians with Cancer
1707 L Street, NW, Suite 1060
Washington, DC 20036
(202) 332-5536
www.mautnerproject.org
   Support services for lesbians who have cancer, their partners, and families. Services include advocacy, counseling, home care, transportation, and legal assistance.

National Alliance for Hispanic Health
1501 16th Street, NW
Washington, DC 20036
(202) 387-5000
www.hispanichealth.org
   Largest and oldest network of health and human service programs serving Hispanic consumers. Provides educational publications and resources.

National Asian Women's Health Organization (NAWHO)
215 Montgomery Street, Suite 900
San Francisco, CA 94104
(415) 989-9747
www.nawho.org
   Works to improve the health status of Asian women and families through research, education, leadership, and public policy programs. Resources for Asian women in English, Cantonese, Laotian, Vietnamese, and Korean.

National Black Leadership Initiative on Cancer
Moorehouse School of Medicine
720 Westview Drive SW
Atlanta, GA 30310
(800) 724-1185
www.nblic.org
   National Cancer Institute program from the Special Populations branch that provides outreach and education with the intention of lowering cancer rates in the African-American community.

National Council of La Raza (NCLR)
1111 19th Street, NW, Suite 1000
Washington, DC 20036
(202) 785-1670
www.nclr.org
   Nonprofit organization dedicated to reducing poverty and discrimination, and to improving opportunities for Hispanics. Provides educational publications and resources.

Office of Minority Health Resource Center
P.O. Box 37337
Washington, DC 20013-7337
(800) 444-6472
www.omhrc.gov/omhhome.htm
    Federal agency whose mission is to improve the health of racial and ethnic populations through effective programs and policies.

Pan American Health Organization (PAHO)
Regional Office of the World Health Organization
525 23rd Street, NW
Washington, DC 20037
(202) 974-3000
www.paho.org
    International public health agency that provides advocacy, educational publications, and resources.

PAIN INFORMATION

American Chronic Pain Association
P.O. Box 850
Rocklin, CA 95677
(800) 533-3231
www.theacpa.org
    Provides peer support and coping skills to anyone with chronic pain.

American Pain Foundation
201 North Charles Street, Suite 710
Baltimore, MD 21201-411
(888) 615-7246
www.painfoundation.org
    An information, education, and advocacy organization that serves people with pain. Accepts telephone calls from individuals with specific pain issues. Publishes the *Pain Care Bill of Rights,* which states that patients have the right to receive information about pain treatments and to receive quality pain management.

PATIENT AND PEER SUPPORT

American Self-Help Group Clearinghouse
100 Hanover Avenue, Suite 202
Cedar Knolls, NJ 07927
(973) 326-6789
www.mentalhelp.net/selfhelp
    Provides lists of self-help groups and information on how to start and manage self-help groups.

CancerCare
275 Seventh Avenue
New York, NY 10001
(800) 813-HOPE or (212) 302-2400
www.cancercare.org
Staffed by oncology social workers and other professionals; provides counseling, education, referrals, publications, and financial assistance.

Cancer Hope Network
Two North Road
Chester, NJ 07930
(877) 467-3638
www.cancerhopenetwork.org
Provides confidential, one-on-one support to survivors and families.

Friends' Health Connection
P.O. Box 114
New Brunswick, NJ 08903
(800) 48FRIEND
www.friendshealthconnection.org
Nonprofit support network that connects people with similar health problems and caregivers for mutual support.

The Wellness Community
919 18th Street, NW, Suite 54
Washington, DC 20006
(888) 793-9355
www.thewellnesscommunity.org
Nonprofit organization that helps survivors deal with the humanistic aspects of living with cancer. Nearly two dozen centers nationwide are staffed with professional support-group leaders, and multifaceted programs targeted at healing body, mind, and spirit conducted in a homelike setting.

LEGAL INFORMATION

STATE INSURANCE DEPARTMENTS

Each state has its own insurance department to oversee all types of insurance. The following offices are responsible for enforcing laws and regulations, and for providing the public with helpful information.

ALABAMA

Alabama Department of Insurance
201 Monroe Street, Suite 1700
P.O. Box 303351

Montgomery, AL 36104
(334) 269-3550
Fax: (334) 241-4192
E-mail: insdept@insurance.state.al.us
www.aldoi.org

ALASKA
Department of Community and Economic Development
Division of Insurance
550 W. 7th Avenue, Suite 1560
Anchorage, AK 99501-3567
(800) INSURAK
Fax: (907) 269-7910
E-mail: insurance@dced.state.ak.us
www.dced.state.ak.us/insurance

ARIZONA
Arizona Department of Insurance
2910 North 44th Street, 2nd Floor
Phoenix, AZ 85018-7256
(602) 912-8444 (Phoenix area) (520) 628-6370 (Tucson area)
Toll free in AZ: (800) 325-2548
Fax: (602) 954-7008 (complaints)
www.id.state.az.us/index

ARKANSAS
Arkansas Department of Insurance
1200 West Third Street
Little Rock, AR 72201-1904
(501) 371-2640
(800) 852-5494
Fax: (501) 371-2749
E-mail: insurance.consumers@mail.state.ar.us
www.state.ar.us/insurance

CALIFORNIA
Department of Insurance
Consumer Communications Bureau
300 South Spring Street, South Tower
Los Angeles, CA 90013
(213) 897-8921 (for out-of-state callers)
Toll free in CA: (800) 927-4357 (consumer hotline)
www.insurance.ca.gov

COLORADO
Division of Insurance
1560 Broadway, Suite 850
Denver, CO 80202
(303) 894-7499, ext. 4311
Toll free in CO: (800) 930-3745
TDD/TTY: (303) 894-7880
Fax: (303) 894-7455
www.dora.state.co.us/Insurance

CONNECTICUT
Consumer Affairs
Department of Insurance
P.O. Box 816
Hartford, CT 06142-0816
(860) 297-3900
Toll free: (800) 203-3447
Fax: (203) 297-3872
www.state.ct.us/cid

DELAWARE
Department of Insurance
841 Silver Lake Boulevard, Rodney Building
Dover, DE 19904
(302) 739-4251
Toll free in DE: (800) 282-8611
Fax: (302) 739-5280
www.state.de.us/inscom

DISTRICT OF COLUMBIA
District of Columbia Department of Insurance and Securities Regulation
810 First Street, NW
Suite 701
Washington, DC 20002
(202) 727-8000
Fax: (202) 535-1196
E-mail: disr@dcgov.org

FLORIDA
Department of Financial Services
Office of Insurance Regulation
200 E. Gaines Street
Tallahassee, FL 32399-0333
(850) 413-3131

Toll free in FL: (800) 342-2762
TDD toll free: (800) 640-0886
www.fldfs.com/companies

GEORGIA
Insurance and Fire Safety
Two Martin Luther King Jr. Drive
Atlanta, GA 30334
(404) 656-2070
Toll free in GA: (800) 656-2298
TDD/TTY: (404) 656-4031
Fax: (404) 651-8719
www.inscomm.state.ga.us

HAWAII
State of Hawaii, Department of Commerce and Consumer Affairs
Insurance Division
250 South King Street, 5th Floor (96813)
P.O. Box 3614
Honolulu, HI 96811-3614
(808) 586-2790
Fax: (808) 586-2806
www.state.hi.us/dcca/ins

IDAHO
State of Idaho Department of Insurance
700 West State Street
P.O. Box 83720
Boise, ID 83720-0043
(208) 334-4250
Toll free in ID: (800) 721-3272
Fax: (208) 334-4398
www.doi.state.id.us

ILLINOIS
Department of Insurance
320 West Washington Street
Springfield, IL 62767
(217) 782-4515
Toll free: (877) 527-9431 (Office of Consumer Health Insurance)
TDD: (217) 524-4872
Fax: (217) 782-5020
E-mail: director@ins.state.il.us
www.state.il.us/ins/

INDIANA
Department of Insurance
311 West Washington Street, Suite 300
Indianapolis, IN 46204-2787
(317) 232-2385
Toll free in IN: (800) 622-4461
Toll free: (800) 452-4800 (in-state senior health insurance information)
Fax: (317) 232-5251
www.state.in.us/idoi/

IOWA
State of Iowa
Division of Insurance
330 Maple Street
Des Moines, IA 50319
(515) 281-5705
(877) 955-1212
Fax: (515) 281-3059
www.iid.state.ia.us

KANSAS
Insurance Department
Topeka Office
420 SW Ninth Street
Topeka, KS 66612-1678
(785) 296-3071
Toll free in KS: (800) 432-2484
Fax: (785) 296-2283
E-mail: webcomplaint@ksinsurance.org
www.kinsurance.org

Wichita Office
130 South Market Street
Suite 1028
Box 3850
Wichita, KS 67201-3850
(316) 337-6010
Toll Free in KS: (800) 432-2484
Fax: (316) 337-6018

KENTUCKY
Department of Insurance
215 West Main Street
Frankfort, KY 40601
(502) 564-3630

Toll free: (800) 595-6053
Fax: (502) 564-1650
http://www.doi.state.ky.us/

LOUISIANA
Department of Insurance
1702 North 3rd Street
Baton Rouge, LA 70802
(225) 343-4834
Toll free: (800) 259-5300
Toll free: (800) 259-5301
Fax: (254) 342-5900
www.ldi.state.la.us

MAINE
Bureau of Insurance
34 State House Station
Augusta, ME 04333
(207) 624-8475
Toll free in ME: (800) 300-5000
TDD: (207) 624-8563
Fax: (207) 624-8599
www.maineinsurancereg.org

MARYLAND
Maryland Insurance Administration
525 St. Paul Place
Baltimore, MD 21202
(410) 468-2000
(410) 468-2340 (property & casualty complaints)
Toll free nationwide: (800) 492-6116
Fax: (410) 468-2020
www.mdinsurance.state.md.us

MASSACHUSETTS
Division of Insurance
South Station, 5th Floor
Boston, MA 02110
(617) 521-7794
TDD: (617) 521-7490
Fax: (617) 521-7772
www.state.ma.us/doi

MICHIGAN
Michigan Office of Financial and Insurance Services
611 West Ottawa Street, 2nd Floor North
P.O. Box 30220 (mailing address)
Lansing, MI 48909-7720
(517) 373-0220
Toll free: (877) 999-6442
Fax: (517) 335-4978
www.michigan.gov/cis (click on Financial and Insurance Services)

MINNESOTA
Department of Commerce
133 East Seventh Street
St. Paul, MN 55101
(651) 296-2488
Toll free: (800) 657-3602
Fax: (651) 296-4328
E-mail: enforcement@state.mn.us
www.commerce.state.mn.us

MISSISSIPPI
Department of Insurance
P.O. Box 79
Jackson, MS 39205
(601) 359-3569
Toll free in MS: (800) 562-2957
Fax: (601) 359-2474
www.doi.state.ms.us

MISSOURI
Missouri Department of Insurance
P.O. Box 690
301 West High Street, Room 530
Jefferson City, MO 65102
(573) 751-4126
(573) 751-2640
Toll free in MO: (800) 726-7390
TTD/TTY: (573) 526-4536
Fax: (573) 751-1165
www.insurance.state.mo.us

MONTANA
Department of Insurance
840 Helena Avenue
P.O. Box 4009
Helena, MT 59601
(406) 444-2040
Toll free in MT: (800) 332-6148
Fax: (406) 444-3497
http://sao.state.mt.us

NEBRASKA
Department of Insurance
941 O Street, Suite 400
Lincoln, NE 68508-3690
(402) 471-2201
TDD toll free: (800) 833-7351
Fax: (402) 471-4610
www.nol.org/home/NDOI

NEVADA
Division of Insurance
Consumer Service Section
788 Fairview Drive, #300
Carson City, NV 89701
(800) 992-0900
www.doi.state.nv.us

NEW HAMPSHIRE
Department of Insurance
56 Old Suncook Road
Concord, NH 03301-7317
(603) 271-2261
Toll free in NH: (800) 852-3416
TDD/TTY toll free in NH: (800) 735-2964
Fax: (603) 271-1406
E-mail: requests@ins.state.nh.us
www.state.nh.us/insurance

NEW JERSEY
Department of Banking and Insurance
20 West State Street
P.O. Box 329
Trenton, NJ 08625
(609) 633-7667

Fax: (609) 292-5865
www.state.nj.us/dobi

NEW MEXICO
Department of Insurance
P.O. Box 1269
Santa Fe, NM 87504-1269
(505) 827-4601
Toll free in NM: (800) 947-4722
Fax: (505) 827-4734
www.nmprc.state.nm.us

NEW YORK
Consumer Services Bureau
NYS Insurance Department
One Commerce Plaza
Albany, NY 12257
(518) 474-6600
www.ins.state.ny.us

Consumer Services Bureau
NYS Insurance Department
65 Court Street
Buffalo, NY 14202
(716) 847-7619
E-mail: consumers@ins.state.ny.us
www.ins.state.ny.us

NORTH CAROLINA
Department of Insurance
Dobbs Building, 430 North Salisbury Street
P.O. Box 26387
Raleigh, NC 27611-6387
(919) 733-2032
Toll free: (800) 546-5664
Fax: (919) 733-6495
www.ncdoi.com

NORTH DAKOTA
North Dakota Insurance Department
600 East Boulevard Avenue
Dept. 401
Bismarck, ND 58505-0320
(701) 328-2440

Toll free in ND: (800) 247-0560
TTY/TDD: (800) 366-6888
Fax: (701) 328-4880
E-mail: insurance@state.nd.us
www.state.nd.us/ndins

OHIO
Department of Insurance
Office of Consumer Services
2100 Stella Court
Columbus, OH 43215-1067
(614) 644-2673
Toll free: (800) 686-1526 (consumer hotline)
Toll free: (800) 686-1527 (fraud hotline)
Toll free: (800) 686-1578 (senior hotline)
TDD: (614) 644-3745
Fax: (614) 644-3744
www.ohioinsurance.gov

OKLAHOMA
Oklahoma Insurance Department
2401 NW 23rd Street, Suite 28
P.O. Box 53408
Oklahoma City, OK 73152-3408
(405) 521-2828
Toll free in OK: (800) 522-0071
www.oid.state.ok.us

OREGON
Oregon Insurance Division
350 Winter Street, NE
Room 440
Salem, OR 97310-3883
(503) 947-7980
Toll free in OR: (888) 877-4894
Fax: (503) 378-4351
E-mail: dcbs.insmail@state.or.us
www.cbs.state.or.us/ins

PENNSYLVANIA
Insurance Department
1326 Strawberry Square
Harrisburg, PA 17120
(717) 787-2317

Toll free: (877) 881-6388
E-mail: consumer@ins.state.pa.us
www.ins.state.pa.us/ins

PUERTO RICO
Office of the Commissioner of Insurance
Call Box 8330
Fernandez Juncos Station
Santurce, PR 00910-8330
(787) 722-8686
(787) 721-5848
Fax: (787) 722-4402
www.ocs.gobierno.pr/

RHODE ISLAND
Department of Business Regulation
Insurance Division
233 Richmond Street, Suite 233
Providence, RI 02903-4233
(401) 222-2223
Fax: (401) 222-5475
www.dbr.state.ri.us/insurance.html

SOUTH CAROLINA
South Carolina Department of Insurance
Consumer Services
1612 Marion Street
P.O. Box 100105 (29202-3105)
Columbia, SC 29201
(803) 737-6180
Toll free in SC: (800) 768-3467
Fax: (803) 737-6231
E-mail: cnsmmail@doe.state.sc.us
www.state.sc.us/

SOUTH DAKOTA
South Dakota Division of Insurance
Department of Commerce and Regulation
445 East Capitol Avenue
Pierre, SD 57501-2000
(605) 773-3563
Fax: (605) 773-5369
www.state.sd.us/insurance

TENNESSEE
Department of Commerce and Insurance
500 James Robertson Parkway
5th Floor
Nashville, TN 37243-0565
(615) 741-6007
Toll free in TN: (800) 342-4029 (consumer insurance services)
Toll free in TN: (800) 525-2816 (counseling for seniors)
Fax: (615) 532-6934
www.state.tn.us/commerce

TEXAS
Texas Department of Insurance
333 Guadalupe (78701) (for special delivery and walk-ins)
P.O. Box 149104
Austin, TX 78614-9104
(512) 463-6169
Toll free in TX: (800) 252-3439 (consumer help line)
Fax: (512) 475-2005
www.tdi.state.tx.us

UTAH
Department of Insurance
State Office Building Room 3110
Salt Lake City, UT 84114
(801) 538-3805
Toll free in UT: (800) 439-3805
TDD: (801) 538-3826
Fax: (801) 538-3829
www.insurance.state.ut.us

VERMONT
Department of Banking, Insurance, Securities, and Health Care Administration
89 Main Street
Drawer 20
Montpelier, VT 05620-3101
(802) 828-3302
Toll free in VT: (800) 964-1784
Fax: (802) 828-3301
www.state.vt.us/bis

VIRGIN ISLANDS
Kongen's Gade #18
St. Thomas, VI 00802

(340) 774-7166
Fax: (340) 774-9458
E-mail: vidoi001@aol.com

VIRGINIA
Bureau of Insurance
State Corporation Commission
P.O. Box 1157
1300 East Main Street (23219) (only for special delivery and walk-ins)
Richmond, VA 23218
(804) 371-9967
Toll free in VA: (800) 552-7945
TDD: (804) 371-9349
www.state.va.us/scc

WASHINGTON
Office of the Commissioner of Insurance
14th Avenue and Water Street
P.O. Box 40255
Olympia, WA 98504-0255
(360) 753-3613
Toll free in WA: (800) 562-6900
TDD: (360) 664-3154
Fax: (360) 586-3535
E-mail: inscomr@aol.com
www.insurance.wa.gov

WEST VIRGINIA
Department of Insurance
1124 Smith St. (25301)
P.O. Box 50540
Charleston, WV 25305-0540
(304) 558-3354
Toll free in WV: (800) 642-9004
Fax: (304) 558-0412
E-mail: wvins@wvnvm.wvnet.edi
www.state.wv.us/insurance

WISCONSIN
Office of the Commissioner of Insurance
125 South Webster Street
P.O. Box 7873
Madison, WI 53707-7873

(608) 266-3585
Toll free in WI: (800) 236-8517
TDD/TTY toll free: (800) 947-3529
Fax: (608) 266-9935
E-mail: information@oci.state.wi.us
http://oci.wi.gov

WYOMING
Wyoming Department of Insurance
Herschler Building, 122 West 25th Street
3rd Floor East
Cheyenne, WY 82002-0440
(307) 777-7401
Toll free in WY: (800) 438-5768
Fax: (307) 777-5895
E-mail: wyinsdep@state.wy.us
http://insurance.state.wy.us/

PUBLIC AGENCIES

Department of Labor
Office of Federal Contract Compliance Programs
(888) 37-OFCCP
www.dol.gov/esa/ofccp
   Provides information on how to enforce rights under Section 503 of the Federal Rehabilitation Act.

Department of Justice
Civil Rights Division
Disability Rights Section-NYAV
950 Pennsylvania Avenue NW
Washington, DC 20035
www.usdoj.gov/crt/drs/drshome.htm
   Provides information on how to enforce rights under Section 504 of the Federal Rehabilitation Act.

Equal Employment Opportunity Commission
1801 L Street NW, Room 9405
Washington, DC 20507
(800) 668-4000 (voice) (to locate regional office)
(800) 669-6820 (TTY) (to locate regional office)
(800) 669-3362 (voice) (for information)
(800) 800-3302 (TTY) (for information)
www.eeoc.gov

Provides information in English and Spanish on how to enforce your rights under the Americans with Disabilities Act. The EEOC can tell you the name and phone number of the state agency that enforces your state employment discrimination law.

Job Accommodation Network
Office of Disability Employment Policy
U.S. Department of Labor
P.O. Box 6080
Morgantown, WV 26506-6080
(800) 526-7234
www.jan.wvu.edu
Provides advice on accommodating employees with disabilities.

National Association of Insurance Commissioners
2301 McGee Street, Suite 800
Kansas City, MO 64108-2662
(816) 842-3600
www.naic.org
Provides the consumer publication, *A Shopper's Guide to Long-Term Care Insurance.*

Pension & Welfare Benefits Administration
United States Department of Labor
(866) 444-3272
www.dol.gov/ebsa
Information on COBRA, the Consolidated Omnibus Budget Reconciliation Act, including the booklet, Health Benefits under the Consolidated Omnibus Budget Reconciliation Act.

PRIVATE ORGANIZATIONS

Cancer Legal Resource Center
A Joint Program of Loyola Law School and the
 Western Law Center for Disability Rights
919 South Albany Street
Los Angeles, CA 90015-1211
(866) 843-2572
Fax: (213) 736-1428
E-mail: clrc@majordomo.lls.edu
www.wlcdr.org
Provides information, education, and resources on cancer-related legal issues, including employment, insurance, government benefits, estate planning, etc. A

volunteer panel of attorneys and other professionals provides additional information as needed.

Council for Responsible Genetics
5 Upland Road, Suite #3
Cambridge, MA 02140
(617) 868-0870
www.gene-watch.org
     Provides information on legal rights related to genetics.

Disability and Business Technical Assistance Center
(800) 949-4322
www.adata.org
     Provides information, materials, technical assistance, and training on the Americans with Disabilities Act.

Health Privacy Project
1120 19th Street NW
8th Floor
Washington, DC 20036
(202) 721-5632
www.healthprivacy.org
     Provides a summary of state health privacy laws.

Life and Health Insurance Foundation for Education
2175 K Street, NW, Suite 250
Washington, DC 20037
(202) 464-5000
www.life-line.org
     Nonprofit consumer organization that provides information on purchasing life insurance.

Medical Care Ombudsman Volunteer Program
Medical Care Management Corporation
5272 River Road
Bethesda, MD 20816-1405
(301) 652-1818
www.mcman.com
     Addresses health care access issues that may involve insurance, discrimination, and underlying employment issues. MCOVP will review as many cases as its panel of over 500 medical experts affiliated with over 100 academic medical centers can

accommodate when physicians have recommended a high-technology or high-risk procedure or complicated medical care.

Medical Information Bureau
P.O. Box 105 Essex Station
Boston, MA 02112
(617) 426-3660
www.mib.com

   Maintains a database on health information of individuals for insurance companies. You can check information on file by writing for or downloading from the Internet a "Request for Disclosure" (Form D-2). A single disclosure report costs $9.

National Employment Lawyers Association
Attorney Listing
44 Montgomery Street, Suite 2080
San Francisco, CA 94104
www.nela.org

   NELA is a specialty bar association for attorneys who exclusively or primarily represent workers in employment disputes. NELA provides help and support to lawyers who protect the rights of workers through networking, educational programs, publications, and technical assistance. To obtain a listing of attorneys in your area, send a self-addressed stamped envelope, with no other information, to NELA.

The National Partnership for Women and Families
1875 Connecticut Avenue, NW, Suite 710
Washington, DC 20009
(202) 986-2600
www.nationalpartnership.org

   A nonprofit, nonpartisan organization dedicated to improving the lives of women and families. The National Partnership for Women and Families provides consumer-friendly information on laws that govern workplace and privacy rights, such as family and medical leave laws and laws that govern genetic information.

Public Citizen's Health Research Group
1600 20th Street, NW
Washington, DC 20009
(202) 588-1000
www.citizen.org/hrg

   The Health Research Group of the watchdog organization Public Citizen publishes a guide to state laws that govern access to medical records.

Financial Information

Public Agencies

Eldercare Locator
(800) 677-1116
www.aoa.dhhs.gov

This nationwide directory-assistance service, part of the Administration on Aging of the U.S. Department of Health and Human Services, is designed to help older persons and their caregivers locate support resources. Eldercare Locator links you with state and local agencies on aging, where you can get information about services such as transportation, meals, home care, housing alternatives, legal issues, and social activities.

Health Insurance Counseling and Advocacy Program (HICAP)
(800) 434-0222
www.cahealthadvocates.org

HICAP is a national Medicare assistance program for the elderly and disabled. HICAP helps people learn about Medicare benefits, including Medicare HMOs, long-term care, Medicare supplemental or long-term care insurance, and other important changes in Medicare. In some locations, HICAP sponsors community education programs on Medicare in addition to counseling and legal services to help answer complex legal questions. The program is part of the U.S. Department of Health and Human Services. It is financed through each state by the state's Insurance Department or Department on Aging.

Hill-Burton Program
Department of Health and Human Services
Health Resources and Services Administration
(800) 638-0742
www.hrsa.gov/osp

Provides information about hospitals that receive Hill-Burton funding.

Medicaid
www.hcfa.gov/medicaid/

Look in your local phone book for the phone number of your state Medicaid office.

Medicare
www.medicare.gov
(800) 633-4227

Office of Minority Health Resource Center
P.O. Box 37337
Washington, DC 20013

(800) 444-6472
www.omhrc.gov

Federal government office that provides information, technical assistance, and referral services on minority health.

Social Security Administration
(800) 772-1213

Manages Social Security, Supplemental Security Income, Medicare, and parts of Medicaid. Social Security provides monthly income for eligible elderly and disabled people. Supplemental Security Income (SSI) adds to Social Security payments for people who have limited income and financial resources. Information about benefits is available by calling the Social Security Administration.

Department of Veterans Affairs
www.va.gov
(800) 827-1000 (Department of Federal Benefits for Veterans and Dependents)
(877) 222-8387 (Uniform Benefits Package Enrollment Service Center)

Veterans can consult with a VA benefits counselor at any VA Medical Center, or call the Department of Federal Benefits for Veterans and Dependents or the Uniform Benefits Package Enrollment Service Center.

PRIVATE AGENCIES

American Cancer Society
1599 Clifton Road NE
Atlanta, GA 30329-4251
(800) ACS-2345
www.cancer.org

Provides publications, counseling, financial assistance, and public education programs. Financial support programs include:

> Hope Lodges: provides free temporary housing for patients and their families.
>
> Road to Recovery: volunteer program that provides local ground transportation.
>
> Look Good Feel Better (www.lookgoodfeelbetter.org): provides free classes to female cancer survivors on beauty techniques to help restore their appearance and self-image during cancer treatment.

AIR TRANSPORTATION PROGRAMS THAT PROVIDE FLIGHT ACCESS FOR PEOPLE IN NEED OF TRANSPORTATION TO HEALTH FACILITIES:

Angel Flight America
(877) 621-7177
www.angelflightamerica.org

AirLife Line
(877) 727-7728
www.airlifeline.org

Corporate Angel Network
(866) 328-1313
www.corpangelnetwork.org

National Patient Air Transport Hotline
P.O. Box 1940
Manassas, VA 20108-0804
(800) 296-1217 or (703) 361-1191
www.npath.org

Blood and Marrow Transplant Information
2900 Skokie Valley Road, Suite B
Highland Park, IL 60035
(847) 433-3313
www.bmtinfonet.org
Provides information and attorney referrals regarding how to obtain insurance coverage for expenses related to bone marrow transplantation.

Health Insurance Association of America
555 13th Street NW
Washington, DC 20004
(202) 824-1600
www.hiaa.org
Advocates for private market-based health care. Publishes a pamphlet, *What You Should Know about Health Insurance.* Web site provides a wealth of consumer information about private insurance, managed care, getting coverage, state insurance departments, and answers to other insurance questions.

Locks of Love
2925 10th Avenue North
Suite 102
Lake Worth, FL 33461
(888) 896-1588 or (561) 963-1677
www.locksoflove.org
A nonprofit organization that provides hairpieces to financially disadvantaged children under the age of 18 suffering from long-term hair loss.

National Association of Community Health Centers, Inc.
1339 New Hampshire Avenue, NW, Suite 122
Washington, DC 20036

(202) 659-8008
www.hachc.com

Provides a listing of local, nonprofit, community-owned health care programs serving low-income and medically underserved urban and rural communities.

National Association of Hospital Hospitality Houses, Inc. (NAHHH)
(800) 542-9730
www.nahhh.org

Nonprofit that provides lodging and other supportive services to patients and families confronted with medical emergencies.

National Association for the Self-Employed (NASE)
NASE Membership Services
P.O. Box 612067
DFW Airport
Dallas, TX 75261-2067
(800) 232-6273
www.membership.com/nase

NASE is a national membership association for small businesses that offers benefits that include affordable health insurance for the self-employed.

Needy Meds
(334) 662-0023
www.needymeds.com

Clearinghouse for information about getting medications from pharmaceutical companies. No charge for the service. Needy Meds makes information about pharmaceutical manufacturers assistance programs more accessible.

Pharmaceutical Research and Manufacturers of America (PhRMA)
1100 15th Street NW
Washington, DC 20005
(202) 835-3400
www.phrma.org

Provides *The Directory of Prescription Drug Patient Assistance Programs,* which is updated yearly. It lists company programs that provide drugs to physicians whose patients could not otherwise afford them. The guide covers how to make a request for assistance, what medicines are covered, and basic eligibility criteria. Available through local libraries and online.

Ronald McDonald House
(630) 623-7048
www.rmhc.com

National nonprofit organization that provides a home-away-from-home for families of children being treated for serious illness.

Sunshine Foundation
(800) 767-1976
www.sunshinefoundation.org
   Attempts to grant the wishes of critically, chronically, and/or terminally ill children whose families are under financial strain.

Y-Me National Breast Cancer Organization
Prosthesis and Wig Bank
212 W. Van Buren Street, Suite 500
Chicago, IL 60607
(800) 221-2141
www.y-me.org
   National breast cancer organization that offers information, support, and free breast prostheses and wigs to women in financial need.

ADVOCACY RESOURCES

Association of Community Cancer Centers
11600 Nebel Street, Suite 201
Rockville, MD 20852
www.accc-cancer.org/publicpolicy
   Provides information on legislation of interest to cancer survivors and how to communicate with elected officials.

Cancer Research Foundation of America: Advocacy
1600 Duke Street, Suite 500
Alexandria, VA 22314
(800) 227-CFRA or (703) 836-4412
www.preventcancer.org/advocates/index.cfm
   Provides information on cancer research legislation.

Families USA
1334 G Street NW
Washington, DC 20005
(202) 628-3030
familiesusa.org
   Nonprofit, nonpartisan organization dedicated to the achievement of high-quality, affordable health and long-term care for all Americans.

The Lance Armstrong Foundation
P.O. Box 161150
Austin, TX 78716-1150
(512) 236-8820

www.laf.org
www.livestrong.org

LAF seeks to promote the optimal physical, psychological, social recovery, and care of cancer survivors and their loved ones through education, comunity programs, national advocacy, and research grants. LAF's project Live Strong provides quality of life information on post-treatment and long-term issues for cancer survivors and their caregivers.

National Coalition for Cancer Survivorship
1010 Wayne Avenue, Suite 770
Silver Spring, MD 20910
(888) 650-9127
www.canceradvocacy.org

The National Coalition for Cancer Survivorship is the only survivor-led organization working exclusively on behalf of all cancer survivors. NCCS's mission is to ensure quality cancer care for all Americans. NCCS provides educational resources and publications, and leads national advocacy efforts on behalf of survivors and those who care for them. Programs include the Cancer Survival Toolbox™, a comprehensive audio program designed to help cancer survivors and caregivers gain practical skills to deal with the diagnosis, treatment, and challenges of cancer. The Toolbox is available for free in several languages and formats at www.cancersurvivaltoolbox.org or (877) TOOLS-4-U (866-5748).

National Partnership for Women and Families
1875 Connecticut Avenue, NW, Suite 650
Washington, DC 20009
(202) 986-2600
www.nationalpartnership.org

Advocates for health and workplace interests of women and families. Provides publications on laws such as the Family and Medical Leave Act and the Health Insurance and Portability Accountability Act.

Patient Advocate Foundation
700 Thimble Shoals Boulevard
Suite 200
Newport News, VA 23606
(800) 532-5274
www.patientadvocate.org

Provides education, legal counseling, and referrals to cancer survivors concerning managed care, insurance, financial issues, job discrimination, and debt crisis.

Vital Options International
15821 Ventura Boulevard, Suite 645

Encino, CA 91436-2946
TeleSupport Cancer Network
(800) 477-7666
Fax: (818) 788-5260
www.vitaloptions.org

A nonprofit cancer communication, support, and advocacy organization that connects survivors to cancer information and resources. Produces The Group Room, a national call-in radio show that provides information to and advocacy for cancer survivors.

HOW TO CONTACT A MEMBER OF CONGRESS

Writing to a Senator:
The Honorable (full name)
United States Senate
Washington, DC 20510
Dear Senator (last name):
www.senate.gov

Writing to a Representative:
The Honorable (full name)
United States House of Representatives
Washington, DC 20515
Dear Representative (last name):
www.house.gov/writerep

Calling all Members of Congress, Committees and Subcommittees
Capitol Hill switchboard
(202) 224-3121

Index

SUPPORT THE NATIONAL COALITION FOR CANCER SURVIVORSHIP

Contact us or make a donation at our Web site: **www.canceradvocacy.org**

Adding your voice to NCCS's advocacy efforts will help NCCS to advocate for patients' access to quality cancer care.

❑ Yes, please add me to NCCS's mailing list.

❑ Yes, I would like to receive NCCS e-mail alerts on important cancer issues and how I can help.

Your donation will help NCCS develop additional tools and programs designed to educate and empower cancer survivors and to advocate for survivors' rights.

❑ $500 ❑ $250 ❑ $100 ❑ $50 ❑ $ _____

This donation is made:

❑ In honor of _____

❑ In memory of _____

❑ In celebration of _____

❑ Please send acknowledgment to _____

_____

Name _____

Affiliation (if any) _____

Address _____

City _____ State _____ Zip _____

Phone _____ E-mail _____

Please make checks payable to NCCS or complete the following credit card information:

Visa/MasterCard Account Number: _____

Expiration Date: _____ Signature: _____

❑ I prefer to remain anonymous. Please do not list my name in NCCS's Annual Report.

NCCS is a 501(c)3 organization. All contributions are tax deductible to the extent permitted by law.

NCCS
1010 Wayne Avenue, Suite 770
Silver Spring, MD 20910
Toll Free: (877) NCCS-YES (877) 622-7937
(301) 565-9670 (fax)
www.canceradvocacy.org

About the Authors

EDITOR

Barbara Hoffman, J.D., is a cofounder of the National Coalition for Cancer Survivorship and has served on its Board of Directors since its inception. She is a member of the Legal Research and Writing Faculty of Rutgers University Law School in Newark, New Jersey. She is the editor of the first two editions of *A Cancer Survivor's Almanac: Charting Your Journey,* and author of numerous book chapters, law review articles, and consumer publications. A survivor of two cancers, Ms. Hoffman has spoken at more than one hundred programs on the legal rights of cancer survivors.

AUTHORS

Irene Card is the president and founder of Medical Insurance Claims, Inc., a health claims processing company that serves individuals throughout the country. She is the insurance advisor to the National Coalition for Cancer Survivorship. She served for seven years as the volunteer consumer representative on the Oncology Nursing Certification Corporation Board of Directors. Ms. Card is a licensed insurance agent (health, life, and long-term care) in New Jersey. She is the author of a weekly newspaper column, *Understanding Health Insurance,* which is available at **www.miconline.com**. Ms. Card is in frequent demand as a speaker on all aspects of health insurance and is a nationally recognized advocate for cancer survivors.

Nancy Chasen, J.D., is a consumer advocate and writer. She was special counsel to President Carter's Consumer Advisor as well as assistant general counsel for legislation of the Federal Trade Commission, and she has handled consumer issues for Senator Thomas Eagleton (D-Mo.). Ms. Chasen has also worked for several consumer organizations, as staff attorney for the Washington office of the Consumers Union, and as a lobbyist for Public Citizen's Congress Watch. She served as a producer and consumer reporter for the PBS program *Modern Maturity.* Ms. Chasen is the author of *Policy Wise: A Guide to Insurance for Older Consumers,* published by the American Association of Retired Persons, and has appeared frequently on panels and before federal agencies to represent consumer interests.

Elizabeth Johns Clark, Ph.D., M.S.W., M.P.H., is the executive director of the National Association of Social Workers—the largest professional organization of social workers in the world. Previously, she was director of diagnostic and thera-peutic services at Albany Medical Center Hospital and an associate professor of medicine in the Department of Medical Oncology at Albany Medical College. She is past-president of the National Coalition for Cancer Survivorship and proj-ect director for the Cancer Survival Toolbox™, a self-advocacy training program. She holds a doctorate in medical sociology. Dr. Clark has lectured and published extensively in the areas of psychosocial oncology, loss and grief, hope, and burnout.

Georgia Decker, M.S., A.N.P., A.O.C.N., has worked as a staff nurse, clini-cal nurse specialist, and nurse practitioner. More than twenty-three years of her thirty-five years in nursing have been in oncology, and her oncology practice has included CAM therapies for over seven years. She is actively involved in the Oncology Nursing Society at the national and local levels. She is the editor of *An Introduction to Complementary and Alternative Therapies* (Oncology Nursing Press), and she is the column editor for *Integrated Care* in the *Clinical Journal of Oncology Nursing*. Ms. Decker has made numerous presentations and written publications on the subject of CAM therapies and cancer care.

Neil Fiore, Ph.D., is a licensed psychologist who provides training for health-care professionals at Stanford Hospital, Kaiser-Permanente, St. Barnabas, and the University of California. He is a cofounder of the National Coalition for Cancer Survivorship and the author of three books, including *The Road Back to Health: Coping with the Emotional Aspects of Cancer* (Celestial Arts). As a cancer survivor himself, Dr. Fiore is dedicated to improving the quality of life for patients, their families, and healthcare professionals. Dr. Fiore can be reached at his website: **www.neilfiore.com.**

Patricia A. Ganz, M.D., is a cofounder of the National Coalition for Cancer Survivorship. A medical oncologist, she has spent the past twenty years doing sys-tematic research on the health-related impact of cancer and its treatment on the quality of life. She currently holds an American Cancer Society Clinical Research Professorship, and is professor in the UCLA Schools of Medicine and Public Health. She serves as an associate editor for the *Journal of Clinical Oncology* and the *Journal of the National Cancer Institute*. She has also been actively involved in measurement of quality of life endpoints in clinical trials, with leadership roles in the Southwest Oncology Group (SWOG) and the National Surgical Adjuvant Breast and Bowel Project (NSBABP). Through her research she has contributed to our understanding of how women adjust to the diagnosis of breast cancer, including its effects on their physical, emotional, social, and sexual well-being.

Susan Leigh, R.N., B.S.N., is a cofounder of the National Coalition for Can-cer Survivorship and served as its president from 1993 to 1995. Drawing on her experience as an oncology nurse and a survivor of Hodgkin's disease, breast can-cer, and bladder cancer, she speaks and writes extensively on survivor issues. Her current interests include awareness, education, and research about long-term cancer survivors, with special emphasis on chronic and delayed effects of the disease and its therapy.

Catherine Logan-Carrillo was diagnosed with cervical cancer in 1979 and breast cancer in 1996. She is the founder of People Living Through Cancer, Inc., in Albuquerque, NM, and was instrumental in the development of the organization's peer support programs and its operations. Logan-Carrillo is cofounder of the National Coalition for Cancer Survivorship and served as its first executive director from 1986 to 1991. Currently she writes and edits health publications.

Gena Love, a twenty-three-year cancer survivor, has been active in survivorship for more than eighteen years. She is the Program Manager for the Comprehensive Cancer Program at the New Mexico Department of Health. She was the director of Support Services of People Living Through Cancer, in Albuquerque, NM, where she served the needs of New Mexico's diverse survivor population. Working in collaboration with leaders in the Native American community, Ms. Love developed a training program designed to assist Native Americans in creating and leading survivorship programs for their own communities. Ms. Love was selected to be one of the charter members of the Director's Consumer Liaison Group, the first consumer advocate panel reporting to the director of the National Cancer Institute.

Jody Pelusi, Ph.D., F.N.P., A.O.C.N., is a community oncology nurse practitioner with more than twenty-five years experience in oncology. She practices in many rural and urban communities in Arizona. Dr. Pelusi works in private practice as well as in community-based oncology programs, giving care to the underinsured and uninsured. In addition, she provides many community and professional presentations, retreats, and programs related to cancer prevention, early diagnosis, treatment, symptom management, long-term follow-up, end-of-life care, and the impact of culture on cancer care. She has served as the Oncology Nursing Society's liaison to the Intercultural Cancer Council and currently sits as the consumer representative on the FDA's Oncological Drug Advisory Council. Dr. Pelusi is on the faculty of Grand Canyon University and the University of Phoenix.

Natalie Davis Spingarn was a prize-winning writer, advocate, and consultant on health and social policy issues. She served on the board of directors of the National Coalition for Cancer Survivorship and edited many of its publications. Her scores of publications include *Hanging in There: Living Well on Borrowed Time* (Stein and Day, 1982) and *The New Cancer Survivors: Living with Grace, Fighting with Spirit* (Johns Hopkins, 1999), which describe her personal experience with metastatic breast cancer and the issues confronting survivors. She was honored at the John Muir Medical Film Festival for her film *Patients and Doctors: Communication is a Two-Way Street.*

Ellen L. Stovall is a thirty-year survivor of two bouts with cancer. In 1992, Ms. Stovall became executive director and subsequently president and CEO of the National Coalition for Cancer Survivorship. She also currently serves as vice-chair of the Institute of Medicine's (IOM) National Cancer Policy Board (NCPB) and as chair of the Robert Wood Johnson Foundation's National Advisory Committee to Promote Excellence in Care at the End of Life. She is frequently called upon to work with administration and congressional staff on a variety of cancer-related policy issues, most notably access to quality cancer care.

Debra Thaler-DeMers, R.N., O.C.N., is a twenty-two-year survivor of cancer. She has served as a member of the board of directors of the National Coalition for Cancer Survivorship, including as the vice chair of the board. Ms. Thaler-DeMers is an oncology nurse at Stanford University Hospital and Clinics. She is the founder of Cancer ACCESS: Advocacy, Counseling, Clinical Education & Survivorship Skills. Ms. Thaler-DeMers writes and speaks frequently on cancer survivorship issues, including sexuality and fertility.